Psychoneuroimmunology

Guest Editor

GREGORY G. FREUND, MD

IMMUNOLOGY AND ALLERGY CLINICS OF NORTH AMERICA

www.immunology.theclinics.com

Consulting Editor
RAFEUL ALAM, MD, PhD

May 2009 • Volume 29 • Number 2

SAUNDERS an imprint of ELSEVIER, Inc.

W.B. SAUNDERS COMPANY
A Division of Elsevier Inc.

1600 John F. Kennedy Blvd., ● Suite 1800 ● Philadelphia, PA 19103-2899.

http://www.theclinics.com

IMMUNOLOGY AND ALLERGY CLINICS OF NORTH AMERICA Volume 29, Number 2
May 2009 ISSN 0889–8561, ISBN-13: 978-1-4377-0865-3, ISBN-10: 1-4377-0865-X

Editor: Patrick Manley

Immunology and Allergy Clinics of North America (ISSN 0889–8561) is published quarterly by Elsevier Inc., 360 Park Avenue South, New York, NY 10010-1710. Months of issue are February, May, August, and November. Business and Editorial Offices: 1600 John F. Kennedy Blvd., Suite 1800, Philadelphia, PA 19103-2899. Customer Service Office: 11830 Westline Industrial Drive, St. Louis, MO 63146. Periodicals postage paid at New York, NY and additional mailing offices. Subscription prices are $233.00 per year for US individuals, $366.00 per year for US institutions, $113.00 per year for US students and residents, $286.00 per year for Canadian individuals, $163.00 per year for Canadian students, $454.00 per year for Canadian institutions, $325.00 per year for international individuals, $454.00 per year for international institutions, $163.00 per year for international students. To receive student/resident rate, orders must be accompanied by name of affiliated institution, date of term, and the *signature* of program/residency coordinator on institution letterhead. Orders will be billed at individual rate until proof of status is received. Foreign air speed delivery is included in all *Clinics* subscription prices. All prices are subject to change without notice. **POSTMASTER:** Send address changes to *Immunology and Allergy Clinics of North America,* Elsevier Journals Customer Service, 11830 Westline Industrial Drive, St. Louis, MO 63146. **Customer Service: 1-800-654-2452 (US and Canada). From outside of the United States and Canada, call 1-314-453-7041. Fax: 1-314-453-5170. For print support, e-mail: JournalsCustomerService-usa@ elsevier.com. For online support, e-mail: JournalsOnlineSupport-usa@elsevier.com.**

Reprints. For copies of 100 or more, of articles in this publication, please contact the Commercial Reprints Department, Elsevier Inc., 360 Park Avenue South, New York, New York 10010-1710. Tel. (212) 633-3812, Fax: (212) 462-1935, e-mail: reprints@elsevier.com.

Immunology and Allergy Clinics of North America is covered in MEDLINE/PubMed (Index Medicus), Current Contents/Life Sciences, Science Citation Index, ISI/BIOMED, Chemical Abstracts, and EMBASE/Excerpta Medica.

Printed and bound by CPI Group (UK) Ltd, Croydon, CR0 4YY
Transferred to Digital Print 2011

Contributors

CONSULTING EDITOR

RAFEUL ALAM, MD, PhD
Veda and Chauncey Ritter Chair in Immunology, Professor, and Director, Division of Immunology and Allergy, National Jewish Health; and University of Colorado Health Sciences Center, Denver, Colorado

GUEST EDITOR

GREGORY G. FREUND, MD
Professor and Head, Department of Pathology, College of Medicine, University of Illinois at Urbana-Champaign, Urbana, Illinois

AUTHORS

RONIT AVITSUR, PhD
School of Behavioral Sciences, The Academic College of Tel Aviv-Yaffo, Yaffo, Israel

WILLIAM A. BANKS, MD
Geriatrics Research Education and Clinical Center, Veterans Affairs Medical Center-St. Louis; and Division of Geriatrics, Department of Internal Medicine, Saint Louis University School of Medicine, St. Louis, Missouri

STEPHAN W. BARTH, DVM
Institute of Nutritional Physiology, Federal Research Center for Nutrition, Karlsruhe, Germany

ROBERT DANTZER, DVM, PhD
Professor of Psychoneuroimmunology, Integrative Immunology and Behavior Program, University of Illinois at Urbana-Champaign, Urbana, Illinois

ERICA J. DOCZY, MS
Department of Psychiatry, University of Cincinnati College of Medicine, Psychiatry North, GRI-E, Cincinnati, Ohio; and Air Force Research Laboratory, Wright Patterson AFB, Ohio

GREGORY G. FREUND, MD
Professor and Head, Department of Pathology, College of Medicine, University of Illinois at Urbana-Champaign, Urbana, Illinois

RACHEL GEORGIOU, MSc
Stroke Services, Hope Hospital, Salford, United Kingdom

RÜDIGER GERSTBERGER, PhD
Faculty of Veterinary Medicine, Department of Veterinary Physiology, Justus-Liebig-University, Giessen, Germany

JONATHAN P. GODBOUT, PhD
Institute for Behavioral Medicine Research; and Department of Molecular Virology, Immunology, and Medical Genetics, the Ohio State University, Columbus, Ohio

STEFAN M. GOLD, PhD
Cousins Center for Psychoneuroimmunology, Semel Institute for Neuroscience, Los Angeles, California; and Multiple Sclerosis Program, Department of Neurology, Geffen School of Medicine, University of California-Los Angeles, Los Angeles, California

CATHERINE R. HARRISON, PhD
Air Force Research Laboratory, Wright Patterson AFB, Ohio

JAMES P. HERMAN, PhD
Professor of Psychiatry, Department of Psychiatry, University of Cincinnati College of Medicine, Psychiatry North, GRI-E, Cincinnati, Ohio

THOMAS HÜBSCHLE, PhD
Faculty of Veterinary Medicine, Department of Veterinary Physiology, Justus-Liebig-Universität, Giessen, Germany

MICHAEL R. IRWIN, MD
Cousins Center for Psychoneuroimmunology, Semel Institute for Neuroscience, Los Angeles, California

DANIEL R. JOHNSON, PhD
Department of Animal Sciences, University of Illinois, Urbana, Illinois

RODNEY W. JOHNSON, PhD
Integrative Immunology and Behavior, Department of Animal Sciences, University of Illinois, Urbana, Illinois

K. TODD KEYLOCK, MS
Department of Kinesiology and Community Health, University of Illinois at Urbana-Champaign, Urbana, Illinois

JASON C. O'CONNOR, PhD
Visiting Assistant Professor, Department of Animal Sciences, University of Illinois, Urbana, Illinois

MARK R. OPP, PhD
Department of Anesthesiology, Department of Molecular and Integrative Physiology, and Neuroscience Graduate Program, University of Michigan, Ann Arbor, Michigan

DAVID A. PADGETT, PhD
Section of Oral Biology; and The Institute for Behavioral Medicine Research, Ohio State University, Columbus, Ohio

NICOLE POWELL, PhD
Section of Oral Biology, Ohio State University, Columbus, Ohio

JOACHIM ROTH, PhD
Faculty of Veterinary Medicine, Department of Veterinary Physiology, Justus-Liebig-Universität, Giessen, Germany

NANCY ROTHWELL, PhD
Faculty of Life Sciences, University of Manchester, Manchester, United Kingdom

CHRISTOPH RUMMEL, PhD, DVM
Faculty of Veterinary Medicine, Department of Veterinary Physiology,
Justus-Liebig-Universität, Giessen, Germany

KIM SEROOGY, PhD
Professor of Neurology, Department of Neurology, University of Cincinnati College of
Medicine, Cincinnati, Ohio

JOHN F. SHERIDAN, PhD
Section of Oral Biology; and The Institute for Behavioral Medicine Research, Ohio State
University, Columbus, Ohio

ROBERT SKINNER, BSc
Faculty of Life Sciences, University of Manchester, Manchester, United Kingdom

PETER THORNTON, BSc
Faculty of Life Sciences, University of Manchester, Manchester, United Kingdom

VICTORIA J. VIEIRA, MS
Department of Kinesiology and Community Health, Division of Nutritional Science,
University of Illinois at Urbana-Champaign, Urbana, Illinois

JEFFREY A. WOODS, PhD
Department of Kinesiology and Community Health, Department of Pathology, Division of
Nutritional Science, University of Illinois at Urbana-Champaign, Urbana, Illinois

Contents

> The term "psychoneuroimmunology" connotes separate compartments that interact. The blood–brain barrier (BBB) is both the dividing line, physical and physiologic, between the immune system and the central nervous system (CNS) and the locale for interaction. The BBB restricts unregulated mixing of immune substances in the blood with those in the CNS, directly transports neuroimmune-active substances between the blood and CNS, and itself secretes neuroimmune substances. These normal functions of the BBB can be altered by neuroimmune events. As such, the BBB is an important conduit in the communication between the immune system and the CNS.

> After defining hyperthermia and fever, this article describes the complete chain of events leading to the genesis of fever, starting with the lipopolysaccharide-induced formation of endogenous pyrogens (cytokines), their interactions with relevant targets in the brain, the induction of enzymes responsible for the formation of prostaglandin E2, the activation of descending neuronal pathways via the EP3 receptor, and the stimulation of thermogenesis via this pathway to support the febrile shift of the thermoregulatory set point. This article also summarizes an alternative hypothesis to account for a rapid induction of the early phase of lipopolysaccharide-induced fever before the release of larger amounts of cytokines into the bloodstream. Other topics discussed include malignant hypothermia, drug-induced hypothermia, and the heat stroke syndrome.

> The psychologic and behavioral components of sickness represent, together with fever response and associated neuroendocrine changes,

a highly organized strategy of the organism to fight infection. This strategy, referred to as *sickness behavior*, is triggered by the proinflammatory cytokines produced by activated cells of the innate immune system in contact with specific pathogen-associated molecular patterns (PAMPs). Interleukin-1 and other cytokines act on the brain via (1) a neural route represented by the primary afferent neurons that innervate the body site where the infectious process takes place and (2) a humoral pathway that involves the production of proinflammatory cytokines. This article presents the current knowledge on the way this communication system is organized and regulated and the implications of these advances for understanding brain physiology and pathology.

Neurologic diseases are often accompanied by significant life stress and consequent increases in stress hormone levels. Glucocorticoid stress hormones are known to have deleterious interactions with neurodegenerative processes, and are hypersecreted in neurologic disorders as well as in comorbid psychiatric conditions, such as depression. This article highlights the state of our knowledge on mechanisms controlling activation and inhibition of glucocorticoid secretion, outlines signaling mechanisms used by these hormones in neural tissue, and describes how endogenous glucocorticoids can mediate neuronal damage in various models of neurologic disease. The article highlights the importance of controlling stress and consequent stress hormone secretion in the context of neurologic disease states.

This article summarizes the endocrine and immune changes induced by an experimental model for social stress characterized by repeated defeat. Data indicate that mice facing a social stressor may use different behavioral coping responses based on the environmental conditions and previous experiences. Although chronic stressors generally suppress immune function and increase a host's susceptibility to disease, this may not be always true in all cases. For example, under conditions in which individuals face the chance of being injured repeatedly, it may be an adaptive advantage to maintain or even enhance an immune response. The development of glucocorticoid resistance after social disruption may be such a mechanism, allowing animals to heal injuries and clear invading microbes in the presence of the anti-inflammatory stress hormones.

The brain uses a variety of mechanisms to survey the immune system constantly. Responses of the immune system to invading pathogens are detected by the central nervous system, which responds by orchestrating complex changes in behavior and physiology. Sleep is one of the behaviors altered in response to immune challenge. The role of cytokines as mediators of responses to infectious challenge and regulators and modulators of sleep is the focus of this article.

An increasing body of evidence suggests that patients who have major depressive disorder show alterations in immunologic markers including increases in proinflammatory cytokine activity and inflammation. Inflammation of the central nervous system is a pathologic hallmark of multiple sclerosis (MS). Patients affected by this disease also show a high incidence of depression. Accumulating evidence from animal studies suggests that some aspects of depression and fatigue in MS may be linked to inflammatory markers. This article reviews the current knowledge in the field and illustrates how the sickness behavior model may be applied to investigate depressive symptoms in inflammatory neurologic diseases.

Aging can impair functional interaction that occurs between the brain and the immune system. Recent findings indicate that microglia and astrocytes, innate immune cells of the brain, become more reactive during normal aging. This age-associated increase in innate immune reactivity sets the stage for an exaggerated inflammatory cytokine response in the brain after activation of the peripheral innate immune system. This elevated neuroinflammatory response may lead to more severe long-lasting behavioral and cognitive deficits. This article discusses new evidence that aging creates a brain environment that is permissive to the occurrence of mental health complications following innate immune activation.

A sizable body of knowledge has arisen demonstrating that type 2 diabetes (T2D) is associated with alterations in the innate immune system. The resulting proinflammatory-leaning imbalance is implicated in the development of secondary disease complications and comorbidities, such as delayed wound healing, accelerated progress of atherosclerosis, and retinopathy, in people who have T2D. New experimental data and the results of recently published health-related quality-of-life surveys indicate that individuals who have T2D experience diminished feelings of happiness, well being, and satisfaction with life. These emotional and psychological consequences of T2D point to altered neuroimmunity as a previously unappreciated complication of T2D. This article discusses recent data detailing the impact of T2D on a person's PNI response.

> Stroke is the major cause of disability in the Western world and is the third greatest cause of death, but there are no widely effective treatments to prevent the devastating effects of stroke. Extensive and growing evidence implicates inflammatory and immune processes in the occurrence of stroke and particularly in the subsequent injury. Several inflammatory mediators have been identified in the pathogenesis of stroke including specific cytokines, adhesion molecules, matrix metalloproteinases, and eicosanoids. An early clinical trial suggests that inhibiting interleukin-1 may be of benefit in the treatment of acute stroke.

> Exercise has beneficial effects on chronic disease, and the drive to understand the mechanisms of these benefits is strong. This article presents several compelling potential mechanisms for the anti-inflammatory effect of exercise, including reduced percentage of body fat and macrophage accumulation in adipose tissue, muscle-released interleukin-6 inhibition of tumor necrosis factor-a, and the cholinergic anti-inflammatory pathway.

RELATED INTEREST

Pediatric Clinics of North America (Volume 56, Issue 1, February 2009)
Common Respiratory Symptoms and Illnesses: A Graded Evidence Based Approach
Anne B. Chang, MBBS, MPHTM, FRACP, PhD, *Guest Editor*

THE CLINICS ARE NOW AVAILABLE ONLINE!
Access your subscription at:
www.theclinics.com

Foreword

Psychoneuroimmunology—The Essence of a Three's Company

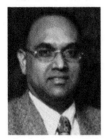

Rafeul Alam, MD, PhD
Consulting Editor

Cogito, ergo sum [I think, therefore I am].
—Rene Descartes

Recognition of self ("what I am") is a fundamental property of biological entities. Brain activity is essential for creating an image of self. The complex process that is used by the brain to create a self-image is still poorly understood. Interestingly, a fundamental task of the immune system is to distinguish self from nonself. The principles and the molecular mechanism by which the immune system makes this distinction have been well delineated. The thymic selection of T cells with moderate affinity for self-antigens illustrates this principle, and it seems to work well. This is just one of many similarities between the central nervous system (CNS) and immune system. Both systems use a unique functional feature called memory. As a matter of fact, memory provides a basic mechanism for distinguishing self from nonself. In this regard, it is quite tantalizing that some of the molecules that are uniquely expressed in the immune system are also expressed in the CNS. The recombination activating gene-1 (RAG-1) is one such example.[1] RAG-1 is critical for generation of the T-cell and B-cell antigen receptors and has been instrumental in the evolution of the adaptive immune system. RAG-1 is expressed at a lower level in the CNS. Its function in the CNS is unclear, but it may be involved in certain neuronal functions.[2] The T-cell–associated molecule CD4 and its kinase Lck are expressed by neurons and microglia.[3] Lck deficiency causes retinal dysplasia.[4] Unc119 (HRG4) is a signaling molecule that is preferentially expressed in the neuron, especially in retinal cells.[5] It is also expressed at a lower level in leukocytes.[6] Unc119 (HRG4) deficiency causes retinal degeneration.[5]

The effect of neuronal molecules on the immune system has been an area of active research for many years. Tachykinins and the proteins of the nerve growth factor family

Supported by NIH grants RO1 AI059719 and AI68088, PPG HL 36577 and N01 HHSN272200700048C.

Immunol Allergy Clin N Am 29 (2009) xiii–xiv
doi:10.1016/j.iac.2009.03.002   immunology.theclinics.com
0889-8561/09/$ – see front matter

directly affect the function of immune cells. Tachykinins, generally released at the nerve endings, are important mediators of neurogenic inflammation. They are also secreted by cells of the immune system, however. Molecules secreted by the immune cells profoundly affect our psyche. Just think how we feel when we have the flu, the common cold, or other minor viral infections. The opposite is also true. We easily succumb to illnesses during times of stress or depression. These are complex issues, and their molecular mechanisms are just beginning to be uncovered. Understanding the mind-body immunity is the fascinating subject of this issue. This is fun to read.

Rafeul Alam, MD, PhD
Division of Allergy and Immunology
National Jewish Health and University of Colorado Denver Health Sciences Center
1400 Jackson Street
Denver, CO 80206

E-mail address:
alamr@njc.org (R. Alam)

REFERENCES

1. Chun JJ, Schatz DG, Oettinger MA, et al. The recombination activating gene-1 (RAG-1) transcript is present in the murine central nervous system. Cell 1991; 64:189–200.
2. Cushman J, Lo J, Huang Z, et al. Neurobehavioral changes resulting from recombinase activation gene 1 deletion. Clin Diagn Lab Immunol 2003;10:13–8.
3. Funke I, Hahn A, Rieber EP, et al. The cellular receptor (CD4) of the human immunodeficiency virus is expressed on neurons and glial cells in human brain. J Exp Med 1987;165:1230–5.
4. Omri B, Blancher C, Neron B, et al. Retinal dysplasia in mice lacking p56lck. Oncogene 1998;16:2351–6.
5. Ishiba Y, Higashide T, Mori N, et al. Targeted inactivation of synaptic HRG4 (UNC119) causes dysfunction in the distal photoreceptor and slow retinal degeneration, revealing a new function. Exp Eye Res 2007;84:473–85.
6. Gorska MM, Stafford SJ, Cen O, et al. Unc119, a novel activator of Lck/Fyn, is essential for T cell activation. J Exp Med 2004;199:369–79.

Preface

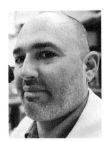

Gregory G. Freund, MD
Guest Editor

In August of 2006 in *Neurologic Clinics of North America*, I asked the question "What is psychoneuroimmunology (PNI)?" I noted that the National Library of Medicine defined PNI as "the field concerned with the interrelationship between the brain, behavior and the immune system." To my chagrin, I discovered that the Encarta World English Dictionary by Microsoft Corporation defined PNI as "a branch of medicine concerned with how emotions affect the immune system." This latter definition seriously misrepresented the field of PNI and colored it as some sort of pseudoscience. In addition, Wikipedia had only 337 words devoted to the subject, and none of them were practically informative, except, perhaps, that the term *psychoneuroimmunology* was "coined by Robert Ader and Nicholas Cohen at the University of Rochester in 1975," which is where I attended medical school and received my postgraduate training in pathology. Today, however, things are different. Wikipedia now has a robust description of the field, and even the publishers of medical education and reference textbooks (usually a lagging indicator of medical advances) are beginning to see the importance of PNI.

In 2006, an all-site content search of McGraw-Hill's AccessMedicine, which contains the contents of 16 respected medical textbooks, including Harrison's Online, provided only one "hit" for the term *psychoneuroimmunology*. This reference was contained in *Adams and Victors' Neurology* in a discussion of the evolution of the study of psychiatric disorders and the apparently deleterious impact that the originating concept of "psychosomatic medicine" in the 1930s had on the treatment of mental illness. Unfortunately, this purported link between PNI and "psychosomatic" disorders is still included. On the positive side, McGraw-Hill's *Current Medical Diagnosis and Treatment 2009* now includes a positive description of PNI in its section on mind-body medicine, noting that "The new field of psychoneuroimmunology has documented, at the physiologic level, the powerful effect of the mind on the nervous, endocrine, and immune systems, and vice versa. Studies have demonstrated that certain forms of mental training, in addition to affecting health, can affect brain function and even structure, leading to a reevaluation of currently held beliefs about neuroplasticity."

Immunol Allergy Clin N Am 29 (2009) xv–xvi
doi:10.1016/j.iac.2009.03.001
0889-8561/09/$ – see front matter © 2009 Elsevier Inc. All rights reserved.

Current clinical practice, especially by means of complementary and alternative medicine approaches, is using and translating the basic science of PNI and capitalizing on the bidirectional communication that occurs between the central nervous system (CNS) and the peripheral immune system. Critical to improving our armamentarium of mind-body–based therapeutics is to recognize that immune organs (lymph nodes, spleen, and thymus) are innervated and communicate with the CNS by means of neuronal pathways. As one example, efferent vagus cholinergic nerve terminals in the spleen are triggered during bacterial infection, and the resultant acetylcholine suppresses macrophage activation, thus forming the "cholinergic anti-inflammatory reflex." Similarly, the afferent vagus conveys proinflammatory cytokine-dependent information about the activation status of the peripheral immune system to the nucleus of the solitary tract, resulting in the classic disease symptoms of fever, lethargy, drowsiness, and loss of appetite. These fundamental biologic concepts are essentially absent from medical texts, including teaching and reference books in anatomy, medicine, neurology, pathology, and surgery, although, *Kaplan and Sadock's Comprehensive Textbook of Psychiatry* notes autonomic nervous system innervation of the peripheral immune organs.

So, what is PNI? It is a rapidly developing field of study dedicated to understanding why illness occurs and why many individuals have trouble recovering from their affliction. As our knowledge of the myriad physiologic pathways activated before, during, and after sickness expands, mind-body medicine should translate these discoveries into innovative new strategies that should ward off, retard, and overcome disease.

I am pleased to present to the readers of *Immunology and Allergy Clinics of North America* this important issue reprinted from *Neurologic Clinics of North America*, with updates included from many of the authors.

Gregory G. Freund, MD
Department of Pathology
190 Medical Sciences Building, MC-714
506 South Mathews Avenue
University of Illinois at Urbana-Champaign
Urbana, IL 61801, USA

E-mail address:
freun@illinois.edu (G.G. Freund)

The Blood–Brain Barrier in Psychoneuroimmunology

William A. Banks, MD[a,b,*]

KEYWORDS

- Blood-brain barrier • Cerebrovascular • Cytokine
- Central nervous system • Brain • Neurovascular unit
- Hormone

Classically, two great communication systems have been described: the nervous system and the endocrine system. Not surprisingly, a role for the nervous system, especially the vagus and sympathetic outflow, was found early in the history of psychoneuroimmunology. Similarly, blood-borne signals were known to be critical for immune cell communication. Increasing evidence also showed that circulating immune signals, including immune cells themselves, somehow exerted an effect on the central nervous system (CNS). It was known that this endocrine-like interaction between the circulating factors of the immune system and the elements of the CNS was complicated by the existence of the blood–brain barrier (BBB). Early work clearly showed that the BBB prevents as free an exchange of the circulating immune elements with the CNS as with the peripheral tissues. The existence of barrier function preventing the unrestricted exchange of immune substances between the blood and CNS raised another, more exciting possibility: that the BBB might preside over a regulated interaction between the immune system and the peripheral tissues.

Work in the last 15 years has shown that the BBB is in fact a regulatory interface between the CNS and peripheral tissues. This interface does not exit in isolation but is modified and affected by circulating substances and, even more, by cells, substances, and events on the CNS side. These intimate interactions of the BBB with events on its luminal (blood) and abluminal (brain) sides have led to the concept of the neurovascular unit (NVU). The concept of the NVU emphasizes that the BBB is in a pivotal position to control the humoral exchanges between the peripheral tissues and the CNS and that such control is modified by CNS and circulatory factors. The

This issue is a repurpose of August 2006 issue of the *Neurologic Clinics* (NCL Volume 24, Issue 3).
[a] Geriatrics Research Education and Clinical Center, Veterans Affairs Medical Center-St. Louis, 915 North Grand Boulevard, St. Louis, MO 63106, USA
[b] Division of Geriatrics, Department of Internal Medicine, Saint Louis University School of Medicine, St. Louis, MO, USA
* Correspondence. Geriatrics Research Education and Clinical Center, Veterans Affairs Medical Center-St. Louis, 915 North Grand Boulevard, St. Louis, MO 63106.
E-mail address: bankswa@slu.edu

roles of the BBB and the NVU in psychoneuroimmunology still are being described, but current thinking can categorize them broadly. This article considers the four functions that are most fundamental to psychoneuroimmunology: (1) barrier functions; (2) permeability functions, further considered here as permeability to cytokines and to immune cells; (3) clearance functions; and (4) secretory functions.

BARRIER FUNCTIONS

The defining characteristic of the BBB is its barrier function **(Fig. 1)**. Experiments by Paul Erlich and others at the end of the nineteenth century found that some dyes could not stain the brain after intravenous injection. Eventually, this lack of staining was found to occur because these dyes bound to circulating albumin and, unlike in peripheral organs and tissues, albumin was unable to leak out of the blood vessels of the CNS. In the late 1960s, electron microscopy studies revealed the anatomic basis for the BBB.[1] Tight junctions cement together the endothelial cells that form capillaries in the brain and spinal cord and that line their arterioles and venules. Other modifications include a lack of intracellular fenestrations and a decreased rate of pinocytosis. Besides the endothelial barrier of the vasculature, there are parallel barriers comprised of epithelial cells at the choroid plexus and tanycytes at the circumventricular organs. Taken together, these modifications prevent the production of a plasma ultrafiltrate and, hence, leakage of serum proteins into the CNS. The barrier formed is the most impressive in biology, with serum/cerebrospinal fluid (CSF) to ratios for restricted proteins of about 200:1.[2]

This lack of leakage no doubt has great benefits to the CNS. Preventing the unrestricted entry of circulating substances into the CNS is one of several ways that the BBB helps provide an ideal environment for the functioning of the CNS. This ultrafiltrate, however, provides much of the nourishment to peripheral tissues. Without it, the CNS must obtain its nutrients by some other means. The BBB serves this need of the CNS as well. The BBB possesses selective saturable transporters for nearly every substance needed for the homeostatic and nutritional maintenance of the CNS. There are, for example, transporters for glucose, amino acids, free fatty acids, vitamins, minerals, and electrolytes. These transporters often have been shown to be modifiable so that they adapt to the needs of the CNS. This dualism of the

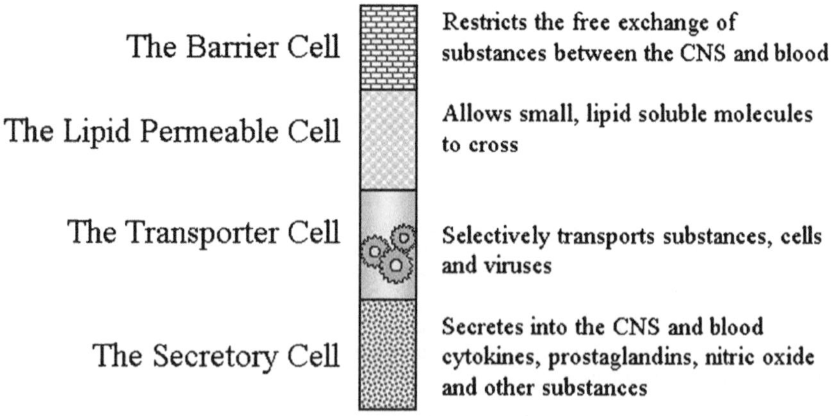

The Barrier Cell	Restricts the free exchange of substances between the CNS and blood
The Lipid Permeable Cell	Allows small, lipid soluble molecules to cross
The Transporter Cell	Selectively transports substances, cells and viruses
The Secretory Cell	Secretes into the CNS and blood cytokines, prostaglandins, nitric oxide and other substances

Fig. 1. Multiple roles are played by the cells that comprise the blood–brain barrier. CNS, central nervous system.

BBB—the power to restrict leakage so severely and to transport substances on a selective basis—makes it a vital player in the interactions between the CNS and the periphery.

Adrenergic compounds are perhaps the most significant class of neuroimmune substances excluded by the BBB. Epinephrine and norepinephrine secreted from the adrenal medulla and adrenergic nerves have been shown to affect immune cell functions.[3] Adrenergic compounds are excluded by the physical presence of the BBB and also by enzymatic degradation by the brain capillaries.[4]

Disruption of the BBB is a highly pathologic event and is associated with many neuroimmune phenomena. The first such phenomenon described was the ability of lipopolysaccharide (LPS) to disrupt the BBB. It is assumed that the release of cytokines such as tumor necrosis factor-α (TNF-α) is the mechanism for such disruption, which also is known to be prostaglandin dependent and independent of nitric oxide. Most events and substances that disrupt the BBB do so not by dissolving the tight junctions of the brain endothelial cells (ie, the paracelluar pathway) but by enhancing pinocytosis and other vesicular-dependent mechanisms (the transcytotic pathway). Recent work, however, has emphasized the role of the paracellular pathway in disease states because of recent advances in understanding how tight junctions work. It is becoming increasingly clear that there are many subtypes of vesicles at the BBB, including those related to transport of viruses across the BBB.

PERMEABILITY FUNCTIONS

If substances could not cross the vascular BBB, the CNS would not survive. As noted previously, numerous classes of substances cross the BBB by way of saturable transporters. Some of these substances act as hormones toward the brain; that is, they are secreted into the blood by peripheral tissues and travel through the bloodstream to affect CNS function.[5] To affect the CNS, these substances must negotiate the BBB. Although there are several indirect ways by which blood-borne substances can influence the CNS, the most direct way is by crossing the BBB. It has long been known that steroid hormones cross the BBB and influence brain function. The idea that peptides and regulatory proteins could cross the BBB was highly controversial when first proposed. It now is clear that many peptides and regulatory proteins can do so. Indeed, consistent with the concept of an NVU, the BBB can be viewed as the crucial intersection in a humoral-based communication between the CNS and peripheral tissues.

Many of the substances that cross the BBB influence the neuroimmune system. The substances that most clearly fit into this category are the cytokines. Currently, more than two dozen cytokines have been examined for their abilities to cross the BBB.[6] Among those found to be transported by a saturable system from blood to brain are interleukin (IL)-1, IL-6, TNF-α, nerve growth factor, neurotensin-3, brain-derived neurotrophic factor, fibroblast growth factor, epidermal growth factor, leukemia inhibitory factor, ciliary neurotrophic factor, gamma interferon, and granulocyte macrophage colony-stimulating factor.

It is increasingly clear that the cytokine transporters are involved in pathologic as well as physiologic states. For example, numerous publications from the laboratory of Pan have shown that the transporters are altered with injuries to the CNS.[7] Those and other studies also show that cytokines with neurotrophic potential can cross the BBB in normal animals as well as in those with injuries to the CNS. At the current time, little or no work is being done to use these transporters to deliver neurotrophic agents to injured brain tissue.

The ability of immune cells to cross the BBB also is of profound importance to neuroimmunology. Trafficking between the CNS and blood occurs under normal circumstances and can be greatly increased in disease conditions.[8] Penetration of the BBB by immune cells does not occur because of a disrupted BBB. Instead, an intimate and orchestrated interaction occurs between the immune cell and the brain endothelial cell. Expression of complementary adhesion molecules by both cells is vital to binding and subsequent interactions. Expression of intercellular adhesion molecule-1 by brain endothelial cells has been identified as a key step in immune cell trafficking in the CNS. The expression of these adhesion molecules is influenced by proinflammatory cytokines. A prominent route by which immune cells cross the BBB is the process of diapedesis in which the immune cell tunnels through the brain endothelial cell, not between the tight junctions between cells. Thus cells programmed or activated by events outside the CNS can enter the brain or spinal cord to secrete substances or otherwise interact with cells within the CNS.

CLEARANCE FUNCTIONS

The role of the movement of substances from the CNS into the blood is an important, but seldom considered, topic for psychoneuroimmunology. Substances enter the blood from the CNS by two broad mechanisms: the efflux of substances from brain interstitial fluid into the blood and the reabsorption of CSF.[9] Efflux from brain interstitial fluid into blood occurs across the capillary wall and can be mediated by saturable efflux systems or by nonsaturable diffusion across the cell membranes comprising the brain endothelial cell. Reabsorption of CSF can occur at the arachnoid villi, in which case the CSF enters the venous drainage of the brain, or at the olfactory bulbs, in which case the CSF enters the lymphatic drainage for the head. Brief examples can show why movement from the CNS to blood is so important in psychoneuroimmunology.

The CNS can be a tremendous source of cytokine production, particularly in states such as meningitis. These cytokines can enter the blood with the reabsorption of the CNS at the arachnoid villi. Only one cytokine has been found to have a saturable transporter directed from the brain to the blood: IL-2. This efflux of cytokine from brain to blood can elevate brain levels, and it is possible that much of the cytokine found in the blood is derived from the CNS.[10]

It seems that much of the methionine enkephalin found in blood is derived from the CNS. Methionine enkephalin is a small opiate peptide produced by both peripheral tissues and the CNS that has neuroimmune functions. It is transported from the CNS to the blood by the saturable peptide transport system-1. It has been estimated that about 30% to 40% of the circulating methionine enkephalin is derived from the CNS.[11]

Substances injected into the CSF can have profound effects on peripheral immune function. This area is understudied, and the mechanisms of action are not clear. The major hypothesis is that the substances are reabsorbed with the CSF and travel to the cervical lymphatics, where they affect immune cell function.[12] In a somewhat similar manner, corticotropin-releasing hormone is transported from brain to blood, where it circulates to the spleen. Once there, it affects splenic production of the opiate neuroimmune modulator β-endorphin.[13]

SECRETORY FUNCTIONS

The BBB can be the conduit by which circulating cytokines affect the CNS through mechanisms other than direct passage. The cytokines, for example, can alter the permeability of the BBB to a variety of substances and through numerous mechanisms. Cytokines also can alter receptor levels on brain endothelial cells. Another mechanism that has received much less attention is the ability of the cells that comprise the BBB to secrete cytokines. In 1993 Fabry and colleagues[14] showed that brain endothelial cells can secrete IL-1 and IL-6. In 1999, Hoffman and colleagues[15] showed that exposure to the HIV-1 protein Tat induced release of IL-8, and Reyes and colleagues[16] showed release of IL-6 on exposure to LPS. Since then, it has been shown that numerous other cytokines are released from brain endothelial cells and the choroid plexus either spontaneously or upon stimulation. Other substances important to the neuroimmune system, including prostaglandins and nitric oxide, also are released from the BBB.

The importance of the BBB release of cytokines in psychoneuroimmunology can be illustrated by the versatility of pathways. First, the brain endothelial cell could receive input from its brain side and secrete substances back into the CNS. As such, it could be the fourth member of the currently popular triad involving cross-talk among neurons, astrocytes, and microglia. Likewise, the BBB could receive neuroimmune stimulation from the blood and respond by secreting substances back into the blood. The most exciting aspect of the BBB secretion of cytokines is that the BBB could receive stimulation from one side and secrete cytokines into the other. For example, a brain endothelial cell might receive an immune signal at its blood side and respond by secreting a cytokine from its brain side. No other part of the immune system, with the exception of immune cells that cross the BBB, can be activated in one compartment of the CNS-immune axis and respond by releasing substances into the other compartment. Recently, it has been shown that brain endothelial cells indeed can receive input from one side and secrete cytokines into the other.[17]

SUMMARY

The very term "psychoneuroimmunology" connotes separate compartments that interact. The BBB is the physical and physiologic dividing line between the immune system and the CNS and is the locale for interaction. Interactions between the immune system and the CNS are mediated at the BBB through a variety of mechanisms. The BBB restricts unregulated mixing of the immune substances in the blood with those in the CNS, directly transports neuroimmune active substances between the blood and the CNS, and secretes neuroimmune substances. All these normal functions of the BBB can be altered in an adaptive or pathologic manner by neuroimmune events. As such, the BBB is an important conduit in the communication of the immune and the central nervous systems.

REFERENCES

1. Reese TS, Karnovsky MJ. Fine structural localization of a blood-brain barrier to exogenous peroxidase. J Cell Biol 1967;34:207–17.
2. Davson H, Segal MB. Blood-brain barrier. Physiology of the CSF and blood-brain barriers. Boca Raton (FL): CRC Press; 1996. p. 49–91.
3. Sanders VM. The role of adrenoceptor-mediated signals in the modulation of lymphocyte function. Adv Neuroimmunol 1995;5:283–98.
4. Hardebo JE, Owman C. Enzymatic barrier mechanisms for neurotransmitter monoamines and their precursors at the blood-brain barrier. In: Johansson BB, Owman C, Widner H, editors. Pathophysiology of the blood-brain barrier. Amsterdam: Elsevier; 1990. p. 41–55.

5. Banks WA, Kastin AJ. Passage of peptides across the blood-brain barrier: pathophysiological perspectives. Life Sci 1996;59:1923–43.

6. Banks WA. Blood-brain barrier transport of cytokines: a mechanism for neuropathology. Curr Pharm Des 2005;11:973–84.

7. Pan W, Kastin AJ. Transport of cytokines and neurotrophins across the blood-brain barrier and their regulations after spinal cord injury. In: Sharma HS, Westman J, editors. Blood-spinal cord and brain barriers in health and disease. Amsterdam: Elsevier; 2004. p. 395–407.

8. Turowski P, Adamson P, Greenwood J. Pharmacological targeting of ICAM-1 signaling in brain endothelial cells: potential for treating neuroinflammation. Cell Mol Neurobiol 2005;25:153–70.

9. Davson H, Segal MB. The return of the cerebrospinal fluid to the blood: the drainage mechanism. In: Physiology of the CSF and blood-brain barriers. Boca Raton (FL): CRC Press; 1996. p. 489–523.

10. Chen G, Reichlin S. Clearance of [^{125}I]-tumor necrosis factor-α from the brain into the blood after intracerebroventricular injection into rats. Neuroimmunomodulation 1998;5:261–9.

11. Banks WA, Kastin AJ. The role of the blood-brain barrier transporter PTS-1 in regulating concentrations of methionine enkephalin in blood and brain. Alcohol 1997;14:237–45.

12. Knopf PM, Cserr HF, Nolan SC, et al. Physiology and immunology of lymphatic drainage of interstitial and cerebrospinal fluid from the brain. Neuropathol Appl Neurobiol 1995;21:175–80.

13. Martins JM, Banks WA, Kastin AJ. Transport of CRH from mouse brain directly affects peripheral production of β-endorphin by the spleen. Am J Physiol 1997; 273:E1083–9.

14. Fabry Z, Fitzsimmons KM, Herlein JA, et al. Production of the cytokines interleukin 1 and 6 by murine brain microvessel endothelium and smooth muscle pericytes. J Neuroimmunol 1993;47:23–34.

15. Hofman F, Chen P, Incardona F, et al. HIV-tat protein induces the production of interleukin-8 by human brain-derived endothelial cells. J Neuroimmunol 1999; 94:28–39.

16. Reyes TM, Fabry Z, Coe CL. Brain endothelial cell production of a neuroprotective cytokine, interleukin-6, in response to noxious stimuli. Brain Res 1999;851: 215–20.

17. Verma S, Nakaoke R, Dohgu S, et al. Release of cytokines by brain endothelial cells: a polarized response to lipopolysaccharide. Brain Behav Immun; 2006. DOI:10.1016/j.bbi.2005.10.005.

Molecular Aspects of Fever and Hyperthermia

Joachim Roth, PhD[a],*, Christoph Rummel, PhD, DVM[a],
Stephan W. Barth, DVM[b], Rüdiger Gerstberger, PhD[a],
Thomas Hübschle, PhD[a]

KEYWORDS

- Innate immunity • Pyrogens • Cytokines
- Immune-to-brain communication • Cyclooxygenase
- Prostaglandins

When heat production or heat gain exceeds heat dissipation or heat loss, the body core temperature rises above its range specified for the normal active state of the species.[1,2] Such a thermal imbalance leads to a state of hyperthermia. This imbalance can occur for several reasons: an increase in metabolic heat production, an impairment of heat-dissipating effector mechanisms, a decrease in heat-absorbing mechanisms by the environment under hot external conditions, or a response to a drug. Usually, an overwhelming of the mechanisms for temperature control causes the resulting hyperthermia.

Fever is a state that also is characterized by an elevation of body temperature, but there is no overwhelming of thermoregulatory control mechanisms. In contrast, the thermoregulatory control system is adjusted to increase body temperature to match a higher set point (ie, the higher body temperature actively is established and defended by the operation of heat-producing and heat-conserving thermoeffectors).[1]

Persons who are hyperthermic have increased skin blood flow to improve convective heat loss and sweat to dissipate heat by evaporation of water. In contrast, at least during the rising phase of fever, skin blood flow is reduced and persons who are febrile do not sweat but rather shiver to increase metabolic heat production. These thermoregulatory effector mechanisms are supported by appropriate behavior. Although a hyperthermic organism seeks a cool environment, the state of fever is characterized

This article is a version of an article previously published in *Neurologic Clinics*: Roth J, Rummel C, Barth SW, Gerstberger R, Hübschle T. Molecular aspects of fever and hyperthermia. Neurol Clin 2006;24(3):421–39.

[a] Department of Veterinary Physiology, Faculty of Veterinary Medicine, Justus-Liebig-University Giessen, Frankfurter Strasse 100, D-35392 Giessen, Germany
[b] Department of Nutritional Physiology and Biochemistry, Federal Research Institute of Nutrition and Food, Haid-und-Neu Strasse 9, D-76131 Karlsruhe, Germany
* Corresponding author.
E-mail address: joachim.roth@vetmed.uni-giessen.de (J. Roth).

by huddling or by the search for warm environmental conditions.[3,4] The strategy to establish fever seems to depend on ambient temperature. In the cold, increased heat production is activated to achieve the febrile state, whereas in warm environments, a suppression of heat-loss mechanisms is typical.[5]

In summary, the rise in core temperature during fever usually is a result of change in the thermocontroller characteristics leading to an elevation of the set point of body temperature. Time course and extent of natural fevers vary, but an upper limit (41°C in humans) rarely is exceeded. At this upper limit, core temperature is maintained for some time and reduced when the set point of body temperature returns to its normal level. Although any rise in body temperature may result from fever, those rises that are not accompanied by supportive changes in thermoeffector activities are termed *hyperthermia*.[1]

FEVER AS A PART OF THE ACUTE-PHASE RESPONSE TO INFECTION OR SYSTEMIC INFLAMMATION

A strong association between fever and infection has been recognized for a long time, which is why fever is frequently called a hallmark of infection.[6] The manifestation of fever, however, is not restricted to infectious diseases of bacterial, viral, protozoal, fungal, or other origin. Fever also is observed in response to injury, such as injuries associated with surgery, trauma, chemicals, or thermal insults. In addition, fever frequently accompanies some endogenous mechanisms. Such mechanisms include autoimmune responses (eg, rheumatoid arthritis) and tumors. The question arises, therefore: What do all these situation that elicit fever have in common?

Inflammation is the general term for changes that may occur in vascularized tissues as part of the response to tissue damage, infection, or immunologic reactions. The aforementioned stimuli that can cause fever are identical to those capable of eliciting inflammatory responses (ie, infection, injury, and endogenous mechanisms). The functions of the inflammatory response include destruction or inactivation of the initiating irritant or agent and then the clearance of the area of debris so that healing can occur. Various cell types activated in the damaged or infected tissue release many soluble mediators, including growth factors, cytokines, chemokines, eicosanoids, kinis, biogenic amines, and neuropepdides. At the site of inflammation, these mediators exert vascular effects (vasodilation, vascular stasis, and increased capillary permeability), promote leukocyte migration from the circulation into the inflamed tissue, and coordinate the still-localized array of defense responses. Some of these mediators have the capacity to stimulate local sensory nerves (discussed later). In cases where the inflammatory response exceeds a certain strength, significant amounts of endogenous mediators and, in case of infection, microbes or microbial products enter the systemic circulation and are disseminated by blood flow to different organs. This results in a complex array of systemic reactions, collectively termed *the acute-phase response*, which is defined as the multifactorial stereotyped response of an organism to infection, injury, or trauma. The acute-phase response comprises changes in plasma concentrations of trace metals, liver proteins (acute-phase proteins), hormones, intermediary metabolism, neutrophilia, and a characteristic set of brain-controlled signs of illness, collectively termed *sickness behavior*.[1,7] Sickness behavior includes development of fever, loss of appetite, increased slow-wave sleep, decreased motor activity, reduced libido, and decreased allertness.[8]

The acute-phase response is considered an early, nonspecific host defense response and is triggered by the release of cytokines, such as interleukin (IL)-1, IL-6, tumor necrosis factor (TNF)-α, and interferons. These cytokines and other inflammatory mediators, which may appear in the blood during infection, injury, or endogenous pathophysiologic reactions (discussed previously), are therefore implicated in fever. They are frequently called *endogenous pyrogens*.[3,6,9–12]

EXPERIMENTAL FEVER

Depending on the disease that causes clinical fever, febrile patterns are categorized into diagnostically valuable groups. A published report from a symposium summarizes clinical fever patterns:[13] sustained fevers of several days with only slight remissions (pneumonia, typhoid fever, or malaria), intermittent fevers with large fluctuations (sepsis), biphasic fevers with two phases lasting several days (many viral infections), weekly periods of fever with equally long afebrile periods and with repetition of this cycle (Hodgkin disease), and several other fever patterns.[13]

Current knowledge of molecular mechanisms of fever derives almost exclusively from experimental fever research performed in animals or, in rare cases, human volunteers. Experimental fever is induced by injection of an exogenous pyrogen, a fever-inducing microbial component or product. Bolus injections of a given exogenous pyrogen usually result in a generalized inflammatory response. In the majority of experimental fever studies, lipopolysaccharide (LPS) from gram-negative bacteria is used to induce a febrile response. Depending on dosage, ambient temperature, and route of administration, LPS, also known as bacterial endotoxin, evokes a stereotypic and reproducible fever that consists of several phases and lasts 6 to 8 hours.[14–17] **Fig. 1** shows the typical thermal responses of rats to intraperitoneal injections of a moderate or a high LPS dose compared with sterile saline at an ambient temperature of 24°C.

In rats, the injection procedure causes a transient stress-induced increase of abdominal temperature, which is measured continuously by means of an intra-abdominally implanted telemetry transmitter. In rats treated with 100 μg/kg LPS, this rise of body temperature is followed by a fever, which is absent in control animals

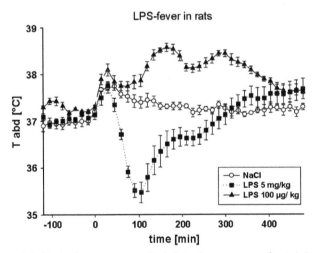

Fig. 1. Changes of abdominal temperature (T abd) in three groups of rats injected intraperitoneally with either sterile saline (NaCl), a moderate dose of 100 μg/kg LPS, or a high dose of 5 mg/kg LPS. Body temperature was recorded continuously by means of an intra-abdominally implanted temperature-sensitive transmitter (remote radiotelemetry) at an ambient temperature of 24°C. The moderate dose of LPS induced a biphasic fever, whereas the high LPS dose caused a septic shock–like state associated with severe hypothermia.

injected with sterile saline. Administration of 5 mg/kg LPS causes a septic shock–like state, characterized by the development of hypothermia rather than fever.

Because most knowledge of molecular aspects of fever is based on studies in which LPS is used as exogenous pyrogen, the majority of the findings presented in this article derive from the experimental model of LPS fever. However, many other products from various microorganisms (gram-positive bacteria, mycoplasmas, viruses, fungi, and parasites) are capable of inducing a pronounced febrile response. The question of whether or not there are common, or rather distinct, molecular mechanisms for the generation of experimental fever in response to all of these exogenous pyrogens is under investigation.[18,19] In addition to microbial products, experimental fever also can be induced by some nonmicrobial agents (different antigens, inflammatory agents, plant lectins, and alcaloids), synthetic products (polynucleotides, antitumor agents, and immunoadjuvants), or even some host-derived substances (destroyed tissue, antigen-antibody complexes, activated complement fragments, certain metabolites, and lymphocyte products). Because most of these fever-inducing pathogenic stimuli are derived from the body's external environment, they generally are termed *exogenous pyrogens*.[11,20]

EXOGENOUS PYROGENS CAUSE THE PRODUCTION OF ENDOGENOUS PYROGENS

The historical discovery of the "endogenous pyrogen" in 1948 led to the hypothesis that exogenous pyrogens do not directly cause fever.[21] This "endogenous pyrogen," obtained from isolated peritoneal macrophages, induced fever in noninfected rabbits. The substance was heat labile and was suggested, therefore, to be a protein. Later studies demonstrated that, after injection of an exogenous pyrogen, such as LPS, endogenous pyrogen appeared in the circulation of the LPS-stimulated animals.[20]

Intensive research has focused on the molecular identification and cloning of putative endogenous pyrogens. These molecules are members of the growing family of cytokines. The term *cytokine* is used as a generic name for a diverse group of soluble proteins acting as humoral regulators that modulate the functional activities of individual cells and tissues. In the context of this article, cytokines of particular interest are those associated with the inflammatory response. With regard to experimentally induced LPS fever (see **Fig. 1**), four sets of observations support a role for inflammatory cytokines in the manifestation of the observed febrile response.

The first set of observations relates to the appearance of several cytokines in the systemic circulation more or less in parallel to the development of fever. In response to injections of LPS, TNF-α is the first cytokine that appears in the bloodstream,[22–24] followed by traces of IL-1[24] and high amounts of IL-6.[23,25,26] From these three cytokines, considered the most important endogenous mediators of LPS fever, only IL-6 can be measured in significant quantities in the blood during the time course of fever, and circulating levels of IL-6 show the best correlation with the febrile changes of body temperature.[23,25,27]

The second body of evidence relates to the repeated observations that systemic injections or infusions of single proinflammatory cytokines can induce fever, as shown for IL-1,[28,29] TNF-α,[30,31] and IL-6.[32,33] In this context, the pyrogenic effects of peripherally administered IL-6 are moderate compared with those of IL-1 or TNF-α. It is a matter of debate whether or not the pyrogenic effects of systemic injections of these cytokines reflect the physiologic conditions induced by administration of LPS.[3]

The third set of observations derives from experimental procedures in which single LPS-induced cytokines were neutralized or antagonized in their biologic activity and a concomitant reduction of LPS fever was observed. Thus, treatments with IL-1 receptor antagonist,[12,26] a TNF-α–neutralizing synthetic form of the P55-soluble TNF-α receptor,[12,34] or IL-6–neutralizing IL-6 antibodies[35] resulted in a significant attenuation of the febrile response to LPS, indicating a role for these cytokines in the manifestation of LPS fever. However, such anticytokine strategies predominantly inhibited the late phases of LPS fever, and there seemed to be some species-specific differences in the role of TNF-α in the LPS-induced febrile response.[3,12,22,34]

Finally, the fourth set of observations derives from studies in cytokine-deficient knockout mice.[36] In IL-1 knockout mice, LPS fever is reduced although not abolished.[37,38] The investigators in these studies conclude that IL-1 contributes to, but is not essential for, the manifestation of a febrile response to LPS. Alternatively, fever in response to a moderate fever–inducing LPS dose is abolished in IL-6 knockout mice,[38,39] suggesting that IL-6 gene expression is essential for fever caused by a moderate LPS challenge.

Thus, a large body of evidence supports the view that the appearance of an exogenous pyrogen (LPS or others) in a host causes fever via the formation of endogenous pyrogens (cytokines). In recent years, our knowledge of how predominantly immune cells are stimulated by foreign molecules to produce a cascade of pyrogenic cytokines has improved substantially. The innate immune system, predominantly associated with neutrophils, monocytes, and macrophages, represents the first defense line against a variety of pathogens. The presence of a given pathogen within an infected host is recognized by endogenous receptors for so-called "pathogen-associated molecular patterns" (PAMPs). Members of the Toll-like receptor (TLR) family are identified as key receptors for the recognition of PAMPs. TLR signal transduction mechanisms in myeloid and possibly other cells finally leads to the production of inflammatory cytokines in the infected host.[19,40,41] LPS from gram-negative bacteria, the best-studied activator of the innate immune system, acts via the TLR4 receptor.[42] Meanwhile, several distinct microbe-associated PAMPs and several specific TLR subtypes recognizing those PAMPs are identified.[40,41] It seems that the activation of various TLRs finally results in similar circulating cascades of proinflammatory cytokines and, thereby, the manifestation of a febrile response.[18,19,34]

HOW DO CIRCULATING CYTOKINES CONVEY A PYROGENIC MESSAGE TO THE BRAIN?

The febrile shift of the thermoregulatory set point to a higher body temperature occurs within the preoptic-anterior hypothalamic area, the most important control center of thermoregulation. Accepting that circulating cytokines are important humoral mediators of fever, the question arises of how these large hydrophilic peptides with a molecular weight of 15 to 25 kd pass the relatively impermeable blood-brain barrier to stimulate the relevant hypothalamic thermoregulatory structures. Three mechanisms for immune-to-brain signaling by circulating pyrogenic cytokines are proposed. Cytokines transported by the bloodstream could act at sites lacking a tight blood-brain barrier, the so-called "circumventricular organs" (CVOs).[43] Alternatively, circulating cytokines could interact with their specific receptors on brain endothelial cells[44] or perivascular cells.[45] Finally, it is proposed that fever-promoting cytokines can pass the blood-brain barrier by active and saturable transport systems specific for individual cytokines.[46] An assumed manifestation of a febrile response by these mechanisms collectively is termed *humoral hypothesis of fever induction*. The article by Banks and colleagues elsewhere in this issue discusses the mechanisms of how endogenous pyrogens are transported from the blood to the brain. Here, a brief look is directed to both of the other humoral fever induction pathways.

INTERACTIONS OF ENDOGENOUS OR EXOGENOUS PYROGENS WITH SENSORY CIRCUMVENTRICULAR ORGANS

CVOs are brain structures that have cells in contact with the cerebroventricular system, have a dense vascularization, and lack a blood-brain barrier. A subgroup of the CVOs is called *sensory CVOs* and includes the vascular organ of the laminae terminalis (OVLT), the subfornical organ, and the area postrema. These brain structures have capillaries with fenestrated endothelia surrounded by perivascular spaces. The parenchyma of these structures is composed of not only glial cells, but also of neuronal soma, dendritic/axonal processes, and terminals that reveal multiple reciprocal connectivities to other hypothalamic and extra-hypothalamic nuclei. Because of the lack of a blood-brain barrier, the cells within the sensory CVOs are exposed directly to circulating signal molecules. The cells may be able to sense the signal molecules via specific receptors.[43] The OVLT and the subfornical organ are located within the anterior wall of the third ventricle, the lamina terminalis. The area postrema is a component of the dorsal vagal motor complex, a major viscerosensory and autonomic center of the medulla oblongata. The locations of the sensory (and other) CVOs are illustrated in **Fig. 2**.

Research suggests that, because of their properties as target structures for circulating inflammatory molecules, each of the three sensory CVOs participates in the manifestation of brain-controlled sickness responses. With regard to fever, the OVLT has special importance because of its location close to the preoptic area. This part of the anterior-preoptic hypothalamic structures, where fever is induced, is activated strongly after intravenous injection of LPS, as demonstrated by a high level of Fos immunoreactivity, which is a neuroanatomic marker for physiologically activated neurons (**Fig. 3**).[47] Because of its high sensitivity to pyrogenic stimulation, this part of the preoptic area is suggested as representing a pyrogenic zone of the brain.[48]

Lesion studies provided the first evidence for a role of the OVLT in the manifestation of fever. Large lesions of the lamina terminalis that completely included the OVLT prevented fever after systemic injections of bacterial LPS.[49,50] At the cellular and molecular levels, three prerequisites must be met for the OVLT to act as a sensor of circulating pyrogenic cytokines: (1) Cellular elements within the OVLT must possess

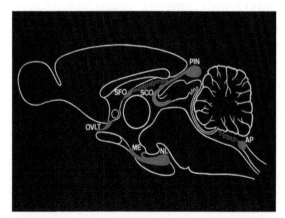

Fig. 2. A midsagittal section through the rat brain. Red indicates areas that lack a tight blood-brain barrier. Blue and yellow indicate parts of the choroid plexus. AP, area postrema; ME, median eminence; NL, neural lobe of the pituitary; PIN, pineal organ; SCO, subcomissural organ; SFO, subfornical organ.

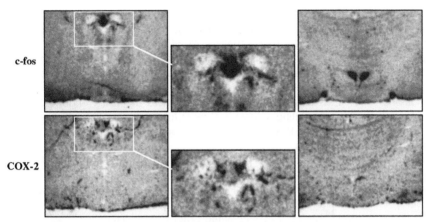

Fig. 3. Expression of the c-fos (*upper three panels*) and the COX-2 gene (*lower three panels*) in the rat brain after LPS treatment (2500 µg/kg) as determined by radioactive in situ hybridization. Strong hybridization signals specific for *c-fos* (*upper panels, left* and *middle*) and *COX-2* mRNA (*lower panels, left* and *middle*) are visible in form of black labeling in the subfornical organ, one of the sensory CVOs. Although *c-fos* signals accumulate in the core region of the subfornical organ, *COX-2*–specific signals are located in the lateral part of the subfornical organ and extend into vascular signals in the surrounding tissue. The paraventricular nucleus shows a strong *c-fos* up-regulation (*upper panels, right*), whereas only scarce vascular *COX-2* signals appear in this region (*lower panels, right*). *COX-2* signals are hardly detectable in control animals injected with sterile saline instead of LPS (not shown).

receptors for IL-1,[51] IL-6,[52] and TNF-α;[53] (2) neurons located in the OVLT must change their firing rate under the influence of pyrogenic cytokines[54] (such electrical activity changes affect adjacent thermosensitive neurons transsynaptically and thereby contribute to the generation of fever), and (3) a direct genomic activation of cellular elements within the OVLT must occur in response to circulating cytokines as revealed by the expression of the c-fos gene[43] or by the nuclear translocation of cytokine-specific transcription factors into the nuclei of cytokine-stimulated cells, such as the acute phase response factor, signal-transducer and activator of transcription 3 (STAT3).[17,33] Thus, much evidence indicates that the OVLT may act as a sensor for circulating endogenous pyrogens and, thus, might be able to transfer febrile signals to the preoptic-hypothalamic structures situated nearby.

In addition to receptors for pyrogenic cytokines, several TLRs are expressed within the sensory CVOs.[41] Consequently, circulating PAMPs (ie, LPS and others) can be sensed by these specialized brain structures even before a peripheral formation of proinflammatory cytokines. We recently reported microglial cells, located in sensory CVOs, directly respond to LPS stimulation with fast transient rises in intracellular calcium concentration and a localized formation of pyrogenic cytokines.[55] This direct and rapid response of brain sites with an incomplete blood-brain barrier, which are implicated in the manifestation of fever, to circulating PAMPs can be interpreted as an alternative possibility for transmission of febrile signals to the brain.

INTERACTIONS OF ENDOGENOUS PYROGENS WITH BRAIN ENDOTHELIAL CELLS AND PERIVASCULAR CELLS

Several lines of arguments support the view that not only sensory CVOs but also the entire brain endothelium is a major target for circulating cytokines implicated in fever.

One such argument points to clear evidence that brain endothelial cells constitutively express receptors for TNF-α[53] and IL-1.[56] Namely, the IL-1 receptor type 1 seems to be predominantly expressed in endothelial cells of brain venules but not in those of arterioles.[56] The accessory signal transduction molecule for the IL-6 receptor, glycoprotein 130, also is expressed constitutively in brain endothelial cells, whereas the expression of the IL-6 receptor itself is induced in these cells under inflammatory conditions.[52] An IL-6–activated signal transduction in the brain endothelium also can be achieved by circulating soluble IL-6 receptors in connection with their ligand (IL-6) and the glycoprotein 130 signal transducer located in the membranes of endothelial cells within the brain.

A genomic activation of the brain endothelium by IL-1[57] or IL-6[58] recently has been demonstrated. IL-1 and IL-6 induce a pronounced nuclear translocation of the transcription factors, nuclear factor κB (NF-κB) (activated by IL-1) or STAT3 (activated by IL-6), in endothelial cells all over the brain.[57,58] **Fig. 4** shows an example from the authors' experiments for IL-6–stimulated brain endothelial cells showing nuclear STAT3 activation.

At least the IL-1 receptor type 1 and its stimulation under inflammatory stimulation also is demonstrated in perivascular cells,[56] a subset of bone marrow–derived brain macrophages. The final response of such a genomic activation of brain endothelial and perivascular cells is the expression of enzymes, which are responsible for the formation of prostaglandin E2 (PGE2). PGE2 is regarded as a key mediator of fever. In this context, there seems to be a critical role for perivascular and endothelial cells in monitoring circulating cytokines. With regard to the capacity of both cell types to respond to such signals with the production of prostaglandins, perivascular cells seem to exhibit an even greater sensitivity to inflammatory stimuli.[45]

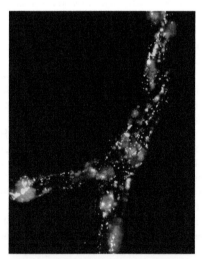

Fig. 4. Guinea pig brain endothelial cells respond to stimulation with bacterial LPS (30 μg/kg, intraperitoneal injection) with a nuclear translocation of the transcription factor STAT3 at 90 minutes after LPS injection. Immunoreactive nuclear STAT3 signals (*red*) are surrounded by immunohistochemically detected von Willebrand factor (*green*), a marker protein of endothelial cells. Nuclear STAT3 activation in brain endothelial cells is detected in LPS-stimulated animals but not in controls injected with sterile saline (not shown).

A CRUCIAL ROLE FOR PROSTAGLANDIN E2 WITHIN THE CENTRAL NERVOUS SYSTEM

Whether or not pyrogenic cytokines are interacting with cells in sensory CVOs or with brain endothelial/perivascular cells or whether or not they are transported into the brain, they have to cause production or release of the final mediators of fever within the preoptic-anterior hypothalamus. For the following reasons, PGE2 traditionally is regarded as the key fever mediator in the brain and as the biologic agent finally responsible for the febrile upward shift of the thermoregulatory set point: (1) Prostaglandins evoke fever when injected into cerebral ventricles,[59] even in very small amounts into the most PGE2-sensitive site within the preoptic-anterior hypothalamic area;[48] (2) the levels of PGE2 in the blood[60] and in the brain[61] rise parallel to the febrile changes of body temperature; and (3) drugs that block prostaglandin synthesis also effectively inhibit fever.[11,12,60] **Fig. 5** shows an example from the authors' experiments on the effects of inhibitors of PGE2 synthesis on LPS-induced fever in rats. Systemic treatments with a nonselective cyclooxygenase (COX) inhibitor (diclofenac) or with a preferential COX-2 inhibitor (meloxicam), which blocks formation of PGE2, result in significant and similar attenuations of LPS-induced fever in rats.

PGE2 is a derivative of arachidonic acid, which is cleaved from membrane phospholipids by phospholipase A2. In a second step, arachidonic acid is converted to prostaglandin H2 by COX enzymes. Finally, prostaglandin H2 is isomerized to PGE2 by prostaglandin E synthase (PGES).[44,62] Several isoenzymes exist for each of these catalytic steps. COX-2 and microsomal PGES-1 (mPGES-1) are inducible enzymes regulated transcriptionally by NF-κB, a transcription factor activated by LPS, IL-1, or TNF-α (ie, under inflammatory conditions).[63] During LPS fever, the expressions of COX-2 and mPGES-1 are up-regulated strongly by pyrogenic cytokines,[64] and the

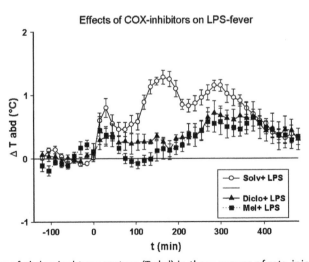

Fig. 5. Changes of abdominal temperature (T abd) in three groups of rats, injected intraperitoneally with 100 μg/kg LPS alone (Solv+ LPS); with 100 μg/kg LPS along with 5 mg/kg of the nonselective COX-inhibitor diclofenac (Diclo+ LPS); or with 100 μg/kg LPS along with 5 mg/kg of the preferential COX-2 inhibitor meloxicam (Mel+ LPS). Body temperature was recorded continuously by means of an intra-abdominally implanted temperature-sensitive transmitter (radiotelemetry). Treatment with both COX-inhibitors (nonselective versus preferential COX-2 inhibitor) resulted in a similar attenuation of LPS-induced fever. t (min), time in minutes.

colocalized expressions of COX-2 and mPGES-1 are suggested as the major source for PGE2 biosynthesis in the brain during fever.[44,63,64] Predominantly brain endothelial cells and perivascular cells express COX-2 under the influence of inflammatory cytokines.[44,45] A strong expression of COX-2 in response to a fever-inducing systemic treatment with LPS occurs in the OVLT and the subfornical organ. An example from the authors' experiments demonstrates this for the subfornical organ (see **Fig. 3**). In contrast, systemic treatment with LPS does not cause a pronounced induction of COX-2 in the hypothalamic paraventricular nucleus, which is known to activate during fever,[47] as shown by the pronounced LPS-induced expression of the c-fos gene (see **Fig. 3**).

The fact that an up-regulation of COX-2/mPGES-1 is observed during LPS fever alone is not proof of a critical role of these inducible enzymes in the manifestation of the febrile response. There is, however, more experimental support for such a hypothesis. Several reports have found that selective COX-2–specific inhibitors block LPS-induced fever.[64–66] Further supporting evidence has come from studies in knockout mice deficient in either COX-2[67,68] or mPGES-1.[69,70] In both cases, the febrile response is depressed. It seems, therefore, that the synthesis of COX-2/mPGES-1 in the brain, which is induced by pyrogenic cytokines, is critical for the brain-intrinsic formation of PGE2 during fever.

PGE2 seems to evoke fever via activation of the prostaglandin receptor subtype EP3, as suggested from studies in knockout mice deficient in this receptor, in which fever in response to LPS is strongly impaired.[71,72] It is suggested that an efferent fever-inducing pathway arises from activated EP3 receptors located in the preoptic-anterior hypothalamic area, namely in the medial preoptic nucleus[73,74] close to the OVLT. Using the viral tracing technique combined with immunocytochemical detection of the EP3 receptor, a complete efferent fever pathway starting from the medial preoptic area and ending finally in the thermogenic brown adipose tissue of the rat is demonstrated neuroanatomically.[75] A colocalization of virus protein with the EP3 receptor also is found in some neurons of the OVLT itself.[75] This neuronal chain thus might be regarded as the efferent part of the thermoregulatory reflexes, which are activated by interactions of circulating endogenous pyrogens with cells located within the OVLT and the adjacent medial preoptic area.

AN ALTERNATIVE AND RAPID MECHANISM OF PYROGENIC SIGNAL TRANSMISSION FROM THE PERIPHERY TO THE BRAIN

This article has described a complete chain of events leading to the genesis of fever, starting with the LPS-induced formation of endogenous pyrogens (cytokines), their interactions with relevant targets in the brain (CVOs and brain endothelial cells), the induction of enzymes responsible for the formation of PGE2 (COX-2 and mPGES-1), the activation of descending neuronal pathways via the EP3 receptor, and the stimulation of thermogenesis via this pathway to support the febrile shift of the thermoregulatory set point. Is this the end of the story? One recent challenge to this hypothesis focuses on the initial or "early" phase of LPS-induced fever (see **Figs. 1** and **5**).[76] The objections to the prevailing view are based mainly on the observation that, at least under some specific experimental conditions, the first phase of LPS-induced fever seems to be initiated before the appearance of cytokines in the blood. Therefore, an alternative and rapid signal pathway for the induction of the early phase of LPS fever is suggested.[77]

Within the past 10 years, several published studies indicate that the humoral hypothesis (described previously) does not represent the only and exclusive pathway by which inflammatory signals from the periphery are transported to the brain. Some evidence suggests that the stimulation of afferent nerves, namely afferents from the vagus nerve but also possibly cutaneous afferent sensory nerves,[78] might participate in the manifestation of brain-controlled sickness responses under specific experimental conditions. Initially, this evidence derived from the observation that such signs of illness, which are regulated by the brain, can be attenuated or even abrogated by surgical section of the abdominal trunks of the vagus nerve.[8,11,12,79,80] In addition to arguments based on these effects of subdiaphragmatic vagotomy, additional arguments support a role of the vagus nerve as a pathway for transmission of immune signals to those parts of the brain where fever, anorexia, or sickness behavior are induced. Injection of IL-1 into the portal vein is shown to increase the firing rate of the vagal hepatic afferent nerve branch[81] and, in primary afferent neurons of the vagus nerve, immediate early genes seem to be activated by cytokines.[82] The role of the vagus nerve in the manifestation of fever is controversial, mainly because studies of vagotomized animals have led to somewhat conflicting results.[83]

Based on several experimental studies, Blatteis[76,77,80] suggests a novel hypothesis, including afferent parts of the vagus nerve. This hypothesis could account for a rapid induction of the early phase of LPS-induced fever before the release of larger amounts of cytokines into the bloodstream. Under some conditions, those larger amounts of cytokines might be involved in the maintenance rather than in the initiation of fever. According to this hypothesis, the febrigenic process is initiated by the arrival of LPS in the liver and its uptake by Kupffer cells, causing an immediate activation of complement. The complement component C5a, in turn, seems to stimulate the Kupffer cells to a rapid release of PGE2, which is suggested as activating local sensory vagal terminals that project to the medulla oblongata of the brainstem. From the medulla, this vagally transmitted excitation is believed to be transmitted to the preoptic-anterior hypothalamic area via the ventral noradrenergic bundle. An intra-hypothalamic release of norepinephrine might cause immediate neuronal activity changes via stimulation of α-adrenoreceptors, which are capable of activating efferent fever-promoting pathways. The aforementioned role for intrahypothalamic COX-2/mPGES-1–dependent release of PGE2 in the manifestation of fever thus might operate only for the longer second phase (see **Figs. 1** and **5**) of the LPS-induced febrile response.[76,77] A critical role for TLR4-bearing hepatic (and pulmonary) macrophages in triggering the earliest phase of LPS fever has also been suggested by Romanovsky and colleagues,[84] who reported a rapid formation of peripheral PGE2 by these cells coinciding with the onset of the febrile response.

In summary, it seems possible that the brain is informed by inflammatory processes in the periphery by rapid neuronal signals and, with some delay, by humoral signals. The combination of both types of signals might allow the brain to better identify the nature of the inflammatory challenge and thereby activate a more appropriate defense strategy. Fever, as a part of many successful defense strategies, thus may be a beneficial component of the acute-phase response, which helps to optimize the responses of the immune system against an infectious insult.

MOLECULAR ASPECTS OF HYPERTHERMIA

As discussed, hyperthermia occurs when temperature regulation against overheating is active as a consequence of the temporary or permanent imbalance between heat load and the capacity to dissipate heat. Molecular aspects of hyperthermia include the description of molecular changes, which occur in the heat-stressed brain and, in some cases, the molecular mechanisms, which are the specific causes for a developing hyperthermia.

MALIGNANT HYPERTHERMIA

Malignant hyperthermia is caused by a rare, genetically fixed mutation of the ryanodine receptor, or calcium release channel, in the sarcoplasmatic reticulum of the striated muscles. Some inhalation anesthetics, such as halothane or isofluorane, cause excessive release of calcium from the sarcoplasmatic reticulum in genetically susceptible subjects. Also, the muscle relaxant succinylcholine or high circulating levels of stress hormones can act as triggering agents. As a consequence, uncoordinated muscle contractions with a tremendous rise in oxygen consumption and metabolic rate induce a severe hyperthermia accompanied by acidosis, tachycardia, or cardiac arrhythmias. The often-fatal hyperthermia is supported by the limitations of active heat dissipation during anesthesia.[1,2]

DRUG-INDUCED HYPERTHERMIA

The use of amphetamine-type stimulants can induce a pronounced and sometimes lethal increase in body temperature. Intoxication with 3,4-methylenedioxymethamphetamine (ecstasy), as a consequence of its worldwide recreational use, results in increasing numbers of hospital cases and deaths.[85] In most cases, lethality results from persistent hyperthermia, which leads to a breakdown of skeletal muscles (rhabdomyolysis) and renal failure. Ecstasy-induced hyperthermia seems to result from a strong activation of the sympathetic nervous system and the hypothalamic-pituitary thyroid/adrenal axes.[86] The excessive release of norepinephrine causes pronounced heat generation via β3-adrenergic activation of uncoupling protein type 3 and α1-adrenergic suppression of heat dissipation resulting from sympathetically mediated vasoconstriction.[86] Ecstasy thus represents an impressive example of a drug-induced manifestation of hyperthermia.

THE HEAT STROKE SYNDROME

During prolonged hyperthermia, with a body temperature of 41°C or higher, the brain suffers severe damage, which frequently leads to death. Alterations in microvascular permeability cause the development of cerebral edema. Postmortem findings show microhemorrhages, tissue softening, and destruction of neurons. Victims exhibit disorientation, delirium, and convulsions. This syndrome is referred to popularly as heat stroke. The precise mechanisms that account for the manifestation of heat stroke are under investigation.[87,88] Several molecular changes that occur in the heat-stressed brain already have been identified.[89] The expression of several molecules is up-regulated in the brain under conditions of severe hyperthermia. Thus, the induction of a specific set of proteins, the so-called "heat-shock proteins," is related closely to damaged brain areas and thus can be used as markers of cell injury. There is some evidence that heat-shock proteins have neuroprotective properties.[89] Hyperthermic brain injury is accompanied further by an activation of glial cells (ie, astrocytes), as indicated by the expression of the cell marker protein, glial fibrillary acidic protein. Under pathologic conditions, such as brain hyperthermia, induction of this protein is associated with a breakdown of the blood-brain barrier and vasogenic edema.

Activation of the immune system during infection or inflammation is characterized not only by a systemic formation of cytokines but also by the expression of cytokines in the brain.[8,90] There is evidence that an increased expression of IL-1 within the central nervous system is associated with brain injury. An increased production of IL-1 in the damaged brain accompanies heat stroke–induced cerebral ischemia and neuronal damage. The survival time of rats can be prolonged by treatment with an IL-1 receptor antagonist. This indicates a role for IL-1 and possibly other cytokines in the manifestation of the heat stroke syndrome.[91] In this context, it recently has been reported that elevated cytokine concentrations occur in human heat stroke and in experimental animal heat stroke models.[87,88] The precise role of the stimulated formation of cytokines in heat stroke, as opposed to fever, still has to be elucidated. It is anticipated that a more detailed understanding of the putative roles of cytokines in the modifications of body core temperature in experimental heat stroke models will provide important insight into the role of these substances in the complex etiology of the long-term consequences of this syndrome.[88]

REFERENCES

1. International Union of Physiological Sciences, Commission for Thermal Physiology. Glossary of terms for thermal physiology. 3rd edition. Jpn J Physiol 2001;51:245–80.
2. Roth J. Hyperthermia. In: Fink G, editor. Encyclopedia of stress, vol. 2. San Diego (CA): Academic Press; 2000. p. 431–8.
3. Kluger MJ. Fever: role of pyrogens and cryogens. Physiol Rev 1991;71:93–127.
4. Moltz H. Fever: causes and consequences. Neurosci Biobehav Rev 1993;17: 237–69.
5. Hellon R, Townsend Y, Laburn H, et al. Mechanisms of fever. In: Schönbaum E, Lomax P, editors. Thermoregulation: pathology, pharmacology and therapy. New York: Pergamon Press; 1991. p. 19–54.
6. Blatteis CM. Fever: pathological or physiological, injurious or beneficial? J Therm Biol 2003;28:1–13.
7. Gabay C, Kushner J. Acute-phase proteins and other systemic responses to inflammation. N Engl J Med 1999;340:448–54.
8. Dantzer R. Cytokine-induced sickness behavior: where do we stand? Brain Behav Immun 2001;15:7–24.
9. Luheshi G, Rothwell NJ. Cytokines and fever. Int Arch Allergy Immunol 1996;109: 301–7.
10. Dinarello CA. Cytokines as endogenous pyrogens. J Infect Dis 1999;179(Suppl 2):S294–304.
11. Zeisberger E. From humoral fever to neuroimmunological control of fever. J Therm Biol 1999;24:287–326.
12. Roth J, de Souza GEP. Fever induction pathways: evidence from responses to systemic or local cytokine formation. Braz J Med Biol Res 2001;34:301–14.
13. Mackowiak PA, Bartlett JG, Borden EC, et al. Concepts of fever: recent advances and lingering dogma. Clin Infect Dis 1997;25:119–38.
14. Romanovsky AA, Szekely M. Fever and hypothermia: two adaptive thermoregulatory responses to systemic inflammation. Med Hypotheses 1998;50:219–26.
15. Rudaya AY, Steiner AA, Robbins JR, et al. Thermoregulatory responses to lipopolysaccharide in the mouse: dependence on the dose and ambient temperature. Am J Physiol 2005;289:R1244–52.
16. Cartmell T, Mitchell D, Lamond FJD, et al. Route of administration differentially affects fevers induced by gram-negative and gram-positive pyrogens in rabbits. Exp Physiol 2002;87(3):391–9.

17. Rummel C, Hübschle T, Gerstberger R, et al. Nuclear translocation of the transcription factor STAT3 in the guinea pig brain during systemic or localized inflammation. J Physiol 2004;557(2):671–87.

18. Fortier ME, Kent S, Ashdown H, et al. The viral mimic, polyinosinic: polycytidylic acid, induces fever in rats via an interleukin-1-dependent mechanism. Am J Physiol 2004;287:R759–66.

19. Hübschle T, Mütze J, Mühlradt PF, et al. Pyrexia, anorexia, adipsia and depressed motor activity in rats during systemic inflammation induced by the Toll-like receptor 2- and 6-agonists MALP-2 and FSL-1. Am J Physiol 2006;290:R180–7.

20. Cooper KE. Fever and antipyresis—the role of the nervous system. Cambridge: University Press; 1995.

21. Beeson PB. Temperature-elevating effect of a substance obtained from polymorphonuclear leucocytes. J Clin Invest 1948;27:524–48.

22. Long NC, Kunkel SL, Vander AL, et al. Antiserum against TNF enhances LPS fever in the rat. Am J Physiol 1990;258:R332–7.

23. Roth J, Conn CA, Kluger MJ, et al. Kinetics of systemic and intrahypothalamic IL-6 and tumor necrosis factor during endotoxin fever in guinea pigs. Am J Physiol 1993; 265:R653–8.

24. Jansky L, Vybiral S, Pospisilova D, et al. Production of systemic and hypothalamic cytokines during the early phase of endotoxin fever. Neuroendocrinology 1995; 62:55–61.

25. LeMay LG, Vander AJ, Kluger MJ. Role of interleukin-6 in fever in the rat. Am J Physiol 1990;258:R798–803.

26. Luheshi G, Miller AJ, Brouwer S, et al. Interleukin-1 receptor antagonist inhibits endotoxin fever and systemic interleukin-6 induction in the rat. Am J Physiol 1996;270:E91–5.

27. Roth J, McClellan JL, Kluger MJ, et al. Attenuation of fever and release of cytokines after repeated injections of lipopolysaccharide in guinea pigs. J Physiol 1994;477(1):177–85.

28. Anforth HR, Bluthe RM, Bristow A, et al. Biological activity and brain actions of recombinant rat interleukin-1α and interleukin-1β. Eur Cytokine Netw 1998;9:279–88.

29. Roth J, Störr B, Voigt K, et al. Inhibition of nitric oxide synthase results in a suppression of interleukin-1 beta-induced fever in rats. Life Sci 1998;62: PL345–50.

30. Dinarello CA, Cannon JG, Wolff SM, et al. Tumor necrosis factor (cachectin) is an endogenous pyrogen and induces production of interleukin-1. J Exp Med 1986; 163:1433–50.

31. Goldbach JM, Roth J, Störr B, et al. Repeated infusions of TNFα cause attenuation of the thermal response and influence LPS-fever in guinea pigs. Am J Physiol 1996;270:R749–54.

32. Blatteis CM, Quan N, Xin L, et al. Neuromodulation of acute phase responses to interleukin-6 in guinea pigs. Brain Res Bull 1990;25:895–901.

33. Harré EM, Roth J, Pehl U, et al. Selected contribution: role of IL-6 in LPS-induced nuclear STAT3 translocation in sensory circumventricular organs during fever in rats. J Appl Physiol 2002;92:2657–66.

34. Roth J, Martin D, Störr B, et al. Neutralization of bacterial pyrogen-induced circulating tumour necrosis factor by its type 1 soluble receptor in guinea pigs: effects on fever and endogenous formation of interleukin-6. J Physiol 1998;509(2): 267–75.

35. Cartmell T, Poole S, Turnbull AV, et al. Circulating interleukin-6 mediates the febrile response to localised inflammation in rats. J Physiol 2000;526(3):653–61.

36. Leon LR. Invited review: cytokine regulation of fever: studies using gene knockout mice. J Appl Physiol 2002;92:2648–55.

37. Kozak W, Zheng H, Conn CA, et al. Thermal and behavioural effects of lipopolysaccharide and influenza in interleukin-1β-deficient mice. Am J Physiol 1995;269:R969–77.

38. Kozak W, Kluger MJ, Soszynski D, et al. IL-6 and IL-1β in fever: studies using cytokine-deficient (knockout) mice. Ann N Y Acad Sci 1998;856:33–47.

39. Chai Z, Gatti S, Toniatti C, et al. Interleukin (IL)-6 gene expression in the central nervous system is necessary for fever in response to lipopolysaccharide or IL-1β: a study on IL-6-deficient mice. J Exp Med 1996;183:311–6.

40. Aderem A, Ulevich RJ. Toll-like receptors in the induction of the innate immune response. Nature 2000;406:782–7.

41. Rivest S. Molecular insights into the cerebral innate immune system. Brain Behav Immun 2003;17:13–9.

42. Poltorak A, Ricciardi-Castagnoli P, Citterio S, et al. Physical contact between LPS and Toll-like receptor 4 revealed by genetic complementation. Proc Natl Acad Sci U S A 2000;97:2163–7.

43. Roth J, Harré EM, Rummel C, et al. Signaling the brain in systemic inflammation: role of sensory circumventricular organs. Front Biosci 2004;9:290–300.

44. Matsumura K, Kobayashi S. Signaling the brain in inflammation: the role of endothelial cells. Front Biosci 2004;9:2819–26.

45. Schiltz JC, Sawchenko PE. Signaling the brain in systemic inflammation: the role of perivascular cells. Front Biosci 2003;8:s1321–9.

46. Banks WA, Kastin AJ, Broadwell RD. Passage of cytokines across the blood-brain barrier. Neuroimmunomodulation 1995;2:241–8.

47. Elmquist JK, Scammell TE, Jacobson CD, et al. Distribution of Fos-like immunoreactivity in the rat brain following intravenous lipopolysaccharide administration. J Comp Neurol 1996;371:85–103.

48. Scammell TE, Elmquist JK, Griffin JD, et al. Ventromedial preoptic prostaglandin E2 activates fever-producing autonomic pathways. J Neurosci 1996;16:6246–54.

49. Blatteis CM, Bealer SL, Hunter WS, et al. Suppression of fever after lesions of the anteroventral third ventricle in guinea pigs. Brain Res Bull 1983;11:519–26.

50. Blatteis CM, Hales JRS, McKinley MJ, et al. Role of the anteroventral third ventricle region in fever in sheep. Can J Physiol Pharmacol 1987;65:1255–60.

51. Ericsson A, Liu C, Hart RP, et al. Type 1 interleukin-1 receptor in the rat brain: distribution, regulation, and relationship to sites of IL-1-induced cellular activation. J Comp Neurol 1995;361:681–98.

52. Valliéres L, Rivest S. Regulation of the genes encoding interleukin-6, its receptor, and gp130 in the rat brain in response to immune activator lipopolysaccharide and the proinflammatory cytokine interleukin-1β. J Neurochem 1997;69:1668–83.

53. Nadeaux S, Rivest S. Effects of circulating tumor necrosis factor on the neuronal activity and expression of the genes encoding the tumor necrosis factor receptors (p55 and p75) in the rat brain: a view from the blood-brain barrier. Neuroscience 1999;93:1449–64.

54. Shibata M, Blatteis CM. Human recombinant tumor necrosis factor and interferon affect the activity of neurons in the organum vasculosum laminae terminalis. Brain Res 1991;562:323–6.

55. Wuchert F, Ott D, Murgott J, et al. Rat area postrema microglial cells act as sensors for the Toll-like receptor-4 agonist lipopolysaccharide. J Neuroimmunol 2008;204:66–74.

56. Konsman JP, Vigues S, Mackerlova L, et al. Rat brain vascular distribution of interleukin-1 type-1 receptor immunoreactivity: relationship to patterns of inducible

cyclooxygenase expression by peripheral inflammatory stimuli. J Comp Neurol 2004;472:113–29.

57. Nadjar A, Combe C, Layé S, et al. Nuclear factor κB nuclear translocation as a crucial marker of brain response to interleukin-1. A study in rat and interleukin-1 type I deficient mouse. J Neurochem 2003;87:1024–36.

58. Rummel C, Voss T, Matsumura K, et al. Nuclear STAT3 translocation in guinea pig and rat brain endothelium during systemic challenge with lipopolysaccharide and interleukin-6. J Comp Neurol 2005;491:1–14.

59. Milton AS, Wendlandt S. Effects on body temperature of prostaglandins of the A, E, and F series on injection into the third ventricle of unanaesthetized cats and rabbits. J Physiol 1971;218:325–36.

60. Milton AS. Prostaglandins and fever. Prog Brain Res 1998;115:129–39.

61. Sehic E, Szekely M, Ungar AL, et al. Hypothalamic prostaglandin E2 during lipopolysaccharide-induced fever in guinea pigs. Brain Res Bull 1996;39:391–9.

62. Ivanov AI, Romanovsky AA. Prostaglandin E2 as a mediator of fever: synthesis and catabolism. Front Biosci 2004;9:1977–93.

63. Turrin NP, Rivest S. Unraveling the molecular details involved in the intimate link between the immune and neuroendocrine systems. Exp Biol Med 2004;229:996–1006.

64. Yamagata K, Matsumura K, Inoue W, et al. Coexpression of microsomal-type prostaglandin E synthase with cyclooxygenase-2 in brain endothelial cells of rats during endotoxin-induced fever. J Neurosci 2001;21:2669–77.

65. Cao C, Matsumura K, Yamagata K, et al. Involvement of cyclooxygenase-2 in LPS-induced fever and regulation of its mRNA by LPS in the rat brain. Am J Physiol 1997;272:R1712–25.

66. Zhang YH, Lu J, Elmquist JK, et al. Specific roles of cyclooxygenase-1 and cyclooxygenase-2 in lipopolysaccharide-induced fever and fos expression in rat brain. J Comp Neurol 2003;463:3–12.

67. Li S, Wang Y, Matsumura K, et al. The febrile response to lipopolysaccharide is blocked in cyclooxygenase-2−/−; but not in cyclooxygenase-1−/− mice. Brain Res 1999;825:86–94.

68. Steiner AA, Rudaya AY, Robbins JR, et al. Expanding the febrigenic role of cyclooxygenase-2 to the previously overlooked responses. Am J Physiol 2005;289:R1253–7.

69. Engblom D, Saha S, Engström L, et al. Microsomal prostaglandin E synthase-1 is the central switch during immune-induced pyresis. Nat Neurosci 2003;6:1137–8.

70. Saha S, Engström L, Mackerlova L, et al. Impaired febrile responses to immune challenge in mice deficient in microsomal prostaglandin E synthase-1. Am J Physiol 2005;288:R1100–7.

71. Ushikubi F, Segi E, Sugimoto Y, et al. Impaired febrile response in mice lacking the prostaglandin E subtype EP3. Nature 1998;395:281–4.

72. Oka T, Oka K, Kobayashi T, et al. Characteristics of thermoregulatory and febrile responses in mice deficient in prostaglandin EP1 and EP3 receptors. J Physiol 2003;551:945–54.

73. Nakamura K, Matsumura K, Kaneko T, et al. The rostral raphe pallidus nucleus mediates pyrogenic transmission from the preoptic area. J Neurosci 2002;22:4600–10.

74. Lazarus M, Yoshida K, Coppari R, et al. EP3 prostaglandin receptors in the median preoptic nucleus are critical for fever response. Nat Neurosci 2007;10:1131–3.

75. Yoshida K, Nakamura K, Matsumura K, et al. Neurons of the rat preoptic area and the raphe pallidus nucleus innervating the brown adipose tissue express prostaglandin E receptor subtype EP3. Eur J Neurosci 2003;18:1848–60.

76. Blatteis CM. The cytokine-prostaglandin cascade in fever production: fact or fancy? J Therm Biol 2004;29:359–68.
77. Blatteis CM. Endotoxic fever: new concepts of its regulation suggest new approaches to its management. Pharm Therap 2006;111:194–223.
78. Ross G, Roth J, Störr B, et al. Afferent nerves are involved in the febrile response to injection of LPS into artificial subcutaneous chambers in guinea pigs. Physiol Behav 2000;71:305–13.
79. Watkins LR, Maier SF, Goehler LE. Cytokine-to-brain communication: a review & analysis of alternative mechanisms. Life Sci 1995;57:1011–26.
80. Blatteis CM, Sehic E. Fever: How may circulating cytokines signal the brain. News Physiol Sci 1997;12:1–9.
81. Niijima A. The afferent discharges from sensors for interleukin 1β in the hepato-portal system in the anesthetized rat. J Auton Nerv Syst 1996;61:287–91.
82. Goehler LE, Gaykema RPA, Hammack SE, et al. Interleukin-1 induces c-Fos immunoreactivity in primary afferent neurons of the vagus nerve. Brain Res 1998;804:306–10.
83. Romanovsky AA. Signaling the brain in the early sickness syndrome: Are sensory nerves involved? Front Biosci 2004;9:494–504.
84. Romanovsky AA, Steiner AA, Matsumura K. Cells that trigger fever. Cell Cycle 2006;5:e1–3.
85. Mills EM, Banks ML, Sprague JE, et al. Uncoupling the agony from ecstasy. Nature 2003;426:403–4.
86. Mills EM, Rusynak DE, Sprague JE. The role of the sympathetic nervous system and uncoupling proteins in the thermogenesis induced by 3,4-methylendioxy-metamphetamine. J Mol Med 2004;82:787–99.
87. Leon LR, Blaha MD, Dubose DA. Time course of cytokine, corticosterone and tissue injury responses in mice during heat strain recovery. J Appl Physiol 2006;100:1400–9.
88. Leon LR. The thermoregulatory consequences of heat stroke: are cytokines involved? J Therm Biol 2006;100:1400–9.
89. Sharma HS, Westman J. Brain function in hot environment. Amsterdam (Netherlands): Elsevier; 1998.
90. Layé S, Parnet P, Goujon E, et al. Peripheral administration of lipopolysaccharide induces the expression of cytokine transcripts in the brain and pituitary of mice. Brain Res Mol Brain Res 1994;27:157–62.
91. Rothwell NJ, Relton JK. Involvement of cytokines in acute neurodegeneration in the CNS. Neurosci Biobehav Rev 1993;17:217–27.

Cytokine, Sickness Behavior, and Depression

Robert Dantzer, DVM, PhD

KEYWORDS

- Inflammation • Cytokine • Sickness • Depression
- Interleukin-1 • Tumor necrosis factor • Brain • Behavior

Anyone who has experienced a viral or bacterial infection knows well the feelings of sickness, in the form of malaise, lassitude, fatigue, numbness, chills, muscle and joint aches, and reduced appetite. Because these symptoms are common, physicians usually ignore them. Physicians dismiss the symptoms as uncomfortable but essentially unhelpful components of the pathogen-induced debilitation process with no benefit to the sufferer's well-being. This view has turned out to be not only simplistic but incorrect.

This simplistic view has turned out to be incorrect. The psychologic and behavioral components of sickness represent, together with fever response and associated neuroendocrine changes, a highly organized strategy of the organism to fight infection.[1] This strategy, referred to as *sickness behavior*, is triggered by the proinflammatory cytokines produced by activated cells of the innate immune system in contact with specific pathogen-associated molecular patterns (PAMPs). These cytokines include mainly interleukin (IL)-1 (IL-1α and IL-1β), IL-6, and tumor necrosis factor α (TNF-α).

The mechanisms that mediate the behavioral effects of peripherally released cytokines have been elucidated over the past 15 years. IL-1 and other cytokines act on the brain via two main communication pathways: (1) a neural route represented by the primary afferent neurons that innervate the body site where the infectious process takes place and (2) a humoral pathway that involves the production of proinflammatory cytokines by phagocytic cells in the circumventricular organs and choroid plexus in response to circulating PAMPs or cytokines, followed by the propagation of these immune signals into the brain parenchyma (**Fig. 1**).[2] This article presents the current knowledge on the way this communication system is organized and regulated and the implications of these advances for understanding brain physiology and pathology.

Supported by National Institutes of Health (MH 71349 and MH 079829).

This article is a version of an article previously published in *Neurologic Clinics*: Dantzer, R. Cytokine, Sickness Behavior, and Depression. Neurol Clin 2006;24(3):441–60.

Integrative Immunology and Behavior Program, University of Illinois at Urbana-Champaign, 212 ERML, 1201 W Gregory Drive, Urbana, IL 61801, USA

E-mail address: dantzer@illinois.edu

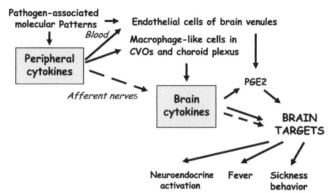

Fig. 1. Mechanisms of brain actions of cytokines. Proinflammatory cytokines are released by activated innate immune cells at the periphery in response to PAMP. PAMP and circulating cytokines act on TLRs on macrophagelike cells in the circumventricular organs (CVOs) and choroid plexus, leading to the production of brain cytokines that diffuse by volume propagation into the brain parenchyma. The action of peripheral proinflammatory cytokines also can be relayed to the brain by afferent nerves, resulting in the production of brain proinflammatory cytokines by microglial cells. In both cases, the action of brain proinflammatory cytokines can be mediated by prostaglandins that diffuse to brain targets or by activation of neural pathways within the brain, which enables the immune message to be transported far away from its site of origin. Prostaglandins can be synthesized only by endothelial cells of brain venules in response to circulating cytokines. Dotted arrows represent instances of neural transmission of the immune message from the periphery to the brain or within the brain itself. PGE2, prostaglandins of the E2 series.

PERIPHERAL PROINFLAMMATORY CYTOKINES INDUCE EXPRESSION OF CYTOKINES IN THE BRAIN
Origin of Peripheral Cytokines

Infectious microorganisms that invade the body encounter a first line of defense represented by monocytes, tissue macrophages, and liver Kupffer cells. These phagocytic cells express Toll-like receptors (TLRs) geared to innately recognize specific PAMPs. TLRs are defined by the presence of a conserved cytoplasmic signaling domain. This domain, the Toll/IL-1 receptor homology domain, signals via the nuclear transcription factor, nuclear factor κB (NF-κB).[3] Thirteen TLRs have been identified, TLR1 through TLR13. Innate immune cells express TLR4s, which recognize lipopolysaccharide (LPS), a component of the cell wall of gram-negative bacteria. The T-cell antigen peptidoglycan, from gram-positive bacteria, is recognized by TLR2s, which are present on the same phagocytic cells. Binding of LPS to TLR4 results in the production of the proinflammatory cytokines IL-1α and IL-1β. IL-1 then is able to induce its own synthesis and the synthesis of other cytokines potentiating its action (TNF-α and IL-6) or antagonizing it (the so-called "anti-inflammatory cytokines," such as IL-10 and the specific antagonist of IL-1 receptors, IL-1Ra). Proinflammatory cytokines do not act as hormones because, aside from IL-6, they are not transported in the circulation to distant cell targets. They act in an autocrine manner on the same cells that have manufactured them, or in a paracrine manner on adjacent cells within the same tissue. Cytokines usually are produced only when needed. Once released, cytokines are biologically active at nano- to picomolar concentrations, and they act on a limited number of receptors per cells that amplify their action via the activation of a large number of genes.

Peripherally Produced Proinflammatory Cytokines Induce Sickness

Peripheral administration of a cytokine inducer, such as LPS, or of recombinant cytokines, such as IL-1β or TNF-α, mimics all nonspecific symptoms of sickness, including fever, activation of the hypothalamic-pituitary-adrenal (HPA) axis, reduction of food intake and other behavioral activities, and withdrawal from the physical and social environment.[1] Conversely, administration of cytokine antagonists abrogates the physiologic and behavioral effects of the cytokine inducer, LPS. In all the experiments examining this question, researchers usually assessed sickness behavior by measuring reduction in food intake of the test animal and by tracking that animal's decreased social investigation of a juvenile conspecific introduced into the test animal's home cage. The findings of these experiments indicate that proinflammatory cytokines mediate the clinical signs of the host response to infection. The physiologic and behavioral changes characteristic of sickness are mediated in the central nervous system (CNS). Fever, for instance, represents a regulated rise in body temperature resulting from increased production of heat (thermogenesis) and decreased thermal loss (thermolysis) in response to an elevated set point for the regulation of body temperature. Given that the body temperature set point is controlled by temperature-sensitive neurons in the preoptic hypothalamus, pyrogenic cytokines, such as IL-1β and IL-6, need to act in the CNS to induce fever.[4] In the same manner, IL-1β acts on the paraventricular nucleus of the hypothalamus where the neurons that contain corticotropin-releasing hormone are located.[5,6] Corticotropin-releasing hormone is released in the portal blood, leading to the release of corticotropin from the pituitary, which in turn increases the release and secretion of glucocorticoids by the adrenal cortex.

The proposed action of IL-1β in the CNS raises the question as to how this cytokine produced at the periphery signals the brain. Like other proinflammatory cytokines, IL-1β is a large hydrophilic peptide that cannot cross the blood-brain barrier passively. In addition, as discussed previously, IL-1β and other cytokines are considered short-range communication molecules that act predominantly in an autocrine or paracrine manner rather than a hormonal manner. For this reason, several pathways of immune-to-brain communication are proposed for the action of these cytokines on the nervous system. These proposals range from one suggesting induction of prostaglandins in those brain areas devoid of a functional blood-brain barrier, to one suggesting the existence of specific saturable transporters.[2] Early studies of the pyrogenic effects of cytokines involved intravenous injection of leukocytic pyrogens. Demonstration of the pyrogenic effects of IL-1β took place with the same mode of administration. Therefore, it was logical to postulate that circulating cytokines act on brain areas devoid of a functional blood-brain barrier. The possibility of intervention of different mechanisms was raised only later, in the mid-1990s, when the brain effects of cytokines were investigated in animals with severed afferent nerves from the abdominal cavity.

Neural Transmission of the Cytokine Message

The hypothesis that cytokines act indirectly on the CNS by activating afferent nerves was based on the recognition that two of the cardinal signs of inflammation, calor (heat) and dolor (pain), require sensory processing, which implies that inflammatory mediators released at the site of injury or infection are able to signal the brain. When LPS or cytokines are injected into the abdominal cavity, they induce inflammation of the peritoneum. One of the major routes of visceral sensibility is represented by the afferent branches of the vagus nerves. These branches contain, in their perineural sheath, macrophages and dendritic cells that express membrane TLRs and produce

IL-1β in response to an intraperitoneal injection of LPS.[7] Sensory neurons of the vagus nerves express IL-1 receptors, and circulating IL-1β stimulates vagal sensory activity.[8]

The role of the vagus nerves in the transmission of information from the periphery to the brain is confirmed by vagotomy experiments in which the vagus nerves were sectioned under the diaphragm so as not to compromise cardiac and pulmonary function. Using this approach, vagal afferents are shown to mediate the activation of the brainstem, hypothalamus, and limbic structures in response to peripherally administered LPS, as demonstrated by the attenuation of the expression of the early activation gene c-fos in the primary and secondary projection areas of the vagus nerves.[9] Sickness behavior also was abrogated in vagotomized animals injected with LPS or IL-1β.[10–12] Because vagotomy did not alter plasma levels of cytokines or the ability of peritoneal macrophages to produce cytokines, the decreased response of vagotomized animals to proinflammatory cytokines was not the result of an inability to mount a peripheral cytokine response to LPS.[10] Furthermore, vagotomized animals still were able to develop a full-blown episode of sickness in response to IL-1β injected by routes other than the intraperitoneal route, including the subcutaneous, intravenous, and intracerebroventricular routes.[11,12] Further evidence for the role of vagal afferents in the induction of sickness behavior was provided by reversible inactivation of the dorsal vagal complex, the primary projection area of the vagus nerves, by a local anesthetic agent. This intervention abrogated LPS-induced sickness behavior and c-fos expression in downstream brain areas.[13]

Other afferent nerves are solicited when the inflammatory response takes place in different parts of the body. For instance, inflammation in the oral cavity is found to give rise to fever via the glossopharyngeal nerves because the transaction of this neural trunk abrogates the fever response to the injection of IL-1β or LPS into the soft palate and the enhanced expression of brain cytokines in response to this peripheral immune stimulus.[14,15]

The importance of the neural pathway in the transmission of the immune message from the periphery to the brain is not the same for all components of sickness behavior. For example, vagotomized rats do not develop the behavioral alterations characteristic of sickness, but they still are able to mount a fever.[16] This demonstrates that vagal afferents are less important for the cytokine-induced fever and activation of the HPA axis than for cytokine-induced sickness behavior. These findings indicate that other pathways of communication function in parallel with the neural pathway.

Humoral Transmission of the Cytokine Message

Besides the relatively fast neural pathway of immune-to-brain communication, there is a slower pathway that involves the action of PAMP or circulating cytokines on macrophagelike cells in circumventricular organs and endothelial cells of brain vessels. This results in the local production of cytokines and molecular intermediates, such as prostaglandins of the E2 series (PGE2) and nitric oxide. PGE2 represent the main mediators of cytokine-induced fever and activation of the HPA axis, as proven through pretreatment with specific inhibitors of the prostaglandin synthesizing enzyme, cyclooxygenase 2, which attenuates these responses.[17,18] The synthesis of PGE2 is dependent on the induction of cyclooxygenase 2 and the enzyme prostaglandin E synthase, both of which are expressed in endothelial cells of cerebral blood vessels and perivascular macrophages after intravenous IL-1β administration. PGE2 diffuse into the brain parenchyma and act on neuronal EP3 or EP4 receptors in the brainstem and hypothalamic neural structures involved in the control of the HPA axis activity and the regulation of body temperature. These brain areas include the catecholaminergic brainstem nuclei, the paraventricular nucleus of the hypothalamus, and the ventromedial pre-optic area.

The reduction in social behavior and the anorexia that develop in response to peripheral LPS and IL-1 are mediated by brain IL-1, as demonstrated when these responses are attenuated by intracerebroventricular administration of the IL-1 receptor antagonist.[19,20] In response to peripheral LPS, IL-1β is synthesized by macrophage-like cells in the circumventricular organs and choroid plexus, where the blood-brain barrier is deficient.[21,22] This synthesis of IL-1β is certainly the result of the action of circulating LPS on TLR4 receptors present on the same cells, and possibly also a response to circulating cytokines and PAMPs. IL-1 can act on neuronal IL-1 receptors in the area postrema, the circumventricular organ of the brainstem.[23] This action results in the activation of a neuronal pathway projecting to the parabrachial nucleus and from there to the central amygdala and the bed nucleus of the stria terminalis. There is evidence that IL-1 also can propagate by volume transmission from the choroid plexus into the surrounding brain parenchyma to reach distant structures, such as the basolateral amygdala, which contains neurons expressing IL-1 receptors.[24] The importance of each of these pathways remains to be fully elucidated. However, they could be responsible for the behaviorally depressing effects of IL-1. In the same manner, diffusion of IL-1 from the median eminence to the arcuate nucleus could mediate IL-1–induced anorexia. However, because lesions of the arcuate nucleus do not disrupt the effects of IL-1 on food intake,[25] the exact mechanisms of the depressive action of cytokines on food intake remain obscure.

Researchers have found that electrical stimulation of the vagus nerve induces the expression of brain IL-1, and vagotomy abrogates the induction of expression of brain IL-1 in response to intraperitoneal LPS and IL-1.[26–28] However, the manner in which the fast neural pathway and the slow humoral pathway converge to promote the brain expression of IL-1 remains unknown. Probably the neural immune-to-brain communication pathway recruits various brain areas and sensitizes them to the action of the slowly propagating cytokine message.[29]

The exact nature of the neurotransmitters responsible for the behavioral effects of IL-1 is unknown. The effects of proinflammatory cytokines on brain neurotransmitters are grossly similar to those of other stressors, but this similarity breaks off at the regional level.[30] More detailed neuroanatomic studies are required to identify the neurotransmitter content of those neuronal structures activated directly or indirectly by cytokines, so that the role of the putative neurotransmitter mediator can be assessed by micropharmacology intervention techniques.

MOLECULAR BASIS OF SICKNESS BEHAVIOR
Role of Interleukin-1

The availability of species-specific recombinant cytokines has enabled assessment of the range of physiologic and behavioral effects of the proinflammatory cytokines produced during an infectious episode. This assessment has been done by administering to healthy animals the cytokine under investigation alone or in combination with other cytokines. As discussed previously, IL-1β is an important cytokine for the induction of sickness behavior. Administration of IL-1β alone at the periphery or into the lateral ventricle of the brain induces all the central components of the acute phase reaction, including fever, HPA axis activation, and behavioral depression.[31] In contrast, IL-6 induces only pyrogenic and corticotropic activities, but no behavioral activity.[32] These findings do not suggest that IL-1β is the sole cytokine that mediates sickness behavior. In accordance with the concept of a cytokine network, a given cytokine never acts alone but in the context of other cytokines that potentiate or oppose its activity. IL-6, for instance, potentiates the behaviorally depressing effects of IL-1β.[32] Such complementary interactions between proinflammatory cytokines can be addressed more easily when one cytokine is missing from the cytokine network because the gene for this cytokine or its receptor has been deleted by the technique of homologous recombination. IL-6 knockout mice, for example, are less sensitive to the behavioral effects of LPS or IL-1β injected peripherally or centrally.[33] In the same manner, type I IL-1 receptor (IL-1RI) knockout mice are responsive to the behaviorally depressing effects of LPS, whereas they do not respond any longer to peripheral or central IL-1.[34] In mice in which the gene coding for the IL-1RI is deleted, the blockade of another proinflammatory cytokine, TNF-α, by a fragment of its soluble receptor injected centrally abrogates the behaviorally depressing effects of LPS, whereas the same blockade has no effect in wild-type mice.[34] These results show that deficiency in one cytokine can be compensated by another cytokine of the network.

As discussed previously, blockade of IL-1 action by central administration of the IL-1 receptor antagonist attenuates cytokine-induced sickness behavior measured by either depression of social exploration[35] or reduction of food intake.[19,35] This shows that IL-1 seems to be the predominant mediator of sickness behavior in the brain. The involvement of brain IL-1 in the depressing effects of LPS on food intake has been confirmed in an experiment using mice deficient in the IL-1β–converting enzyme. This enzyme, also known as caspase 1, processes inactive pro–IL-1β into mature IL-1β. IL-1β–converting enzyme knockout mice are less sensitive to the depressing effects of LPS on food intake when LPS is injected into the lateral ventricle of the brain, whereas they do not differ from controls in their response to intraperitoneal LPS.[36]

Receptor Mechanisms of the Effect of Interleukin 1 in the Brain

Interleukin-1 receptors

Several receptor subtypes mediate the effects of IL-1 on its cellular targets. These subtypes feature an extracellular domain with three immunoglobulinlike domains, a single transmembrane domain, and an intracellular domain that involves adaptor proteins and kinase cascades. The IL-1RI that mediates all of the known biologic effects of IL-1 uses the adaptor molecule MyD88 to mediate a complex pathway involving a cascade of kinases organized by multiple adapter molecules into signaling complexes, leading to activation of the transcription factor NF-κB.[37] The type II IL-1 receptor (IL-1RII) is a negative regulator of the IL-1 system and functions as a decoy receptor. Its intracellular domain is short and has no signaling function. The additional IL-1 receptor accessory protein (IL-1RacP) is necessary for IL-1 signal transduction because binding of IL-1 to the IL-1RI leads to the formation of a heterodimeric complex with this accessory protein, whereas binding of IL-1Ra to the IL-1RI prevents the formation of this complex.[38] This explains why IL-1RacP knockout mice behave like IL-1RI knockout mice.

Brain interleukin-1 receptors

All the biochemistry techniques used to date to characterize IL-1 receptors on neurons, glial cells, and endothelial cells of brain venules show a striking similarity between brain IL-1 receptors and those found on peripheral immune and nonimmune cells. Most of the members of the IL-1Rs family are cloned from transformed lines of blood cells. The descriptive work on the type and localization of IL-1 receptors present in the brain is based on autoradiographic detection of radioiodinated ligands, such as IL-1α, IL-1β, or IL-1Ra; polymerase chain reaction detection of a small fragment of the complementary DNA–encoding IL-1 receptors; and immunohistochemical detection with antibodies raised against epitopes of IL-1 receptors from peripheral blood cells. While these techniques cannot conclusively determine whether or not brain IL-1Rs and peripheral IL-1Rs are the same, the difficulty of cloning new brain-specific IL-1Rs favors the likelihood that peripheral and brain receptors are identical. In agreement with this assumption, detection of IL-1Rs in the brain using in situ hybridization or ribonuclease protection assay with full-length complementary DNA or long riboprobes[23] indicates that the same IL-1RI messenger RNA (mRNA) is present in peripheral and central nervous tissue. Moreover, autoradiography studies of knockout mice for IL-1RI confirm that this receptor is responsible for all IL-1–binding sites in the mouse brain.[34] Yet, this last result was unexpected in view of the presence of IL-1RI and IL-1RII in the mouse brain. The most likely explanation for the lack of IL-1RII binding in the brain of IL-1RI knockout mice is the low amount of IL-1RII and the low sensitivity of in vitro binding techniques. Consistent with this interpretation, immunohistochemistry studies reveal the expression of IL-1RII, but not IL-RI, in the mouse hypothalamus, even though this expression of IL-1RII is undetected with the use of binding techniques.[39] These results emphasize the need for multiple methods to study brain cytokine receptors to be able to confirm their presence or absence in this organ.

Localization of brain interleukin-1 receptors
In the rat, the first study performed to localize IL-1 binding sites made use of quantitative autoradiography to show that IL-1 receptors are spread widely across the brain, with the highest level in the granular layer of the dentate gyrus, in the granule cell layer of the cerebellum, in the hypothalamus, and in the pyramidal cell layer of the hippocampus.[40] These findings are interpreted as an indication of a neuronal localization. Seven years after that study, Ericsson and coworkers[23] used in situ hybridization with a 1.35-kilobase complementary DNA probe to determine the distribution of IL-1RI in rat brain. IL-1RI mRNA expression was localized in nonneuronal cells in structures at the interface between the brain parenchyma and its fluid environments, such as the choroid plexus and the endothelial cells of the brain vasculature. Neuronal expression appeared mostly in the hippocampus and also was detected in a few cell groups of the basolateral nucleus of the amygdala and the basomedial nuclei of the hypothalamus. It was not possible to determine the exact nature of the few labeled cells observed in the arcuate nucleus and the area postrema.

Compared with IL-1RI, much less is known about the expression of IL-1RII mRNA in the rat brain. IL-1RII mRNA seems to be undetectable in the normal adult brain but is induced in the dentate gyrus, the hippocampus, and the basolateral amygdaloid nucleus in response to a systemic injection of kainic acid.[41] IL-1RII mRNA also can be observed 24 hours later in neurons of the medial and median preoptic area, the dorsomedial and paraventricular hypothalamic nuclei, and various thalamic nuclei. When distinct inflammatory lesions are induced in the rat brain by localized injection of IL-1β, IL-1RII expression is found to be restricted to brain endothelial cells and infiltrating neutrophils.[42]

In contrast to the localized expression of IL-1RI and IL-1RII mRNA, rat IL-1RacP mRNA detected by ribonuclease protection assay is ubiquitous and expressed at high levels in many brain regions (eg, hypothalamus, cortex, hippocampus, and cerebellum).[43] The presence of IL-1RacP in brain areas devoid of IL-1RI raises the question of what is the exact role of this accessory protein in the rat brain.

In the mouse, the first evidence for the presence of IL-1 receptors in the brain was obtained by demonstration of the expression of IL-1RI and IL-1RII mRNA and by radioactive IL-1α binding affinity.[44–46] Later, immunohistochemistry allowed confirmation of the protein expression and neuronal localization of the two subtypes of IL-1 receptors.[39] IL-1RI and IL-1RII were found to be expressed on neuronal soma in the granular cell layer of the dentate gyrus and the CA1 through CA4 pyramidal cell fields of Ammon's horn of the hippocampus. Similarly, both IL-1R isoforms are expressed on ependymal epithelial cells, choroid plexus epithelial cells, and Purkinje's cells of the cerebellum. IL-RII, but not IL-RI, is detected on neuronal soma and proximal cell processes in the hypothalamic paraventricular gray matter. No clear evidence of immunolabeling on vascular endothelial cells and meninges has been found. Choroid plexus epithelial cells and ventricular ependidymal epithelial cells expressed easily detectable IL-1RI and IL-1RII, however, which is in accordance with their role in the entrance of IL-1 into the brain. Only limited immunoreactivity for IL-1RI and IL-1RII was detected on astroglial cells of normal adult mouse brain, although in mice previously infected with Moloney murine leukemia, an abundant expression of IL-1RI was observed on reactive astrocytes. In the intact rat brain, IL-1RI expression is much more localized and restricted to nonneuronal cells, especially endothelial cells of brain venules, as assessed by immunohistochemistry with antibodies directed against the extracellular domain of IL-1RI or the p65 subunit of NF-κB.[47,48]

IL-1RacP localization is similar in the mouse and rat brains.[49,50] Surprisingly, 125I-IL-1–binding studies in IL-1RacP knockout mice do not reveal a lower affinity of the binding sites, indicating that IL-1RI and IL-1RacP do not necessarily form in this organ the heterodimeric complex that normally is required for high-affinity binding. Again, these findings argue for a role of IL-1RacP in the rodent brain that has not yet been defined.

Functionality of brain interleukin-1 receptors

Administration of IL-1β or IL-1α into the lateral ventricle of the brain or directly into the brain parenchyma induces the typical signs of sickness behavior. Local administration of IL-1Ra into the brain abrogates these effects, thus demonstrating the role of brain IL-1 receptors in mediating the effects.[1]

To determine which IL-1 receptor subtype mediates the behavioral effects of IL-1, researchers use passive immunization experiments, antisense technology, and mouse knockout strategies. Blockade of IL-1RI with a specific neutralizing antibody totally abrogates the behavioral effects of centrally and peripherally injected IL-1β in mice.[51] Blockade of IL-1RII potentiates the suppressing effect of IL-1β on food intake.[51] Blockade of brain IL-1RI by antisense oligonucleotides abrogates the anorexic but not the adipsic effects of intracerebroventricular IL-1β.[52] Following blockade, these IL-1RI–deficient mice no longer were responsive to the behaviorally depressing effects of IL-1β injected at the periphery or directly into the brain. However, these mice were responsive to LPS.[34] Thus, the lack of response to IL-1β did not stem from an inability to mount a sickness response. In the same manner, IL-1RacP knockout mice did not respond any longer to IL-1β injected into the lateral ventricle of the brain.[53]

The signaling pathways that mediate the behavioral effects of IL-1 have been recently investigated. Because IκBα is expressed strongly in the circumventricular organs and choroid plexus during peripheral immune stimulation,[54] and this response is associated with NF-κB translocation, the effects of IL-1 at this level are likely to be dependent on the transcription factor NF-κB. In accordance with this hypothesis, central administration of an NF-κB inhibitor peptide is found to block the somnogenic and pyrogenic effects of peripheral IL-1β in rabbits.[55] In the same manner, blockade of NF-κB activation by intracerebroventricular administration of a cell permeant peptide that blocks the interaction of the NF-kB essential modulator with the IκB kinase complex abrogates sickness behavior elicited by intraperitoneal IL-1β.[56] In contrast to the predominant role of NF-κB in IL-1 signaling at the blood-brain interface, activation of pathways for mitogen-activated protein kinases seems to be involved in the neural effects of IL-1, including IL-1β–induced inhibition of long-term potentiation in perforant path-granule cell synapses and IL-1β–induced elevation in intracellular free calcium levels in rat cortical synaptosomes.[57]

ENDOGENOUS ANTI-INFLAMMATORY MOLECULES

Because of the tight regulation of the expression and action of cytokines at the periphery and in the brain, cytokine-induced sickness behavior normally is a fully reversible phenomenon. The molecular factors involved in this regulation include mainly anti-inflammatory cytokines that target IL-1 specifically, such as IL-1Ra and soluble IL-1RII, or have more generalized antagonist effects on a wide variety of proinflammatory cytokines, such as IL-10 and transforming growth factor β. Molecules that do not belong to the network of cytokines include glucocorticoids, neuropeptides (such as vasopressin and alpha-melanotropin), and growth factors (such as insulin-like growth factor I).[1] Any alteration in the balance between proinflammatory and anti-inflammatory cytokines, in the sense of a predominance of proinflammatory cytokines over anti-inflammatory cytokines, results in an exaggerated sickness response to activation of the peripheral immune system or direct activation of the brain cytokine system. This is shown to be the case in aged mice[58] and in obese mice.[59] These two conditions are associated with a low-grade inflammation status that, because of the immune-to-brain communication, leads to priming or sensitization of brain microglial cells.[60] Superimposed on this low-grade inflammation status, a peripheral infectious episode leads to exaggerated synthesis of inflammatory cytokines and other mediators in the brain, which in turn have an impact on behavior and mood or exacerbate the progression of chronic neurodegenerative disease.

PATHOPHYSIOLOGIC IMPLICATIONS

Based on previous evidence, sickness behavior seems to be only the outward expression of a reversible episode of cytokine expression and action in the brain in response to peripheral immune stimulation. Sickness behavior, however, is not a passive response in the form of a temporary disappearance of the usual activities of the host. The proinflammatory cytokines produced by activated innate immune cells serve as sensory signals recognized and interpreted by the brain. The brain representation of peripheral immune activation resets the organism's priorities to enable the subjects at risk to deal with infection in the most efficient way. The expression of sickness behavior is not simply the result of the changes in internal state experienced by sick subjects, but rather the joint function of the changes in their internal state and the environmental constraints to which they are exposed.[1,61] This is characteristic of motivated behavior. An experiment performed on sickness behavior in lactating mice, in which caring for their pups is the predominant motivation, provides a good example of the motivational conflict that can take place in sick individuals. Lactating mice were made sick by an appropriate dose of systemic LPS. They remained inactive and indifferent to the solicitations of their pups until the pups were dispersed in the cage and the nest was removed. In this situation, their maternal motivation took over their sickness motivation, and they engaged in pup retrieval. Furthermore, when provided with cotton wool, which they normally use to build a nest, they did not engage in nest building in addition to pup retrieval unless the ambient temperature dropped to 6°C.[62]

Because cytokine-induced sickness behavior is the expression of a motivational state triggered by activation of the peripheral innate immune system, it is not pathologic per se but as normal as the fear response that occurs in individuals exposed to the threat of a predator (**Fig. 2**). Like fear, sickness behavior can become abnormal or pathologic when it occurs out of context (ie, in the absence of any inflammatory stimulus) or when it is exaggerated in intensity or duration. Several conditions can be responsible for an abnormal or pathologic sickness behavior: (1) when proinflammatory cytokines are produced in higher quantities and for a longer duration than normal; (2) when the regulatory molecules that normally down-regulate activation of the molecular and cellular components of the sickness response are faulty; or (3) when the neuronal circuits that are the targets of inflammatory mediators and organize sickness behavior become sensitized. Because of the similarities between symptoms of sickness and clinical signs of depression, any of these conditions is likely a risk factor for the occurrence of major depressive disorders. Evidence for the possibility of a shift from sickness behavior to depression is available from two different sources, clinical research and experimental studies on animal models of depressive disorders.

At the clinical level, a growing volume of evidence shows that major depression is associated with significant elevations in circulating levels of proinflammatory cytokines, in particular IL-6.[63–68] (See the article by Irwin and colleagues elsewhere in this issue for further discussion of the relationship between depression and immunity.) Conversely, chronic activation of the innate immune system can precipitate the development of depressive disorders, as exemplified by the psychopathologic alterations that occur in patients receiving repeated injections of recombinant cytokines, mainly IL-2 or interferon alfa, for the treatment of viral infections (hepatitis C) or cancer. During the first stages of cytokine therapy, all patients usually develop a full-blown episode of sickness behavior, characterized by the symptoms of fever, malaise, anorexia, pain, and fatigue. At later stages of treatment, up to one third of patients develop mood alterations characteristic of depression, including sadness, inability to feel, depressed mood, and even suicidal ideation.[69] The onset of depressive symptoms depends on the cytokine and treatment modalities (eg, dosage and administration route). Depression can be prevented by pretreatment with paroxetine, a selective serotonin reuptake inhibitor with antidepressant properties. Nevertheless, pretreatment with paroxetine has a minimal or null effect on the development of neurovegetative symptoms of sickness, including fever, fatigue, and anorexia, confirming the dissociation between sickness behavior and depression.[70]

These findings can be interpreted to suggest that depressive disorders develop from cytokine-induced sickness behavior only in vulnerable patients (**Fig. 3**). Vulnerability, in the present context, refers to an innate or acquired predisposition to develop

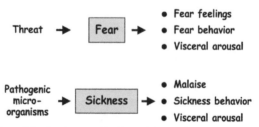

Fig. 2. Motivational model of sickness. Like fear, sickness has motivational properties in the sense that it organizes the organism's functioning at three levels—subjective, behavioral, and visceral—so as to cope with the threat to which the organism is exposed.

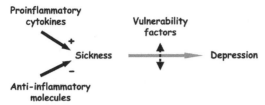

Fig. 3. The two-hit model of cytokine-induced depression. Production of proinflammatory cytokines induces sickness behavior that usually is terminated by endogenous anti-inflammatory molecules. Sustained production of proinflammatory cytokines in the context of insufficient production of anti-inflammatory molecules can lead to depression in vulnerable individuals. Many factors, acquired or genetic, can contribute to vulnerability.

a given pathology when causal factors are present. Dysfunction in genes controlling key proteins in cytokine production (eg, IL-6[71]) and serotoninergic neurotransmission (eg, activity of the serotonin transporter[71] or serotonin receptor subtype[72]) are identified as vulnerability factors for cytokine-induced depression. Psychologic features can reveal vulnerability to cytokine-induced depression. Patients who have high scores on depression scales (including the Montgomery-Asberg Depression Rating Scale and the Hamilton Depression Rating Scale) at the start of cytokine treatment are more likely to develop depressive syndrome in response to immunotherapy than patients who have a low score at baseline.[73,74] Vulnerability also can be revealed by physiologic features. Patients who respond to the first injection of interferon alfa with an exaggerated pituitary-adrenal response are more likely to become depressed in response to repeated administration of interferon alfa than patients who display a lower pituitary-adrenal response.[75] These two different characteristics are markers of vulnerability. They can help to identify patients at risk, but they do not explain why patients who have these characteristics are more vulnerable than those who do not have them.

The model of cytokine-induced depression has the advantage of providing clinicians with the possibility of observing development of depressive symptoms over time in a large number of patients who can be monitored closely from the time they start receiving immunotherapy. Furthermore, patients who develop depression can be compared transversally to patients who remain free of any mood disorder. The model of cytokine-induced depression, therefore, provides valuable insights into the relationship between cytokines and depression. At the clinical level, there is evidence that symptoms of mood disorder are more polymorphic than just depression. A study of patients who had hepatitis C and were treated with interferon alfa shows, for instance, that dysphoria and mixed states dominate the clinical presentation of patients, with increases in irritability and anxiety as the main symptoms.[76] No one yet understands why patients who have hepatitis C become irritable in response to interferon alfa while patients with cancer become depressed. The differences may stem from medical context (cytokine immunotherapy is palliative only for patients who have cancer, whereas it usually is curative for patients who have hepatitis C), immunologic context (immune responses of patients infected by a virus are different from those of patients who have cancer), or simply variations in treatment modalities (high doses of interferon alfa administered intravenously and daily to patients who have malignant melanoma versus low doses of pegylated interferon alfa administered together with ribavirin once a week to patients who have chronic hepatitis C). These variations also could be related to differences in affective and psychiatric background, because many patients who have chronic hepatitis C have a history of substance abuse.

At the pathophysiologic level, an insight into the chain of events linking cytokines to mood alterations has emerged from the observation that patients who have cancer and are treated with cytokines develop a drastic decrease in plasma tryptophan levels that correlates with depression scores at 4 weeks of treatment.[77] This decrease in plasma tryptophan levels previously was noted but in a qualitative rather than quantitative manner.[78] These findings are important because bioavailability of tryptophan is the limiting factor for the synthesis of serotonin. The acute depletion of tryptophan produced by feeding excess amounts of large neutral amino acids that compete with tryptophan for entry into the brain results in the development of depressed mood in subjects at risk for depression. A likely candidate for this decrease in plasma tryptophan in patients submitted to cytokine immunotherapy is the enzyme indoleamine 2,3-dioxygenase (IDO), which degrades tryptophan into kynurenine and quinolinic acid (**Fig. 4**). IDO is present in macrophages and monocytes, endothelial cells, and brain glial cells. It is potently activated by proinflammatory cytokines, such as TNF-α and interferon gamma, both at the periphery and in the brain.[79] Its activation results in a decrease in tryptophan bioavailability for the synthesis of serotonin and in the formation of neuroactive compounds, such as kynurenine, which acts as an antagonist of glutamate receptors, and quinolinic acid, which acts as an agonist of glutamate receptors. Experiments carried out in mice submitted to acute inflammation in response to LPS or to chronic inflammation with bacille Calmette-Guérin, an attenuated form of *Mycobacterium bovis*, reveal the gradual emergence of depressivelike behavior after waning of the sickness response.[80,81] The emergence of depressivelike behavior is associated with activation of IDO.[82] Furthermore, blockade of IDO, by

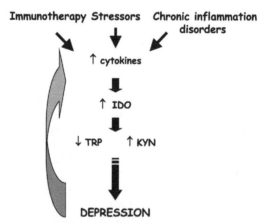

Fig. 4. Mechanisms of the depressing effects of cytokines on mood. Cytokine immunotherapy or psychosocial stressors (via a β2-adrenergic receptor), by causing overproduction of proinflammatory cytokines, triggers activation of the innate immune system. The same condition occurs during chronic inflammation. Cytokines, such as TNF-α and interferon gamma, increase activity of the enzyme IDO, which degrades tryptophan along the kynurenine/quinolinic acid metabolic pathway, resulting in a decrease in tryptophan and an increase in kynurenine. The decreased tryptophan bioavailability leads to decreased serotoninergic neurotransmission and depressed mood. Depression itself can be accompanied by altered immunity, including activation of the innate immune system, further increasing the proinflammatory cytokine load.

interfering with the cytokine response or directly inhibiting IDO, results in the abrogation of depressivelike behavior.[83] In the same manner, blockade of TNF-α in psoriasis patients results in an attenuation of fatigue and depression symptoms before the medical condition resolves.[84] The interference of proinflammatory cytokines with serotoninergic neurotransmission can explain some of the clinical signs, such as impulsivity and depressed mood, that develop in vulnerable patients. Another possible mechanism is the production of kynurenine metabolites that act as agonists of the glutamate receptors.[85,86] The interference of cytokines with serotoninergic neurotransmission does not account, however, for the anhedonia, fatigue, and psychomotor retardation observed in patients treated with cytokine.[69] These symptoms probably reflect a decrease in dopaminergic neurotransmission. This hypothesis is supported by neuroimaging studies showing alterations in the activity of basal ganglia during cytokine therapy.[87,88]

Despite its heuristic value, the clinical relevance of the model of cytokine-induced depression could be questioned because it is a rather extreme situation. There is evidence, however, that overproduction of proinflammatory cytokines also is associated with mood disorders in chronic inflammatory medical conditions, including coronary heart disease. Of course, because patients who have such medical conditions are examined at different stages of their disease process, the relationship between cytokines and depression for them is more difficult to reveal and medical conditions may result in much higher interindividual variability. Despite these constraints, it is possible to observe higher levels of myocardial cytokines and higher antibody titers against microbial pathogens possibly involved in the pathophysiology of coronary heart disease in patients suffering from vital exhaustion at the time of coronary bypass.[89] In the same manner, depressive disorders that develop over time in post-ischemic coronary patients are associated with endothelial cell activation and probably inflammation, although the therapeutic use of statins that have anti-inflammatory actions attenuates differences betweens cases and controls.[90]

SUMMARY

Sufficient evidence is now available to support the concept that the brain recognizes cytokines as molecular signals of sickness. Progress in elucidating the cellular and molecular components of the intricate system that mediates cytokine-induced sickness behavior has helped to clarify our understanding of the way the brain processes information generated by the innate immune system. We are still far, however, from understanding the system as a whole. Among the hundreds of genes that proinflammatory cytokines can induce in their cellular targets, only a handful have been examined functionally. In addition, a dynamic view of the cellular interactions that occur at the brain sites of cytokine production and action is missing, and the mechanisms that favor the transition toward pathology remain to be clarified.

REFERENCES

1. Dantzer R, O'Connor JC, Freund GG, et al. From inflammation to sickness and depression: when the immune system subjugates the brain. Nat Rev Neurosci 2008;9:46–56.
2. Konsman JP, Parnet P, Dantzer R. Cytokine-induced sickness behaviour: mechanisms and implications. Trends Neurosci 2002;25:154–9.
3. Barton GM, Medzhitov R. Toll-like receptor signaling pathways. Science 2003; 300:1524–5.

4. Romanovsky A, Almeida MC, Aronoff DM, et al. Fever and hypothermia in systemic inflammation: recent discoveries and revisions. Front Biosci 2005;10: 2193–216.

5. Berkenbosch F, van Oers J, del Rey A, et al. Corticotropin-releasing factor-producing neurons in the rat activated by interleukin-1. Science 1987;238:524–6.

6. Ericsson A, Kovacs KJ, Sawchenko PE. A functional anatomical analysis of central pathways subserving the effects of interleukin-1 on stress-related neuro-endocrine neurons. J Neurosci 1994;14:897–913.

7. Goehler LE, Gaykema RP, Nguyen KT, et al. Interleukin-1beta in immune cells of the abdominal vagus nerve: a link between the immune and nervous systems? J Neurosci 1999;19:2799–806.

8. Ek M, Kurosawa M, Lundeberg T, et al. Activation of vagal afferents after intrave-nous injection of interleukin-1beta: role of endogenous prostaglandins. J Neurosci 1998;18:9471–9.

9. Wan W, Wetmore L, Sorensen CM, et al. Neural and biochemical mediators of endotoxin and stress-induced c-fos expression in the rat brain. Brain Res Bull 1994;34:7–14.

10. Bluthe RM, Walter V, Parnet P, et al. Lipopolysaccharide induces sickness behav-iour in rats by a vagal mediated mechanism. C R Acad Sci III 1994;317:499–503.

11. Bluthe RM, Michaud B, Kelley KW, et al. Vagotomy attenuates behavioural effects of interleukin-1 injected peripherally but not centrally. Neuroreport 1996;7:1485–8.

12. Bluthe RM, Michaud B, Kelley KW, et al. Vagotomy blocks behavioural effects of interleukin-1 injected via the intraperitoneal route but not via other systemic routes. Neuroreport 1996;7:2823–7.

13. Marvel FA, Chen CC, Badr N, et al. Reversible inactivation of the dorsal vagal complex blocks lipopolysaccharide-induced social withdrawal and c-Fos expres-sion in central autonomic nuclei. Brain Behav Immun 2004;18:123–34.

14. Romeo HE, Tio DL, Taylor AN. Effects of glossopharyngeal nerve transection on central and peripheral cytokines and serum corticosterone induced by localized inflammation. J Neuroimmunol 2003;136:104–11.

15. Romeo HE, Tio DL, Rahman SU, et al. The glossopharyngeal nerve as a novel pathway in immune-to-brain communication: relevance to neuroimmune surveil-lance of the oral cavity. J Neuroimmunol 2001;115:91–100.

16. Konsman JP, Luheshi GN, Bluthe RM, et al. The vagus nerve mediates behaviou-ral depression, but not fever, in response to peripheral immune signals; a func-tional anatomical analysis. Eur J Neurosci 2000;12:4434–46.

17. Rivest S, Lacroix S, Vallieres L, et al. How the blood talks to the brain parenchyma and the paraventricular nucleus of the hypothalamus during systemic inflamma-tory and infectious stimuli. Proc Soc Exp Biol Med 2000;223:22–38.

18. Romanovsky AA. Thermoregulatory manifestations of systemic inflammation: lessons from vagotomy. Auton Neurosci 2000;85:39–48.

19. Laye S, Gheusi G, Cremona S, et al. Endogenous brain IL-1 mediates LPS-induced anorexia and hypothalamic cytokine expression. Am J Physiol Regul In-tegr Comp Physiol 2000;279:R93–8.

20. Kent S, Bluthe RM, Dantzer R, et al. Different receptor mechanisms mediate the pyrogenic and behavioral effects of interleukin 1. Proc Natl Acad Sci USA 1992; 89:9117–20.

21. van Dam AM, Brouns M, Louisse S, et al. Appearance of interleukin-1 in macro-phages and in ramified microglia in the brain of endotoxin-treated rats: a pathway for the induction of non-specific symptoms of sickness? Brain Res 1992;588: 291–6.

22. Konsman JP, Kelley K, Dantzer R. Temporal and spatial relationships between lipopolysaccharide-induced expression of Fos, interleukin-1beta and inducible nitric oxide synthase in rat brain. Neuroscience 1999;89:535–48.
23. Ericsson A, Liu C, Hart RP, et al. Type 1 interleukin-1 receptor in the rat brain: distribution, regulation, and relationship to sites of IL-1-induced cellular activation. J Comp Neurol 1995;361:681–98.
24. Vitkovic L, Konsman JP, Bockaert J, et al. Cytokine signals propagate through the brain. Mol Psychiatry 2000;5:604–15.
25. Reyes TM, Sawchenko PE. Involvement of the arcuate nucleus of the hypothalamus in interleukin-1-induced anorexia. J Neurosci 2002;22:5091–9.
26. Laye S, Bluthe RM, Kent S, et al. Subdiaphragmatic vagotomy blocks induction of IL-1 beta mRNA in mice brain in response to peripheral LPS. Am J Physiol 1995; 268(5 Pt 2):R1327–31.
27. Hansen MK, Nguyen KT, Goehler LE, et al. Effects of vagotomy on lipopolysaccharide-induced brain interleukin-1beta protein in rats. Auton Neurosci 2000; 85:119–26.
28. Hosoi T, Okuma Y, Nomura Y. Electrical stimulation of afferent vagus nerve induces IL-1beta expression in the brain and activates HPA axis. Am J Physiol Regul Integr Comp Physiol 2000;279:R141–7.
29. Dantzer R, Konsman JP, Bluthe RM, et al. Neural and humoral pathways of communication from the immune system to the brain: parallel or convergent? Auton Neurosci 2000;85:60–5.
30. Dunn AJ, Wang J, Ando T. Effects of cytokines on cerebral neurotransmission. Comparison with the effects of stress. Adv Exp Med Biol 1999;461:117–27.
31. Anforth HR, Bluthe RM, Bristow A, et al. Biological activity and brain actions of recombinant rat interleukin-1alpha and interleukin-1beta. Eur Cytokine Netw 1998;9:279–88.
32. Lenczowski MJ, Bluthe RM, Roth J, et al. Central administration of rat IL-6 induces HPA activation and fever but not sickness behavior in rats. Am J Physiol 1999; 276(3 Pt 2):R652–8.
33. Bluthe RM, Michaud B, Poli V, et al. Role of IL-6 in cytokine-induced sickness behavior: a study with IL-6 deficient mice. Physiol Behav 2000;70:367–73.
34. Bluthe RM, Laye S, Michaud B, et al. Role of interleukin-1beta and tumour necrosis factor-alpha in lipopolysaccharide-induced sickness behaviour: a study with interleukin-1 type I receptor-deficient mice. Eur J Neurosci 2000;12:4447–56.
35. Konsman JP, Tridon V, Dantzer R. Diffusion and action of intracerebroventricularly injected interleukin-1 in the CNS. Neuroscience 2000;101:957–67.
36. Burgess W, Gheusi G, Yao J, et al. Interleukin-1beta-converting enzyme-deficient mice resist central but not systemic endotoxin-induced anorexia. Am J Physiol 1998;274(6 Pt 2):R1829–33.
37. Li X, Qin J. Modulation of Toll-interleukin 1 receptor mediated signaling. J Mol Med 2005;83:258–66.
38. Cullinan EB, Kwee L, Nunes P, et al. IL-1 receptor accessory protein is an essential component of the IL-1 receptor. J Immunol 1998;161:5614–20.
39. French RA, VanHoy RW, Chizzonite R, et al. Expression and localization of p80 and p68 interleukin-1 receptor proteins in the brain of adult mice. J Neuroimmunol 1999;93:194–202.
40. Katsuura G, Gottschall PE, Arimura A. Identification of a high-affinity receptor for interleukin-1 beta in rat brain. Biochem Biophys Res Commun 1988;156:61–7.
41. Nishiyori A, Minami M, Takami S, et al. Type 2 interleukin-1 receptor mRNA is induced by kainic acid in the rat brain. Brain Res Mol Brain Res 1997;50:237–45.

42. Docagne F, Campbell SJ, Bristow AF, et al. Differential regulation of type I and type II interleukin-1 receptors in focal brain inflammation. Eur J Neurosci 2005;21:1205–14.
43. Ilyin SE, Plata-Salaman CR. In vivo regulation of the IL-1 beta system (ligand, receptors I and II, receptor accessory protein, and receptor antagonist) and TNF-alpha mRNAs in specific brain regions. Biochem Biophys Res Commun 1996;227:861–7.
44. Takao T, Tracey DE, Mitchell WM, et al. Interleukin-1 receptors in mouse brain: characterization and neuronal localization. Endocrinology 1990;127:3070–8.
45. Ban E, Milon G, Prudhomme N, et al. Receptors for interleukin-1 (alpha and beta) in mouse brain: mapping and neuronal localization in hippocampus. Neuroscience 1991;43:21–30.
46. Parnet P, Amindari S, Wu C, et al. Expression of type I and type II interleukin-1 receptors in mouse brain. Brain Res Mol Brain Res 1994;27:63–70.
47. Konsman JP, Vigues S, Mackerlova L, et al. Rat brain vascular distribution of interleukin-1 type-1 receptor immunoreactivity: relationship to patterns of inducible cyclooxygenase expression by peripheral inflammatory stimuli. J Comp Neurol 2004;472:113–29.
48. Nadjar A, Combe C, Laye S, et al. Nuclear factor kappaB nuclear translocation as a crucial marker of brain response to interleukin-1. A study in rat and interleukin-1 type I deficient mouse. J Neurochem 2003;87:1024–36.
49. Gabellec MM, Jafarian-Tehrani M, Griffais R, et al. Interleukin-1 receptor accessory protein transcripts in the brain and spleen: kinetics after peripheral administration of bacterial lipopolysaccharide in mice. Neuroimmunomodulation 1996;3:304–9.
50. Liu C, Chalmers D, Maki R, et al. Rat homolog of mouse interleukin-1 receptor accessory protein: cloning, localization and modulation studies. J Neuroimmunol 1996;66:41–8.
51. Cremona S, Goujon E, Kelley KW, et al. Brain type I but not type II IL-1 receptors mediate the effects of IL-1 beta on behavior in mice. Am J Physiol 1998;274(3 Pt 2):R735–40.
52. Sonti G, Flynn MC, Plata-Salaman CR. Interleukin-1 (IL-1) receptor type I mediates anorexia but not adipsia induced by centrally administered IL-1beta. Physiol Behav 1997;62:1179–83.
53. Liege S, Laye S, Li KS, et al. Interleukin 1 receptor accessory protein (IL-1RAcP) is necessary for centrally mediated neuroendocrine and immune responses to IL-1beta. J Neuroimmunol 2000;110:134–9.
54. Quan N, Whiteside M, Kim L, et al. Induction of inhibitory factor kappaBalpha mRNA in the central nervous system after peripheral lipopolysaccharide administration: an in situ hybridization histochemistry study in the rat. Proc Natl Acad Sci USA 1997;94:10985–90.
55. Kubota T, Kushikata T, Fang J, et al. Nuclear factor-kappaB inhibitor peptide inhibits spontaneous and interleukin-1beta-induced sleep. Am J Physiol Regul Integr Comp Physiol 2000;279:R404–13.
56. Nadjar A, Bluthe RM, May MJ, et al. Inactivation of the cerebral NFkappaB pathway inhibits interleukin-1beta-induced sickness behavior and c-Fos expression in various brain nuclei. Neuropsychopharmacology 2005;30:1492–9.
57. Kelly A, Vereker E, Nolan Y, et al. Activation of p38 plays a pivotal role in the inhibitory effect of lipopolysaccharide and interleukin-1 beta on long term potentiation in rat dentate gyrus. J Biol Chem 2003;278:19453–62.
58. Godbout JP, Chen J, Abraham J, et al. Exaggerated neuroinflammation and sickness behavior in aged mice following activation of the peripheral innate immune system. FASEB J 2005;19:1329–31.

59. O'Connor JC, Satpathy A, Hartman ME, et al. IL-1beta-mediated innate immunity is amplified in the db/db mouse model of type 2 diabetes. J Immunol 2005;174:4991–7.
60. Perry VH. The influence of systemic inflammation on inflammation in the brain: implications for chronic neurodegenerative disease. Brain Behav Immun 2004; 18:407–13.
61. Hart BL. Biological basis of the behavior of sick animals. Neurosci Biobehav Rev 1988;12:123–37.
62. Aubert A, Goodall G, Dantzer R, et al. Differential effects of lipopolysaccharide on pup retrieving and nest building in lactating mice. Brain Behav Immun 1997;11: 107–18.
63. Lutgendorf SK, Garand L, Buckwalter KC, et al. Life stress, mood disturbance, and elevated interleukin-6 in healthy older women. J Gerontol A Biol Sci Med Sci 1999;54:M434–9.
64. Kiecolt-Glaser JK, Glaser R. Depression and immune function: central pathways to morbidity and mortality. J Psychosom Res 2002;53:873–6.
65. Alesci S, Martinez PE, Kelkar S, et al. Major depression is associated with significant diurnal elevations in plasma interleukin-6 levels, a shift of its circadian rhythm, and loss of physiological complexity in its secretion: clinical implications. J Clin Endocrinol Metab 2005;90:2522–30.
66. Maes M, Bosmans E, Meltzer HY. Immunoendocrine aspects of major depression. Relationships between plasma interleukin-6 and soluble interleukin-2 receptor, prolactin and cortisol. Eur Arch Psychiatry Clin Neurosci 1995;245: 172–8.
67. Maes M, Bosmans E, De Jongh R, et al. Increased serum IL-6 and IL-1 receptor antagonist concentrations in major depression and treatment resistant depression. Cytokines 1997;9:853–8.
68. Brambilla F, Maggioni M. Blood levels of cytokines in elderly patients with major depressive disorder. Acta Psychiatr Scand 1998;97:309–13.
69. Capuron L, Ravaud A, Miller AH, et al. Baseline mood and psychosocial characteristics of patients developing depressive symptoms during interleukin-2 and/or interferon-alpha cancer therapy. Brain Behav Immun 2004;18:205–13.
70. Capuron L, Gumnick JF, Musselman DL, et al. Neurobehavioral effects of interferon-alpha in cancer patients: phenomenology and paroxetine responsiveness of symptom dimensions. Neuropsychopharmacology 2002;26:643–52.
71. Bull SJ, Huezo-Diaz P, Binder EB, et al. Functional polymorphisms in the interleukin-6 and serotonin transporter genes, and depression and fatigue induced by interferon-alpha and ribavirin treatment. Mol Psychiatry 2008, May 6 [Epub ahead of print].
72. Kraus MR, Al-Taie O, Schäfer A, et al. Serotonin-1A receptor gene HTR1A variation predicts interferon-induced depression in chronic hepatitis C. Gastroenterology 2007;132:1279–86.
73. Capuron L, Ravaud A. Prediction of the depressive effects of interferon alfa therapy by the patient's initial affective state. N Engl J Med 1999;340:1370.
74. Miyaoka H, Otsubo T, Kamijima K, et al. Depression from interferon therapy in patients with hepatitis C. Am J Psychiatry 1999;156:1120.
75. Capuron L, Neurauter G, Musselman DL, et al. Interferon-alpha-induced changes in tryptophan metabolism. Relationship to depression and paroxetine treatment. Biol Psychiatry 2003;54:906–14.
76. Constant A, Castera L, Dantzer R, et al. Mood alterations during interferon-alfa therapy in patients with chronic hepatitis C: evidence for an overlap between manic/hypomanic and depressive symptoms. J Clin Psychiatry 2005;66:1050–7.

77. Capuron L, Ravaud A, Neveu PJ, et al. Association between decreased serum tryptophan concentrations and depressive symptoms in cancer patients undergoing cytokine therapy. Mol Psychiatry 2002;7:468–73.
78. Maes M, Bonaccorso S, Marino V, et al. Treatment with interferon-alpha (IFN alpha) of hepatitis C patients induces lower serum dipeptidyl peptidase IV activity, which is related to IFN alpha-induced depressive and anxiety symptoms and immune activation. Mol Psychiatry 2001;6:475–80.
79. Lestage J, Verrier D, Palin K, et al. The enzyme indoleamine 2,3-dioxygenase is induced in the mouse brain in response to peripheral administration of lipopolysaccharide and superantigen. Brain Behav Immun 2002;16:596–601.
80. Frenois F, Moreau M, O'Connor J, et al. Lipopolysaccharide induces delayed FosB/DeltaFosB immunostaining within the mouse extended amygdala, hippocampus and hypothalamus, that parallel the expression of depressive-like behavior. Psychoneuroendocrinology 2007;32:516–31.
81. Moreau M, Andre C, O'Connor JC, et al. Inoculation of Bacillus Calmette-Guerin to mice induces an acute episode of sickness behavior followed by chronic depressive-like behavior. Brain Behav Immun 2008;22:1087–95.
82. Andre C, O'Connor JC, Kelley KW, et al. Spatio-temporal differences in the profile of murine brain expression of proinflammatory cytokines and indoleamine 2,3 dioxygenase in response to peripheral lipopolysaccharide administration. J Neuroimmunol 2008;200:90–9.
83. O'Connor JC, Lawson MA, Andre C, et al. Lipopolysaccharide-induced depressive-like behavior is mediated by indoleamine 2,3 dioxygenase activation in muce. Mol Psychiatry 2008;Jan 15 [Epub ahead of print].
84. Tyring S, Gottlieb A, Papp K, et al. Etanercept and clinical outcomes, fatigue, and depression in psoriasis: double-blind placebo-controlled randomized phase III trial. Lancet 2006;367:29–35.
85. Schwarcz R, Pellicciari R. Manipulation of brain kynurenines: glial targets, neuronal effects, and clinical opportunities. J Pharmacol Exp Ther 2002;303: 1–10.
86. Wichers MC, Koek GH, Robaeys G, et al. IDO and interferon-alpha-induced depressive symptoms: a shift in hypothesis from tryptophan depletion to neurotoxicity. Mol Psychiatry 2005;10:538–44.
87. Juengling FD, Ebert D, Gut O, et al. Prefrontal cortical hypometabolism during low-dose interferon alpha treatment. Psychopharmacology (Berl) 2000;152: 383–9.
88. Capuron L, Pagnoni G, Fornwalt FB, et al. Brain metabolic changes and neurovegetative symptoms in medically ill patients undergoing interferon-alpha therapy. Abstr Soc Neurosci 2005;660:23.
89. Appels A, Bar FW, Bar J, et al. Inflammation, depressive symptomatology, and coronary artery disease. Psychosom Med 2000;62:601–5.
90. Lesperance F, Frasure-Smith N, Theroux P, et al. The association between major depression and levels of soluble intercellular adhesion molecule 1, interleukin-6, and C-reactive protein in patients with recent acute coronary syndromes. Am J Psychiatry 2004;161:271–7.

Hypothalamo-Pituitary-Adrenocortical Axis, Glucocorticoids, and Neurologic Disease

Erica J. Doczy, MS[a,c], Kim Seroogy, PhD[b], Catherine R. Harrison, PhD[c], James P. Herman, PhD[a,*]

KEYWORDS

- Stress • Glucocorticoid
- Hypothalamo-pituitary-adrenocortical axis
- Neurologic disease • Cortisol • Neurotrama

The role of stress in neurologic disease is often overlooked. Several chronic neurologic disease states (eg, Alzheimer disease[1]) are associated with elevated secretion of stress hormones (such as cortisol), resulting from overactivity of the hypothalamo-pituitary-adrenocortical (HPA) axis. Stress can also trigger or exacerbate symptom onset and perhaps progression of chronic illness, such as Parkinson disease.[2] Stress hormones can also mediate the impact of acute neurotrauma. For example, there is a positive correlation between cortisol levels and mortality following head injury. Thus, neurologic disease states can occur within a context of elevated glucocorticoids, which may have profound influences on recovery and neuroplasticity. In addition, abnormal regulation of glucocorticoid release is associated with numerous affective disorders, such as depression and posttraumatic stress disorder, that are overrepresented in populations with neurologic disease (eg, Parkinson disease).[2]

This article is a version of an article previously published in *Neurologic Clinics*: Herman J. Hypothalamo-pituitary-adrenocortical axis, glucocorticoids, and neurologic disease. Neurol Clin 2006;24(3):461–81.

This article was supported by NIH grants AG12962 (Herman), AG10836 (Herman), and NS060114 (Seroogy).

[a] Departments of Psychiatry, University of Cincinnati College of Medicine, Psychiatry North, GRI-E, ML 0506, 2170 East Galbraith Road, Cincinnati, OH 45237-0506, USA
[b] Departments of Neurology, University of Cincinnati College of Medicine, Cincinnati, OH 45237-0506, USA
[c] Air Force Research Laboratory, 711th HPW/RHPA, Wright Patterson AFB, OH 45433, USA
* Corresponding author. Department of Psychiatry, Psychiatry North, GRI-E, ML 0506, 2170 East Galbraith Road, Cincinnati, OH 45237-0506, USA.
E-mail address: james.herman@uc.edu (J.P. Herman).

Acute and sustained glucocorticoid release can also precipitate changes in both peripheral and central immune signaling,[2] resulting in cytokine/chemokine profiles that may be deleterious for functional recovery in the face of neurologic challenge.

This article describes the basic organization of the HPA loop controlling glucocorticoid release, the central circuits that control glucocorticoid release, glucocorticoid signaling mechanisms, and the overall importance of this system to central nervous system function in the face of challenge or damage.

THE HYPOTHALAMO-PITUITARY-ADRENOCORTICAL AXIS

The HPA stress axis plays a major role in control of systemic homeostasis. Stimulation of this axis causes secretion of glucocorticoid hormones (cortisol in humans, corticosterone in rats), which act in both the brain and periphery to promote adaptation. Glucocorticoids function primarily to redistribute energy resources, and are intimately involved in restoration or defense of homeostasis following challenge.[3]

Activation of the HPA axis can be triggered by stimuli signaling disruption of internal homeostasis, such as blood loss, hypoglycemia, infection, or tissue damage (signaled by pain). However, release of glucocorticoids can also occur in anticipation of adverse events, a mechanism that is particularly relevant to neurologists and psychoneuroimmunologists. Keyed by either prior experience (memories) or instinctual predispositions, anticipatory release of glucocorticoids occurs in the absence of a frank physical stimulus. The relevance of the anticipatory response is likely to be associated with the predicted occurrence of physical challenge. The HPA axis tries to "head off" threats before they disrupt normal physiologic functions.

Stimulus-induced HPA axis activation is commonly associated with the concept of stress. For practical purposes, stress can be broadly defined as "a real or perceived threat to homeostasis." Stressors, in addition to activating the HPA axis, also induce a very rapid and short-lived sympathoadrenomedullary response. In addition, stressors cause behavioral responses that may or may not occur in concert with physiologic changes. Thus, the glucocorticoid response is a component of the stress response, but is not synonymous with it.

The general organization of the HPA axis is presented in **Fig. 1**. The hypothalamic paraventricular nucleus (PVN) is the prime mover of glucocorticoid responses to stress (see **Fig. 1**).[4,5] Stimulation of hypophysiotrophic neurosecretory neurons in the medial parvocellular PVN initiates activation of the HPA axis. These neurons project to blood vessels in the median eminence and release numerous corticotropin "secretagogues," including corticotropin-releasing hormone (CRH) and arginine vasopressin (AVP).[4,5] These travel by way of the pituitary portal system to the anterior pituitary and cause release of corticotropin, which subsequently causes synthesis and secretion of glucocorticoids at the adrenal gland.

While stress clearly drives the HPA axis, a powerful circadian glucocorticoid rhythm also plays a role. In most organisms, glucocorticoids peak immediately before the onset of waking and are highest early in the behaviorally active period.[6] Glucocorticoid levels attained during the diurnal peak are not trivial. Typically, in rats, circadian peak levels of corticosterone can approach values that rival those seen in a stress response. This contrasts markedly with extremely low levels seen during the nadir, which are at or near the limit of detectability. As a result, there is a roughly 40- to 50-fold fluctuation in glucocorticoid levels every day. Accordingly, daily corticosterone variations have a potentially profound impact on brain (and body) glucocorticoid signaling across the day.

The acute glucocorticoid response to stress is clearly an adaptive mechanism, causing a variety of physiologic (and perhaps psychological) changes that aid in

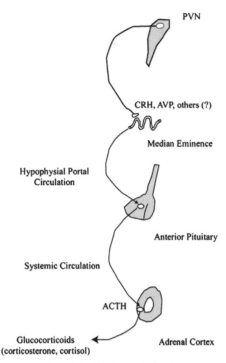

PVN

CRH, AVP, others (?)

Median Eminence

Hypophysial Portal
Circulation

Anterior Pituitary

Systemic Circulation

ACTH

Glucocorticoids   Adrenal Cortex
(corticosterone, cortisol)

Fig. 1. HPA axis. Neurons located within the hypothalamic paraventricular nucleus (PVN) drive pituitary corticotrophs via release of secretagogues (such as corticotropin-releasing hormone [CRH] and arginine vasopressin [AVP]) into the portal vasculature, stimulating corticotropin (ACTH). Corticotropin, in turn, mediates the synthesis and release of corticosteroids from the adrenal glands.

restoring homeostasis.[3] However, if glucocorticoid release is left unchecked, numerous deleterious processes can occur in the body and brain, including immune dysfunction, bone and muscle wasting, and depression. Thus, in healthy organisms, negative-feedback inhibition maintains control of glucocorticoid secretion. Negative feedback is mediated by glucocorticoids acting via both rapid (likely nongenomic) and delayed (likely genomic) mechanisms (discussed below).[7]

Chronic drive of the HPA axis with prolonged stress precipitates long-term changes in both central and peripheral effector systems. These changes include adrenal hypertrophy, which is associated with prolonged exposure of the adrenal cortex to corticotropin, and thymic atrophy, which is a cumulative result of repeated glucocorticoid elevation.[8] Chronic glucocorticoid release consequent to stress may also have an impact on other endocrine systems (eg, inhibition of testosterone).[9] Elevated glucocorticoid levels have been linked to chronic stress-induced hippocampal damage and cognitive deficits,[10,11] and also contribute to decreased appetite,[12] behavioral anhedonia,[13] and altered cardiovascular tone,[14] which are characteristics of prolonged stress exposure.

The net impact of chronic stress regimens on the HPA axis is dependent on stressor modality, duration, and intensity. Chronic stress designs create some degree of long-term increases in basal corticosterone release.[8,15,16] Enhanced release is observed as long as 24 hours after the last stress exposure, indicating that the HPA system has undergone long-term up-regulation. At the pituitary, chronic stress increases pro-opiomelanocortin mRNA expression and pituitary corticotropin stores.[17] However, CRH-receptor binding is decreased,[18,19] indicative of an adaptive, down-regulatory response to enhanced CRH secretion. In the hypothalamus, chronic stress increases central indicators of PVN drive, including CRH and AVP mRNA expression,[8,20–23] PVN and median eminence CRH peptide levels,[24] and the extent of CRH/AVP co-localization in the median eminence.[25] Enhanced PVN CRH expression is negatively correlated with PVN glucocorticioid receptor levels,[8,22,26] suggesting reduced hypothalamic glucocorticoid feedback efficacy following chronic stress.

Chronic stress also causes changes in extrahypothalamic regulators of HPA axis function. For example, chronic regimens can reduce hippocampal expression of glucocorticoid and mineralocorticoid receptors[8,15,22,27] and increase expression of tyrosine hydroxylase in locus coeruleus.[28] The overall connection between these mRNA changes in stress regulatory regions and stress-induced drive of the HPA axis remains to be determined.

Repeated exposure to some stressors (eg, restraint, cold) can cause habituation of HPA axis responses.[29,30] Animals exposed to repeated, "homotypic" stress still respond to an individual stressor, and are therefore still subject to the cumulative impact of multiple episodes of glucocorticoid secretion. The habituation rate depends on the severity of the repeated stressor. For example, HPA axis responses to total immobilization do not show response decrements.[31] While responses to homotypic stressors diminish over time, responses to stressors of different modality (heterotypic stressors) are sensitized,[29,32] indicating that the cumulative effect of repeated stress can make the animal more vulnerable to subsequent insults (eg, acute neurologic trauma or disease).

Chronic stress results in numerous physiologic and behavioral changes similar to human disease or aging pathology. For example, chronic stress-induced adrenal hypertrophy, weight loss, anhedonia, and dexamethasone feedback resistance are highly reminiscent of melancholic depression,[13] a disease with clear links to glucocorticoid hypersecretion and stress.

NEURAL CONTROL OF HYPOTHALAMO-PITUITARY-ADRENOCORTICAL AXIS INTEGRATION

Multiple brain regions mediate control of HPA axis activation. Forebrain limbic structures are thought to be responsible in large part for anticipatory stress responses, which are responses that do not involve an overt challenge to homeostasis. The limbic structures involved include the hippocampus, prefrontal cortex, and amygdala, all of which are frequently affected in psychiatric and neurologic disease states. Accordingly, disorders of forebrain HPA control sites may be responsible for glucocorticoid dyshomeostasis seen in these diseases.

The hippocampus is believed to be involved in inhibition of the HPA axis.[33–35] Stimulation of the hippocampus decreases glucocorticoid secretion in rats and humans,[36,37] whereas lesions of the hippocampus increase release of corticosterone, or corticotropin, or both corticosterone and corticotropin.[38–41] Hippocampal damage also increases PVN CRH and AVP gene expression[42–44] and the extent of PVN neural activation (as measured by c-fos induction) following stress, suggesting that the hippocampal inhibition of the HPA is mediated via the PVN. The impact of hippocampal lesions on HPA excitability is stressor specific: Hippocampal damage exacerbates anticipatory stress responses, but does not enhance reactive responses to stimuli, such as hypoxia or ether inhalation.[45–47]

Like the hippocampus, the medial prefrontal cortex is implicated in HPA axis inhibition. Lesions of the prelimbic and anterior cingulate subregions of the medial prefrontal cortex increase corticotropin and corticosterone secretion and PVN *c-fos* mRNA induction following restraint stress.[48,49] Medial prefrontal cortex lesions do not affect responses to ether inhalation, again suggesting a role in inhibition of anticipatory responses. However, recent studies suggest that the role of the prefrontal cortex in HPA integration may be dependent on both subregion and hemisphere. Lesions restricted to the right infralimbic cortex decrease, rather than increase, corticosterone responses to restraint stress, whereas left-sided lesions do not affect glucocorticoid secretion.[50] In addition, the infralimbic part of the medial prefrontal complex cortex may be more keyed to regulation of reactive responses. This is suggested because lesions of this region attenuate corticotropin secretion following interleukin-1 beta injection, but those same lesions do not affect response to noise.[51] Taken together, these observations suggest an intricate topographic organization of prefrontal cortex output to HPA regulatory circuits.

The amygdala is clearly involved in activating the HPA axis, principally by way of the medial and central amygdaloid nuclei. Large amygdaloid lesions or lesions of the central or medial amygdaloid nuclei attenuate stress-induced corticotropin and corticosterone secretion in rats,[52–56] whereas stimulation enhances release of HPA hormones.[57–59] The HPA-stimulatory effects of amygdaloid subnuclei are consistent with the role of the amygdala in autonomic activation, fear, and anxiety.[60,61]

The excitatory influence of the amygdala on the HPA axis is stressor- and region-specific. The medial amygdala is intensely activated during anticipatory stress responses (eg, restraint, social stress, predator exposure),[62–64] but shows considerably less activation during reactive responses (inflammatory stimuli, hypoxia, hemorrhage).[63,65,66] Lesions of this amygdalar region also attenuate corticotropin release following restraint.[67] The central amygdaloid nucleus shows an opposite response pattern, being preferentially *c-fos* responsive during reactive responses.[65,66] Furthermore, lesions of this region attenuate HPA activation following inflammatory cytokine administration[68] but not restraint.[8,53,67]

Despite profound actions of all of the above limbic structures on the HPA axis, none send direct projections to the PVN. The influence of these regions on the HPA axis require relay through basal forebrain (bed nucleus of the stria terminalis), hypothalamic, and brainstem cell populations, which in turn innervate the medial parvocellular PVN. Thus, information from the limbic system requires an intermediary synapse to influence HPA activation.

Neuroanatomical tracing studies indicate that, in the bed nucleus of the stria terminalis and hypothalamus, the majority of these intermediary neurons contain the inhibitory neurotransmitter γ-aminobutyric acid (GABA).[69,70] GABA neurons in PVN-projecting zones of these regions are stress-activated,[71] consistent with involvement in HPA-axis inhibition. Interactions of various limbic stress regulatory regions with GABA neurons largely explain the nature of their influence on the PVN. Projections of both the hippocampus and prefrontal cortex are predominantly excitatory (ie, glutamate-containing).[72,73] Thus, inhibition of the HPA axis is likely mediated through excitation of GABAergic relay neurons. In contrast, central and medial amygdala projection neurons contain GABA.[74] Amygdalar "activation" of the HPA axis may actually reflect disinhibition, mediated through sequential inhibitory neurons (**Fig. 2**).

Direct excitation of the HPA axis is likely mediated via the brainstem. The nucleus of the solitary tract (NTS) provides rich innervation of the PVN by both catecholaminergic (norepinephrine) and noncatecholaminergic (eg, glucagonlike peptide-1) neurons.[75–77] Both of these transmitter systems are thought to be stress-excitatory via direct activation of PVN CRH neurons.[78] Catecholamines appear to contribute primarily to reactive stress responses. For example, destruction of NTS inputs to the PVN attenuates

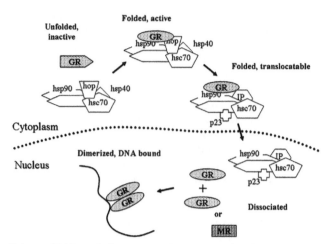

Fig. 2. Intracellular trafficking of glucocorticoid receptors. The glucocorticoid (GR) or miner-alocorticoid receptors (MR) require association with heat shock protein (hsp) 90 before hormone binding. The presence of heat shock cognate protein (hsc70) and other cellular chaperones (hsp40, hop) is required to maintain the GR/MR in a state suitable for hormone binding. Nuclear trafficking of the ligand bound GR/MR is accomplished in association with the hsp90 complex, p23, and an immunophilin (IP) moiety. Once in the nucleus, the recep-tors are released from the hsp complex, whereupon they can homodimerize (or heterodi-merize with the glucocorticoid receptor or other steroid receptor species) to bind DNA. Downstream effects on transcription are likely mediated through interaction with nuclear coactivator or co-repressor proteins.

HPA responses to hypoglycemia but does not affect the HPA response to restraint. In contrast, central inhibition of glucagonlike peptide-1 receptors using a peptide frag-ment (exendin 9-36) inhibits corticotropin and corticosterone release in response to either novelty or visceral illness,[79] suggesting that this noncatecholaminergic cell pop-ulation may be involved in both anticipatory and reactive responses. Notably, the NTS receives input from limbic structures, such as the central amygdaloid nucleus and in-fralimbic cortex, which may in part explain the ability of this region to be an excitatory mediator of stress responses.

GLUCOCORTICOID SIGNALING IN THE CENTRAL NERVOUS SYSTEM

The endpoint of HPA-axis activation is the release of glucocorticoids, which cause a variety of transcriptional and nontranscriptional events to occur in both body and brain. At least two distinct receptors mediate glucocorticoid action in the central nervous system. The "traditional" glucocorticoid receptor (GR) binds glucocorticoids with 5- to 10-nM affinity.[80] The binding characteristics of this receptor are quite intriguing. It is extensively unbound during periods of low glucocorticoids (late at night in humans, early morning in rodents), and becomes 50% to 70% occupied during the circadian peak.[80,81] The GR will become fully occupied under conditions of severe stress. In the mid-80s, Reul and deKloet[80] and Spencer and colleagues[81] discovered an additional adrenocorticosteroid receptor in the brain. Somewhat surprisingly, this receptor was found to be identical to the mineralocorticoid receptor (MR), which medi-ates biologic effects of aldosterone in the kidney.[80] Subsequent work revealed that 11 beta-hydroxysteroid dehydrogenase in the kidney breaks down corticosterone, allowing recognition of aldosterone, which circulates at low levels in blood. Meanwhile, the levels of aldosterone in the central nervous system are so low that it does not fully occupy the MR, thus allowing it to be a receptor for both glucocorticoids and mineralocorticoids.[82] The binding characteristics of MRs are quite different from those of GRs. The MR binds cortisol and corticosterone with higher affinity (0.5–1 nM), making it extensively bound even at the circadian trough (>70%), and fully bound at the circadian peak and during stress.[80,81]

Both GRs and MRs exert primary biologic actions via gene transcription. Both are members of the steroid hormone receptor superfamily, possessing DNA-binding domains that become available after ligand binding.[83] The receptors are cytosolic when unbound, and are associated with a macromolecular chaperone complex that includes heat shock protein 90 dimers in association with other heat shock proteins and immunophilins (**Fig. 3**).[84] When bound, a nuclear localization signal is revealed that allows the receptors to be transported to the cell nucleus. Once in the nucleus, the receptors can modulate transcription in one of two ways: (1) by direct binding with DNA response elements as homodimers or possibly as GR-MR heterodimers[85] or (2) via protein-protein interactions with other transcription factor complexes.[86] Transcriptional effects can be either excitatory or inhibitory.

Considerable evidence indicates the existence of a membrane GR responsible for rapid actions of glucocorticoids. This receptor has yet to be isolated.

GLUCOCORTICOID RECEPTORS AND INHIBITION OF THE HYPOTHALAMO-PITUITARY-ADRENOCORTICAL AXIS

Glucocorticoids have powerful negative-feedback action on corticotropin release, and are prime points of HPA axis control. These actions are believed to be mediated via binding to both nuclear and membrane GRs.

Because it takes only very low levels of circulating glucocorticoids to extensively occupy neuronal MRs, the neuronal MR is thought to be important in basal inhibition of the HPA axis. A role for MR in basal HPA regulation is further supported by data indicating that spironolactone, a potent MR antagonist, can increase morning corticotropin release in rats[87] and enhance basal cortisol and corticotropin levels in humans.[88] Intracerebroventricular injection of MR antagonist treatment increases morning corticosterone levels in rats. Meanwhile, however, intracerebroventricular injection of GR antagonist treatment has no effect on morning corticosterone levels in rats. This suggests that endogenous corticosterone inhibits basal HPA activity via central MRs.[89,90] Inhibition of MRs also prohibits inhibitory actions of corticosterone on rising levels of glucocorticoids in the evening,[91] and combined treatment with GR and MR antagonists is required to inhibit circadian peak corticosterone secretion. Thus, it is likely that the two receptors work together to control peak daily secretory rhythms.[87]

Glucocorticoid inhibition of acute HPA axis stress responses may also involve both GRs and MRs. Combined injection of GR (RU45055) or MR (RU28318) antagonists increases peak corticosterone responses to novelty, whereas injection of either alone is ineffective, indicating that binding of both receptors is required for normal stress inhibition.[87] Notably, blockade of GRs but not MRs produces long-term elevation of corticosterone observed following an acute stress, suggesting a selective role for GR in terminating corticosteroid secretory responses.[92] Central administration of the GR antagonist RU486 enhances the magnitude of the corticosteroid response to novelty, whereas both MR and GR antagonists prolong the magnitude of the HPA response to this stimulus, again suggesting a role for both receptors in stress control by the central nervous system.[89]

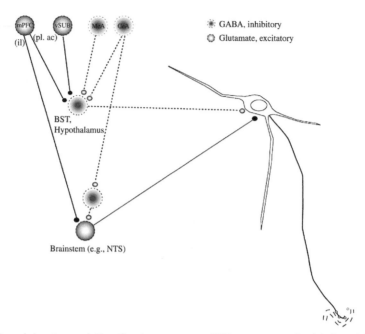

Fig. 3. Neural circuits regulating the stress response. PVN neurons receive (1) direct inhibitory (GABA-containing) input from neurons in the bed nucleus of the stria terminalis (BST) and numerous hypothalamic nuclei and (2) excitatory input from the brainstem, including neurons of the nucleus of the solitary tract (NTS). These direct pathways are heavily influenced by input from limbic structures, which likely fuel anticipatory stress responses and underlie HPA pathology associated with affective disease or chronic stress. Inhibitory circuits receive excitatory input from such regions as the hippocampus (via the ventral subiculum [vSUB] and medial prefrontal cortex [mPFC], anterior cingulate [ac], and prelimbic [pl] regions), which results in a net inhibition of the stress response. In contrast, inhibitory PVN inputs receive GABAergic (ie, inhibitory) input from the medial amygdaloid (MeA) and central amygdaloid (CeA) nuclei, resulting in disinhibition at the level of the PVN (and thus activation of the HPA axis). PVN excitatory regions receive direct innervation from glutamate neurons of the infralimbic (il) region of the medial prefrontal cortex, which may enhance HPA activity. Brainstem excitatory regions also receive input from the central amygdaloid nuclei, which may disinhibit brainstem neurons by way of local inhibitory interneurons.

The loci mediating GR or MR control of the HPA axis have yet to be definitively identified. Previous studies suggest that the hippocampus alone, or the prefrontal cortex alone, or both the hippocampus and the prefrontal cortex mediate corticosteroid-dependent termination of stress responses. However, there is considerable conflicting data on this topic.[34,93] Notably, recent studies employing a mouse line with selective deletion of GRs in the hippocampus and cortex reveal elevated corticosterone and corticotropin at both the trough and nadir of the circadian rhythm and resistance to dexamethasone suppression,[94] suggesting that glucocorticoids work through the hippocampal GR, the cortical GR, or both to inhibit basal HPA tone.

Chronic exposure to homotypic stressors results in habituation of stress responses.[95–97] Acute treatment with MR or combined MR-GR antagonists prevents habituation, whereas GR antagonist alone does not,[30] indicating that the MR may also be involved in adjusting the long-term responsiveness of the HPA system.

It is also critical to consider possible nongenomic mechanisms of HPA axis inhibition. Exogenous glucocorticoids can inhibit HPA axis stress responses within minutes, a process known as "fast" or "rate-sensitive" feedback. This process occurs at least in part at the level of the PVN, as local injections of glucocorticoids inhibit PVN neurons within seconds to minutes of exposure.[98] Genomic actions of corticosteroids cannot account for such rapid inhibition of the HPA axis. In accordance with these findings, electrophysiological studies indicate that fast feedback effects of corticosteroids on PVN neurons are mediated through inhibition of presynaptic glutamate release. This mediation occurs by way of a G-protein–coupled receptor activating synthesis of endocannabinoids (acting as retrograde messengers).[99] A membrane corticosteroid receptor with appropriate characteristics has been detected in amphibians,[100] but mammalian analogs have yet to be identified and cloned.

GLUCOCORTICOIDS, STRESS, AND NEURODEGENERATION

Studies in experimental animals indicate that high doses of systemic steroids can have toxic effects on neurons in select regions of the brain, most notably the hippocampus. Studies in the mid-80s indicated that intense and prolonged stress exposure can result in death of hippocampal neurons, with the cornu ammonis (CA) 3 subfield being particularly vulnerable.[35] These results have not been extensively replicated in other models,[101] suggesting that overt toxicity may be relegated to intense stress exposure. However, fairly good evidence indicates that exogenous glucocorticoids can endanger neurons, particularly in the hippocampus.[102] High-dose glucocorticoid treatment greatly exacerbates neuronal damage following concomitant insults (eg, excitotoxin exposure[103]). Prolonged glucocorticoid treatment causes retraction of apical dendrites in the hippocampal CA3 region,[104] a process thought to be associated with glucocorticoid modulation of glutamate signaling.[105] The mechanism of glucocorticoid action may involve a number of factors, including inhibition of glucose transport,[106] enhancement of glutamate toxicity[102] or reduced expression of neurotrophic factors (eg, brain-derived neurotrophic factor[107]). Glucocorticoids damage the hippocampal pyramidal neurons by inhibiting their glucose uptake and reducing the production of adenosine triphosphate, leading to atrophy and ultimately cell death.[108] This inhibits long-term potentiation in the hippocampus, decreasing neuronal plasticity and contributing to memory impairments.[109] Glucocorticoids also reduce neurogenesis (birth of new neurons) in the dentate gyrus.[110] While the link between neurogenesis and neurodegeneration/regeneration has yet to be clearly defined, it stands to reason that loss of the capacity to make new neurons may reduce the capacity for neuroplastic responses in the face of adverse events.

The GR is thought to mediate the glucocorticoid effects on neurotoxicity. Most toxic effects occur only at high doses of glucocorticoids, which are sufficient to bind GRs. In vitro studies indicate that glucocorticoid enhancement of neurotoxicity is inhibited by the GR antagonist RU486, but not by MR antagonists.[111,112] In addition, administration of GR (but not MR) agonists are sufficient to enhance neurotoxic damage in the hippocampus.[113]

Stimulation of endogenous release by stress replicates many of the neurotoxic and neuroadaptive effects of exogenous glucocorticoids. For example, chronic severe social stress is reported to result in hippocampal neurodegeneration in primates.[114] In rodents, chronic restraint stress can cause CA3 dendritic atrophy,[115] exacerbate excitotoxic damage,[103] and impair neurogenesis,[116] all of which are also seen with glucocorticoid administration.

Glucocorticoids also play an important, supportive role in cell survival. Elimination of glucocorticoids by adrenalectomy produces neurodegeneration in the dentate gyrus,[117] indicating a trophic role in this region. Very low doses of glucocorticoids or administration of MR agonist are sufficient to block this degeneration,[118] indicating that the trophic actions of glucocorticoids are likely mediated by occupation of the MR.

ENDOGENOUS GLUCOCORTICOIDS AND NEUROLOGIC DISEASE

The HPA axis is a dynamic system that responds to adverse physiologic and psychological stimuli. Chronic neurologic disease states clearly qualify as adverse situations, and can be accompanied by elevations in circulating glucocorticoids.[119] In addition, patients with neurologic diseases can also exhibit comorbid depression,[2] which can also elevate glucocorticoid levels. In either case, elevations in glucocorticoids may be relevant to the progression of neurodegenerative events. Likewise, acute neurologic crises also cause secretion of endogenous glucocorticoids.[120] Thus, the possible contribution of glucocorticoids to underlying pathology needs to be considered in all cases where neurologic conditions are associated with pronounced stress.

Animal studies indicate that acute neurotoxic or neurotraumatic events can elicit pronounced increases in endogenous glucocorticoid release. For example, in rats, a single systemic kainate injection produces profound elevations in glucocorticoids as long as 24 hours post-insult.[121] These levels rival those seen following the most intense stressors and likely cause extensive and total occupation of the GRs for a prolonged period of time. Traumatic brain injury also produces marked glucocorticoid release. However, the response to this insult shows more substantial recovery over time.[122] Even the act of brain surgery alone can have effects on the HPA axis: Rats receiving sham surgery for intracranial injection procedures manifest physiologic changes consistent with long-term effects of perioperative glucocorticoid secretion.[8]

Animal studies indicate that endogenous glucocorticoids play a role in neurodegeneration and recovery of neural tissue following insults. Our group has investigated this contribution by studying the effects of selective MR and GR antagonism on cell survival following in vivo insult. In these studies, rats received twice-daily injections of GR or MR antagonist for 3 days before challenge. Rats treated with MR antagonist showed, in subfield CA3 of the hippocampus, substantial exacerbation of kainate neurotoxicity in terms of frank neuronal loss and incidence of damaged neurons. In contrast, GR blockade did not affect cell loss (**Fig. 4**).[121] The increased neurodegeneration following MR antagonism was associated with a decrease in expression of Bcl-2, an antiapoptotic protein, in this same subregion.[123] The overall data suggest that the profound increases in endogenous glucocorticoids do not play a major role in the degenerative process. However, MR binding is required for normal cell survival following excitotoxic damage. The data suggest that glucocorticoids retain a beneficial trophic action on hippocampal neurons even under conditions of marked HPA axis challenge, but do not contribute to neurodegeneration in response to this type of insult.

In contrast, glucocorticoid secretion may be a major factor in modulating cell death following traumatic brain injury. The hippocampus undergoes substantial cell loss following controlled cortical contusion, likely as a secondary effect of the compression injury. Prior exposure to the GR antagonist RU486 effectively blocks hippocampal cell loss in subfield CA1 of the hippocampus, as measured by stereological analysis of cell counts (**Fig. 5**).[124] This loss is neither exacerbated nor attenuated by administration of spironolactone (MR antagonist).[124] Thus, the posttraumatic surge in glucocorticoids (shown to be present at least 6 hours following injury in this model) plays an important role in degeneration of CA1 pyramidal neurons following this type of neural insult.

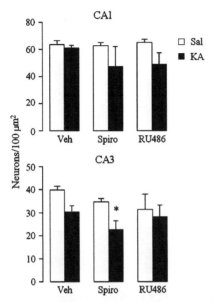

Fig. 4. Effects of MR blockade and GR blockade on kainate neurotoxicity in the hippocampus. MR blockade with spironolactone significantly decreased the number of viable CA3 neurons following systemic kainate injection. Pretreatment with RU486 did not affect CA3 cell death, and neither antagonist modulated kainate-induced cell loss in CA1 (*asterisk P* ≤ .05). KA, kainic acid; Sal, saline; Spiro, spironolactone; Veh, vehicle. (*Data from* Cunningham Jr. ET, Sawchenko PE. Anatomical specificity of noradrenergic inputs to the paraventricular and supraoptic nuclei of the rat hypothalamus. J Comp Neurol 1988;274:60.)

Additional research is required to determine whether blocking the neuronal GR with RU486 can have beneficial effects on behavioral outcomes following trauma.

Recent evidence shows that the dysregulation of the HPA axis caused by traumatic brain injury can be long-lasting. Following mild controlled cortical impact, stress-induced corticosterone levels remain enhanced 70 days following injury.[125] In contrast, corticosterone responses are attenuated through day 70 following a moderate controlled cortical impact, indicating that severity of injury has differential effects on the long-term stress-induced HPA responses.[125]

Stress and inflammation may work together to exacerbate clinical symptoms following injury. Stress causes cytokine dysregulation, as seen by stress-induced increases in IL-1β in rats.[126] With glucocorticoids increasing in neurotrauma patients,[127] the already deleterious inflammatory response may be aggravated by glucocorticoid modulation of cytokine production and signaling. In addition, inflammation can activate the HPA axis, as seen by increased corticotropin and glucocorticoids following lipopolysachharide-induced proinflammatory cytokines,[128] thereby increasing the capacity for toxic actions of glucocorticoids on neurons. There is also evidence for direct effects of stress on neurotoxic immune factors. For example, following ischemic brain damage, subacute stress can increase damage by mechanisms involving Toll-like receptor 4, a receptor that mediates the inflammatory response.[129]

Several of the clinical symptoms that manifest after brain injury are mediated by disruption of feedback through the HPA axis.[130] Traumatic brain injury can produce adrenal insufficiency through direct injury to the hypothalamus or pituitary, with

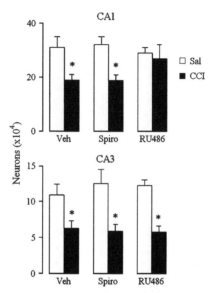

Fig. 5. Effects of MR blockade and GR blockade on hippocampal neuron viability following controlled cortical impact (CCI) injury, as measured by the optical fractionator method. CCI significantly decreased the number of viable neurons in CA1 and CA3 of vehicle-pretreated animals. Pretreatment with RU486 protected CA1 pyramidal neurons from CCI-induced cell loss. CCI decreased the number of viable neurons in CA3 in both spironolactone- and RU486-pretreated animals (*asterisk* $P \leq$ .05). Sal, saline; Spiro, spironolactone; Veh, vehicle. (*Data from* Rinaman L. Interoceptive stress activates glucagon-like peptide-1 neurons that project to the hypothalamus. Am J Phys 1999;277:R582.)

associated symptoms that may include weakness, fatigue, weight loss, and depression. Hypoadrenalism during the late phase of injury occurs in a significant portion of traumatic brain injury patients.[131] A recent clinical trial reported 23.6% of traumatic brain injury patients in the early phase of injury presented with adrenal insufficiency.[132] Disruptions in the HPA axis may also lead to disorders of arousal, for example. Sleep-wake cycle disturbance is common in traumatic brain injury patients.[133]

The effects of stress can be differentiated from the effects of exogenous glucocorticoids in some neurologic illnesses. For example, stress has been hypothesized to contribute to the neuropathology of Parkinson disease and to exacerbate parkinsonian symptoms, possibly by increasing the vulnerability of mesencephalic dopamine neurons to degeneration.[2] However, recent evidence raises the possibility that glucocorticoid therapy may be considered in patients with the disorder. For example, dexamethasone prevented the degeneration of nigrostriatal dopaminergic neurons in two different rodent models of Parkinson disease,[134,135] probably due to its anti-inflammatory actions, although neuroprotective mechanisms cannot be ruled out. Thus, the comingling of stress and stress-related disorders (such as depression) in Parkinson disease and other related neurodegenerative disorders warrants further investigation.

INTEGRATION: GLUCOCORTICOID SYSTEMS AND NEUROLOGY

The HPA axis plays a powerful role in disorders of the nervous system. Normally, the HPA exerts tight control of circulating glucocorticoid levels. By doing so, it maintains glucocorticoid signaling capacity, ensuring that beneficial effects on nervous tissue (mediated perhaps by the MR) are permitted, whereas the potential damage caused by major stress responses are temporally limited. However, neurologists may frequently be confronted by situations in which HPA control is tenuous at best. Such situations include, for example, those involving severe distress associated with acute or prolonged neural dysfunction, inflammatory processes that command major activation of the HPA system, and patients whose HPA axis is compromised by other conditions (eg, depression). Thus, understanding and considering the endogenous regulatory systems in place for control of glucocorticoids may be appropriate to consider in future treatment strategies. Issues of most relevance include the following:

Many, if not most, neurologic conditions occur within the context of profound psychogenic stress (eg, hospitalization, anxiety). These states are powerful stimulants to the HPA axis, whose hormones have a role in neurodegenerative and inflammatory processes.

Many brain regions targeted by neurologic disorders and dementias, such as the hippocampus, amygdala, and prefrontal cortex, are also responsible for control of HPA function. Thus, damage to these areas has the potential to promote further glucocorticoid release and perhaps contribute to neurodegenerative processes.

Neurologic disorders may be accompanied by clinical depression, which is associated with impaired negative-feedback regulation of the HPA axis. Impaired feedback may permit a cumulative negative influence of glucocorticoids on neuronal growth and survival.

While glucocorticoids are of clear benefit for some neurologic disorders (eg, brain edema associated with tumors[136]), the use of glucocorticoids as an adjunct treatment for stroke or trauma may not be mandated. Indeed, reviews of the literature find glucocorticoid treatment in association with stroke or trauma to be of no clear benefit,[136] and in some cases may even worsen prognosis (the CRASH [Corticosteroid Randomisation After Significant Head Injury] study).[137]

In sum, glucocorticoids play a significant role in neurologic outcomes. While the extent to which endogenous glucocorticoids participate in the neurodegenerative process remains to be definitively established, it is prudent to consider strategies designed to limit the extent of stress experienced by neurologic patients.

ACKNOWLEDGMENTS

The authors thank laboratory members who have contributed to this work.

REFERENCES

1. Martignoni E, Costa A, Sinforiani E, et al. The brain as a target for adrenocortical steroids: cognitive implications. Psychoneuroendocrinology 1992;17:343–54.
2. Smith AD, Castro SL, Zigmond MJ. Stress-induced Parkinson's disease: a working hypothesis. Physiol Behav 2002;77:527–31.
3. Munck A, Guyre PM, Holbrook NJ. Physiological functions of glucocorticoids in stress and their relations to pharmacological actions. Endocr Rev 1984;5:25–44.
4. Antoni FA. Hypothalamic control of adrenocorticotropin secretion: Advances since the discovery of 41-residue corticotropin-releasing factor. Endocr Rev 1986;7:351–78.
5. Whitnall MH. Regulation of the hypothalamic corticotropin-releasing hormone neurosecretory system. Prog Neurobiol 1993;40:573–629.

6. Dallman MF, Akana SF, Cascio CS, et al. Regulation of ACTH secretion: variations on a theme of B. Recent Prog Horm Res 1987;43:113–73.
7. Keller-Wood M, Dallman MF. Corticosteroid inhibition of ACTH secretion. Endocr Rev 1984;5:1–24.
8. Prewitt CM, Herman JP. Hypothalamo-pituitary-adrenocortical regulation following lesions of the central nucleus of the amygdala. Stress 1997;1:263–80.
9. Tamashiro KL, Nguyen MM, Sakai RR. Social stress: from rodents to primates. Front Neuroendocrinol 2005;26:27–40.
10. McEwen BS, Sapolsky RM. Stress and cognitive function. Curr Opin Neurobiol 1995;5:205–16.
11. Sapolsky RM. Glucocorticoids and hippocampal atrophy in neuropsychiatric disorders. Arch Gen Psychiatry 2000;57:925–35.
12. Dallman MF, Pecoraro N, Akana SF, et al. Chronic stress and obesity: a new view of "comfort food". Proc Natl Acad Sci U S A 2003;100:11696–701.
13. Willner P, Muscat R, Papp M. Chronic mild stress-induced anhedonia: a realistic animal model of depression. Neurosci Biobehav Rev 1992;16:525–34.
14. Grippo AJ, Moffitt JA, Johnson AK. Cardiovascular alterations and autonomic imbalance in an experimental model of depression. Am J Phys Regul Integr Comp Physiol 2002;282:R1333–41.
15. Gomez F, Lahmame A, de Kloet ER, et al. Hypothalamic-pituitary-adrenal response to chronic stress in five inbred rat strains: differential responses are mainly located at the adrenocortical level. Neuroendocrinology 1996;63:327–37.
16. Ottenweller JE, Servatius RJ, Tapp WN, et al. A chronic stress state in rats: effects of repeated stress on basal corticosterone and behavior. Physiol Behav 1992;51:689–98.
17. Shiomi H, Watson SJ, Kelsey JE, et al. Pretranslational and posttranslational mechanisms for regulating beta-endorphin-adrenocorticotropin of the anterior pituitary lobe. Endocrinology 1986;119:1793–9.
18. Anderson SM, Kant GJ, De Souza EB. Effects of chronic stress on anterior pituitary and brain corticotropin-releasing factor receptors. Pharmacol Biochem Behav 1993;44:755–61.
19. Fuchs E, Flugge G. Modulation of binding sites for corticotropin-releasing hormone by chronic psychosocial stress. Psychoneuroendocrinology 1995;20:33–51.
20. DeGoeij DC, Jezova D, Tilders FJ. Repeated stress enhances vasopressin synthesis in CRF neurons in the paraventricular nucleus. Brain Res 1992;577:165–8.
21. DeGoeij DC, Kvetnansky R, Whitnall MH, et al. Repeated stress-induced activation of corticotropin-releasing factor neurons enhances vasopressin stores and colocalization with corticotropin-releasing factor in the median eminence of rats. Neuroendocrinology 1991;53:150–9.
22. Herman JP, Adams D, Prewitt CM. Regulatory changes in neuroendocrine stress-integrative circuitry produced by a variable stress paradigm. Neuroendocrinology 1995;61:180–90.
23. Imaki T, Nahan JL, Rivier C, et al. Differential regulation of corticotropin-releasing factor mRNA in rat brain regions by glucocorticoids and stress. J Neurosci 1991;11:585–99.
24. Chappell PB, Smith MA, Kilts CD, et al. Alterations in corticotropin-releasing factor-like immunoreactivity in discrete brain regions after acute and chronic stress. J Neuroscic 1986;6:2908–14.
25. Whitnall MH. Stress selectively activates the vasopressin-containing subset of corticotropin-releasing hormone neurons. Neuroendocrinology 1989;50:702–7.

26. Makino S, Smith MA, Gold PW. Increased expression of corticotropin-releasing hormone and vasopressin messenger ribonucleic acid (mRNA) in the hypothalamic paraventricular nucleus during repeated stress: association with reduction in glucocorticoid receptor mRNA levels. Endocrinology 1995; 136:3299–309.

27. Sapolsky RM, Krey LC, McEwen BS. Stress down-regulates corticosterone receptors in a site-specific manner in the brain. Endocrinology 1984;114: 287–92.

28. Mamalaki E, Kvetnansky R, Brady LS, et al. Repeated immobilization stress alters tyrosine hydroxylase, corticotropin-releasing hormone and corticosteroid receptor ribonucleic acid levels in rat brain. J Neuroendocrinol 1993;4:689–99.

29. Akana SF, Dallman MF, Bradbury MJ, et al. Feedback and facilitation in the adrenocortical system: unmasking facilitation by partial inhibition of the glucocorticoid response to prior stress. Endocrinology 1992;131:57–68.

30. Cole MA, Kalman BA, Pace TW, et al. Selective blockade of the mineralocorticoid receptor impairs hypothalamic-pituitary-adrenal axis expression of habituation. J Neuroendocrinol 2000;12:1034–42.

31. Dobrakovova M, Kvetnansky R, Torda T, et al. Changes of plasma and adrenal catecholamines and corticosterone in stressed rats with septal lesions. Physiol Behav 1982;29:41–5.

32. Bhatnagar S, Dallman M. Neuroanatomical basis for facilitation of hypothalamic-pituitary-adrenal responses to a novel stressor after chronic stress. Neuroscience 1998;84:1025–39.

33. Herman JP, Cullinan WE. Neurocircuitry of stress: central control of the hypothalamo-pituitary-adrenocortical axis. Trends Neurosci 1997;20:78–83.

34. Jacobson L, Sapolsky RM. The role of the hippocampus in feedback regulation of the hypothalamo-pituitary-adrenocortical axis. Endocr Rev 1991;12:118–34.

35. Sapolsky RM, Krey LC, McEwen BS. The neuroendocrinology of stress and aging: the glucocorticoid cascade hypothesis. Endocr Rev 1986;7:284–301.

36. Dunn JD, Orr SE. Differential plasma corticosterone responses to hippocampal stimulation. Exp Brain Res 1984;54:1–6.

37. Rubin RT, Mandell AJ, Crandall PH. Corticosteroid responses to limbic stimulation in man: localization of stimulation sites. Science 1966;153:1212–5.

38. Fendler K, Karmos G, Telegdy G. The effect of hippocampal lesion on pituitary-adrenal function. Acta Physiol Scand 1961;20:293–7.

39. Knigge KM. Adrenocortical response to stress in rats with lesions in hippocampus and amygdala. Proc Soc Exp Biol Med 1961;108:18–21.

40. Knigge KM, Hays M. Evidence of inhibitive role of hippocampus in neural regulation of ACTH release. Proc Soc Exp Biol Med 1963;114:67–9.

41. Sapolsky RM, Krey LC, McEwen BS. Glucocorticoid-sensitive hippocampal neurons are involved in terminating the adrenocortical stress response. Proc Natl Acad Sci U S A 1984;81:6174–7.

42. Herman JP, Cullinan WE, Morano MI, et al. Contribution of the ventral subiculum to inhibitory regulation of the hypothalamo-pituitary-adrenocortical axis. J Neuroendocrinol 1995;7:475–82.

43. Herman JP, Cullinan WE, Young EA, et al. Selective forebrain fiber tract lesions implicate ventral hippocampal structures in tonic regulation of paraventricular nucleus CRH and AVP mRNA expression. Brain Res 1992;592:228–38.

44. Herman JP, Schäfer MK-H, Young EA, et al. Evidence for hippocampal regulation of neuroendocrine neurons of the hypothalamo-pituitary-adrenocortical axis. J Neurosci 1989;9:3072–82.

45. Bradbury MJ, Strack AM, Dallman MF. Lesions of the hippocampal efferent pathway (fimbria-fornix) do not alter sensitivity of adrenocorticotropin to feedback inhibition by corticosterone in rats. Neuroendocrinology 1993;58:396–407.

46. Herman JP, Dolgas CM, Carlson SL. Ventral subiculum regulates hypothalamo-pituitary-adrenocortical and behavioural responses to cognitive stressors. Neuroscience 1998;86:449–59.

47. Mueller NK, Dolgas CM, Herman JP. Stressor-selective role of the ventral subiculum in regulation of neuroendocrine stress responses. Endocrinology 2004; 145:3763–8.

48. Diorio D, Viau V, Meaney MJ. The role of the medial prefrontal cortex (cingulate gyrus) in the regulation of hypothalamo-pituitary-adrenal responses to stress. J Neurosci 1993;13:3839–47.

49. Figueiredo HF, Bruestle A, Bodie B, et al. The medial prefrontal cortex differentially regulates stress-induced c-fos expression in the forebrain depending on type of stressor. Eur J Neurosci 2003;18:2357–64.

50. Sullivan RM, Gratton A. Lateralized effects of medial prefrontal cortex lesions on neuroendocrine and autonomic stress responses in rats. J Neurosci 1999;19: 2834–40.

51. Crane JW, Ebner K, Day TA. Medial prefrontal cortex suppression of the hypothalamic-pituitary-adrenal axis response to a physical stressor, systemic delivery of interleukin-1beta. Eur J Neurosci 2003;17:1473–81.

52. Allen JP, Allen CF. Role of the amygdaloid complexes in the stress-induced release of ACTH in the rat. Neuroendocrinology 1974;15:220–30.

53. Beaulieu S, DiPaolo T, Barden N. Control of ACTH secretion by the central nucleus of the amygdala: implication of the serotonergic system and its relevance to the glucocorticoid delayed negative feedback mechanism. Neuroendocrinology 1986;44:247–54.

54. Dayas CV, Day TA. Opposing roles for medial and central amygdala in the initiation of noradrenergic cell responses to a psychological stressor. Eur J Neurosci 2002;15:1712–8.

55. Feldman S, Conforti N, Itzik A, et al. Differential effect of amygdaloid lesions of CRF-41, ACTH and corticosterone responses following neural stimuli. Brain Res 1994;658:21–6.

56. Van de Kar LD, Piechowski RA, Rittenhouse PA, et al. Amygdaloid lesions: differential effect on conditioned stress and immobilization-induced increases in corticosterone and renin secretion. Neuroendocrinology 1991;54:89–95.

57. Dunn JD, Whitener J. Plasma corticosterone responses to electrical stimulation of the amygdaloid complex: cytoarchitectonic specificity. Neuroendocrinology 1986;42:211–7.

58. Matheson GK, Branch BJ, Taylor AN. Effects of amygdaloid stimulation on pituitary-adrenal activity in conscious cats. Brain Res 1971;32:151–67.

59. Redgate ES, Fahringer EE. A comparison of the pituitary adrenal activity elicited by electrical stimulation of preoptic, amygdaloid and hypothalamic sites in the rat brain. Neuroendocrinology 1973;12:334–43.

60. Davis M. The role of the amygdala in fear and anxiety. Annu Rev Neurosci 1992; 15:353–75.

61. Gray TS. Amygdaloid CRF pathways. Role in autonomic, neuroendocrine, and behavioral responses to stress. Ann N Y Acad Sci 1993;697:53–60.

62. Cullinan WE, Herman JP, Battaglia DF, et al. Pattern and time course of immediate early gene expression in rat brain following acute stress. Neuroscience 1995;64:477–505.

63. Figueiredo HF, Bodie BL, Tauchi M, et al. Stress integration after acute and chronic predator stress: differential activation of central stress circuitry and sensitization of the hypothalamo-pituitary-adrenocortical axis. Endocrinology 2003;144:5249–58.
64. Kollack-Walker S, Watson SJ, Akil H. Social stress in hamsters: defeat activates specific neurocircuits within the brain. J Neurosci 1997;17:8842–55.
65. Sawchenko PE, Brown ER, Chan RWK, et al. The paraventricular nucleus of the hypothalamus and the functional neuroanatomy of visceromotor responses to stress. Prog Brain Res 1996;107:201–22.
66. Thrivikraman KV, Su Y, Plotsky PM. Patterns of fos-immunoreactivity in the CNS induced by repeated hemorrhage in conscious rats: correlations with pituitary-adrenal axis activity. Stress 1997;2:145–58.
67. Dayas CV, Buller KM, Day TA. Neuroendocrine responses to an emotional stressor: evidence for involvement of the medial but not the central amygdala. Eur J Neurosci 1999;11:2312–22.
68. Xu Y, Day TA, Buller KM. The central amygdala modulates hypothalamic-pituitary-adrenal axis responses to systemic interleukin-1beta administration. Neuroscience 1999;94:175–83.
69. Cullinan WE, Herman JP, Watson SJ. Ventral subicular interaction with the hypothalamic paraventricular nucleus: evidence for a relay in the bed nucleus of the stria terminalis. J Comp Neurol 1993;332:1–20.
70. Roland BL, Sawchenko PE. Local origins of some GABAergic projections to the paraventricular and supraoptic nuclei of the hypothalamus of the rat. J Comp Neurol 1993;332:123–43.
71. Cullinan WE, Helmreich DL, Watson SJ. Fos expression in forebrain afferents to the hypothalamic paraventricular nucleus following swim stress. J Comp Neurol 1996;368:88–99.
72. Broman J, Hassel B, Rinvik E, et al. Biochemistry and anatomy of transmitter glutamate. In: Otterson OP, Storm-Mathisen J, editors. Glutamate. vol. 18. Amsterdam: Elsevier; 2000. p. 1–44.
73. Walaas I, Fonnum F. Biochemical evidence for glutamate as a transmitter in hippocampal efferents to the basal forebrain and hypothalamus in the rat brain. Neuroscience 1980;5:1691–8.
74. Swanson LW, Petrovich GD. What is the amygdala? Trends Neurosci 1998;21:323–31.
75. Cunningham ET Jr, Sawchenko PE. Anatomical specificity of noradrenergic inputs to the paraventricular and supraoptic nuclei of the rat hypothalamus. J Comp Neurol 1988;274:60–76.
76. Cunningham ET Jr, Bohn MC, Sawchenko PE. Organization of adrenergic inputs to the paraventricular and supraoptic nuclei of the hypothalamus in the rat. J Comp Neurol 1990;292:651–67.
77. Rinaman L. Interoceptive stress activates glucagon-like peptide-1 neurons that project to the hypothalamus. Am J Phys 1999;277:R582–90.
78. Plotsky PM, Cunningham ET Jr, Widmaier EP. Catecholaminergic modulation of corticotropin-releasing factor and adrenocorticotropin secretion. Endocr Rev 1989;10:437–58.
79. Kinzig KP, D'Alessio DA, Herman JP, et al. CNS glucagon-like peptide-1 receptors mediate endocrine and anxiety responses to interoceptive and psychogenic stressors. J Neurosci 2003;23:6163–70.
80. Reul JM, deKloet ER. Two receptor systems for corticosterone in rat brain: microdistribution and differential occupation. Endocrinology 1985;117:2505–11.

81. Spencer RL, Young EA, Choo PH, et al. Adrenal steroid type I and type II receptor binding: estimates of in vivo receptor number, occupancy, and activation with varying level of steroid. Brain Res 1990;514:37–48.

82. Edwards CR, Stewart PM, Burt D, et al. Localisation of 11 beta-hydroxysteroid dehydrogenase–tissue specific protector of the mineralocorticoid receptor. Lancet 1988;2:986–9.

83. Evans RM. The steroid and thyroid hormone receptor superfamily. Science 1988; 240:889–95.

84. Pratt WB, Toft DO. Steroid receptor interactions with heat shock protein and immunophilin chaperones. Endocr Rev 1997;18:306–60.

85. Trapp T, Holsboer F. Heterodimerization between mineralocorticoid and glucocorticoid receptors increases the functional diversity of corticosteroid action. Trends Pharmacol Sci 1996;17:145–9.

86. Smoak KA, Cidlowski JA. Mechanisms of glucocorticoid receptor signaling during inflammation. Mech Ageing Dev 2004;125:697–706.

87. Spencer RL, Kim PJ, Kalman BA, et al. Evidence for mineralocorticoid receptor facilitation of glucocorticoid receptor-dependent regulation of hypothalamic-pituitary-adrenal axis activity. Endocrinology 1998;139:2718–26.

88. Deuschle M, Weber B, Colla M, et al. Mineralocorticoid receptor also modulates basal activity of hypothalamus-pituitary-adrenocortical system in humans. Neuroendocrinology 1998;68:355–60.

89. Ratka A, Sutanto W, Bloemers M, et al. On the role of brain mineralocorticoid (type I) and glucocorticoid (type II) receptors in neuroendocrine regulation. Neuroendocrinology 1989;50:117–23.

90. van Haarst AD, Oitzl MS, de Kloet ER. Facilitation of feedback inhibition through blockade of glucocorticoid receptors in the hippocampus. Neurochem Res 1997;22:1323–8.

91. Bradbury MJ, Akana SF, Dallman MF. Roles of type I and II corticosteroid receptors in regulation of basal activity in the hypothalamo-pituitary-adrenal axis during the diurnal trough and the peak: evidence for a nonadditive effect of combined receptor occupation. Endocrinology 1994;134:1286–96.

92. Moldow RL, Beck KD, Weaver S, et al. Blockage of glucocorticoid, but not mineralocorticoid receptors prevents the persistent increase in circulating basal corticosterone concentrations following stress in the rat. Neurosci Lett 2005;374:25–8.

93. Herman JP, Figueiredo H, Mueller NK, et al. Central mechanisms of stress integration: hierarchical circuitry controlling hypothalamo-pituitary-adrenocortical responsiveness. Front Neuroendocrinol 2003;24:151–80.

94. Boyle MP, Brewer JA, Funatsu M, et al. Acquired deficit of forebrain glucocorticoid receptor produces depression-like changes in adrenal axis regulation and behavior. Proc Natl Acad Sci U S A 2005;102:473–8.

95. Campmany L, Pol O, Armario A. The effects of two chronic intermittent stressors on brain monoamines. Pharmacol Biochem Behav 1996;53:517–23.

96. Gadek-Michalska A, Bugajski J. Repeated handling, restraint, or chronic crowding impair the hypothalamic-pituitary-adrenocortical response to acute restraint stress. J Physiol Pharmacol 2003;54:449–59.

97. Keim KL, Sigg EB. Physiological and biochemical concomitants of restraint stress in rats. Pharmacol Biochem Behav 1976;4:289–97.

98. Saphier D. Catecholaminergic projections to tuberoinfundibular neurones of the paraventricular nucleus: I. Effects of stimulation of A1, A2, A6 and C2 cell groups. Brain Res Bull 1989;23:389–95.

99. Di S, Malcher-Lopes R, Halmos KC, et al. Nongenomic glucocorticoid inhibition via endocannabinoid release in the hypothalamus: a fast feedback mechanism. J Neurosci 2003;23:4850–7.

100. Orchinik M, Murray TF, Moore FL. A corticosteroid receptor in neuronal membranes. Science 1991;252:1848–51.

101. Reagan LP, McEwen BS. Controversies surrounding glucocorticoid-mediated cell death in the hippocampus. J Chem Neuroanat 1997;13:149–67.

102. Sapolsky RM. The physiological relevance of glucocorticoid endangerment of the hippocampus. Ann N Y Acad Sci 1994;746:294–304.

103. Stein-Behrens B, Mattson MP, Chang I, et al. Stress exacerbates neuron loss and cytoskeletal pathology in the hippocampus. J Neurosci 1994;14:5373–80.

104. Magarinos AM, Orchinik M, McEwen BS. Morphological changes in the hippocampal CA3 region induced by non-invasive glucocorticoid administration: a paradox. Brain Res 1998;809:314–8.

105. Magarinos AM, McEwen BS. Stress-induced atrophy of apical dendrites of hippocampal CA3c neurons: involvement of glucocorticoid secretion and excitatory amino acid receptors. Neuroscience 1995;69:89–98.

106. Virgin CE, Ha TP-T, Packan DR, et al. Glucocorticoids inhibit glucose transport and glutamate uptake in hippocampal astrocytes: implications for glucocorticoid neurotoxicity. J Neurochem 1991;57:1422–8.

107. Smith MA, Makino S, Kvetnansky R, et al. Stress and glucocorticoids affect the expression of brain-derived neurotrophic factor and neurotrophin-3 mRNAs in the hippocampus. J Neurosci 1995;15:1768–77.

108. Sapolsky RM. Glucocorticoids, hippocampal damage and the glutamatergic synapse. Prog Brain Res 1990;86:13–23.

109. Kim JJ, Song EY, Kosten TA. Stress effects in the hippocampus: synaptic plasticity and memory. Stress 2006;9:1–11.

110. Cameron HA, Gould E. Adult neurogenesis is regulated by adrenal steroids in the dentate gyrus. Neuroscience 1994;61:203–9.

111. Behl C, Lezoualc'h F, Trapp T, et al. Glucocorticoids enhance oxidative stress-induced cell death in hippocampal neurons in vitro. Endocrinology 1997;138: 101–6.

112. Talmi M, Carlier E, Bengelloun W, et al. Synergistic action of corticosterone on kainic acid-induced electrophysiological alterations in the hippocampus. Brain Res 1995;704:97–102.

113. Goodman Y, Bruce AJ, Cheng B, et al. Estrogens attenuate and corticosterone exacerbates excitotoxicity, oxidative injury, and amyloid beta-peptide toxicity in hippocampal neurons. J Neurochem 1996;66:1836–44.

114. Uno H, Tarara R, Else JG, et al. Hippocampal damage associated with prolonged and fatal stress in primates. J Neurosci 1989;9:1705–11.

115. Magarinos AM, McEwen BS. Stress-induced atrophy of apical dendrites of hippocampal CA3 neurons: comparison of stressors. Neuroscience 1995;69: 83–8.

116. Gould E, Tanapat P. Stress and hippocampal neurogenesis. Biol Psychiatry 1999;46:1472–9.

117. Sloviter RS, Sollas AL, Dean E, et al. Adrenalectomy-induced granule cell degeneration in the rat hippocampal dentate gyrus: characterization of an in vivo model of controlled neuronal death. J Comp Neurol 1993;330:324–36.

118. Woolley CS, Gould E, Sakai RR, et al. Effects of aldosterone or RU28362 treatment on adrenalectomy-induced cell death in the dentate gyrus of the adult rat. Brain Res 1991;554:312–5.

119. Dodt C, Dittmann J, Hruby J, et al. Different regulation of adrenocorticotropin and cortisol secretion in young, mentally healthy elderly, and patients with senile dementia of Alzheimer's type. J Clin Endocrinol Metab 1991;72:272–6.

120. Cernak I, Savic VJ, Lazarov A, et al. Neuroendocrine responses following graded traumatic brain injury in male adults. Brain Inj 1999;13:1005–15.

121. McCullers DL, Herman JP. Adrenocorticosteroid receptor blockade and excitotoxic challenge regulate adrenocorticosteroid receptor mRNA levels in hippocampus. J Neurosci Res 2001;64:277–83.

122. McCullers DL, Sullivan PG, Scheff SW, et al. Traumatic brain injury regulates adrenocorticosteroid receptor mRNA levels in rat hippocampus. Brain Res 2002;947:41–9.

123. McCullers DL, Herman JP. Mineralocorticoid receptors regulate Bcl2 and p53 mRNA expression in rat hippocampus. Neuroreport 1998;9:3085–9.

124. McCullers DL, Sullivan PG, Scheff SW, et al. Mifepristone protects CA1 hippocampal neurons following traumatic brain injury in rat. Neuroscience 2002;109:219–30.

125. Taylor AN, Rahman SU, Sanders NC, et al. Injury severity differentially affects short- and long-term neuroendocrine outcomes of traumatic brain injury. J Neurotrauma 2008;25:311–23.

126. Pugh CR, Nguyen KT, Gonyea JL, et al. Role of interleukin-1 beta in impairment of contextual fear conditioning caused by social isolation. Behav Brain Res 1999;106:109–18.

127. Narayan RK, Povlishock JT, Wilberger JE, editors Neurotrauma. New York: McGraw-Hill Professional; 1996.

128. Dunn AJ, Wang J, Ando T. Effects of cytokines on cerebral neurotransmission. Comparison with the effects of stress. Adv Exp Med Biol 1999;461:117–27.

129. Caso JR, Pradillo JM, Hurtado O, et al. Toll-like receptor 4 is involved in subacute stress-induced neuroinflammation and in the worsening of experimental stroke. Stroke 2008;39:1314–20.

130. Powner DJ, Boccalandro C, Alp MS, et al. Endocrine failure after traumatic brain injury in adults. Neurocrit Care 2006;5:61–70.

131. Tsagarakis S, Tzanela M, Dimopoulou I. Diabetes insipidus, secondary hypoadrenalism and hypothyroidism after traumatic brain injury: clinical implications. Pituitary 2005;8:251–4.

132. Llompart-Pou JA, Raurich JM, Perez-Barcena J, et al. Acute hypothalamic-pituitary-adrenal response in traumatic brain injury with and without extracerebral trauma. Neurocrit Care 2008;9:230–6.

133. Makley MJ, English JB, Drubach DA, et al. Prevalence of sleep disturbance in closed head injury patients in a rehabilitation unit. Neurorehabil Neural Repair 2008;22:341–7.

134. Castano A, Herrera AJ, Cano J, et al. The degenerative effect of a single intranigral injection of LPS on the dopaminergic system is prevented by dexamethasone, and not mimicked by rh-TNF-alpha, IL-1beta and IFN-gamma. J Neurochem 2002;81:150–7.

135. Kurkowska-Jastrzebska I, Litwin T, Joniec I, et al. Dexamethasone protects against dopaminergic neurons damage in a mouse model of Parkinson's disease. Int Immunopharmacol 2004;4:1307–18.

136. Gomes JA, Stevens RD, Lewin JJ 3rd, et al. Glucocorticoid therapy in neurologic critical care. Crit Care Med 2005;33:1214–24.

137. Roberts I, Yates D, Sandercock P, et al. Effect of intravenous corticosteroids on death within 14 days in 10008 adults with clinically significant head injury (MRC CRASH trial): randomised placebo-controlled trial. Lancet 2004;364:1321–8.

Social Interactions, Stress, and Immunity

Ronit Avitsur, PhD[a],*, Nicole Powell, PhD[b], David A. Padgett, PhD[b,c],
John F. Sheridan, PhD[b,c]

KEYWORDS

• Social defeat • GC resistance • Hierarchy • Splenomegaly

Stressors generally are defined as external or internal challenges that disrupt homeostasis.[1] Thus, potential stressors are all around us. For example, stressors can include changes in the environment, such as temperature extremes; physiologic difficulties, such as scarcity of food or water; and psychosocial burdens, such as social subordination or loneliness. Some of these stressors may be acute, posing a short-term demand on individuals. Others may reoccur or may be long-lasting, creating a chronic burden for the organism.

The response to a stressor typically consists of physiologic and behavioral changes to help reestablish homeostasis. These are somewhat predictable and were recognized as early as 1936 when Selye[2,3] coined the term *general adaptation syndrome* to describe the "nonspecific response of the body to any demand." In other words, each of the variety of stressors in people's lives elicits a similar collection of stress responses. These include activation of the hypothalamic-pituitary-adrenal (HPA) axis and the sympathetic nervous system. Products of these systems, which include glucocorticoids and catecholamines, change cardiovascular tone and respiration rate and increase the flow of blood to muscle tissue.[4]

Although it generally is agreed that a set of core stress responses are activated nonspecifically by threats to homeostasis, it is now understood that there is a wide variety of stress-specific responses. Recent studies show considerable individual differences in the response to a similar stressor. A closer inspection of those studies

This article is a version of an article previously published in *Neurologic Clinics*: Avitsur R, Padgett DA, Sheridan JF. Social interactions, stress, and immunity. Neurol Clin 2006;24(3):483–91.

Supported by NIH grants R01 MH 046801 (JFS) and T32 DE 014320 (JFS), The Israel Science Foundation (RA), and The United States-Israel Binational Science Foundation (RA and JFS).

[a] School of Behavioral Sciences, The Academic College of Tel Aviv-Yaffo, 14 Rabenu Yerucham Street, PO Box 8401, Yaffo 68114, Israel

[b] Section of Oral Biology, College of Dentistry, Ohio State University, 305 W. 12th Avenue, Columbus, OH 43210, USA

[c] The Institute for Behavioral Medicine Research, College of Medicine, Ohio State University, 300 W. 10th Avenue, Columbus, OH 43210, USA

* Corresponding author.

E-mail address: avitsur@mta.ac.il (R. Avitsur).

suggests that personality traits and psychosocial factors play an important role in modulating the overall stress response.[4,5]

The association between distinctive stress responses and a specific stressor can be demonstrated using social disruption, a model of social stress in mice. Although many aspects of the response to social disruption are similar to those of other chronic stressors, social disruption also elicits a unique set of endocrine and immune responses that, to the best of current knowledge, are characteristic of this particular stressor. In addition, social disruption invokes a range of individual differences in genetically similar inbred mice.

This article presents an overview of the endocrinologic and immunologic responses to social disruption. It discusses the possible implications of these stress responses as survival advantages or consequences for the host, particularly in terms of resistance to infection. This article finishes with comments on possible behavioral factors that contribute to individual behavioral and physiologic differences elicited by social disruption.

THE SOCIAL DISRUPTION STRESS MODEL

Male mice caged together form social hierarchies. These hierarchies usually consist of (1) a dominant alpha male, (2) codominant cage mates, and (3) subordinate cage mates. The status of the animals in a group typically is determined by fighting over dominance or by passive acceptance of subordination.[6] In the model of social disruption stress, naturally occurring social hierarchies in groups of male mice are disrupted daily by introducing an aggressive intruder into a cage with an established hierarchy. Social disruption is repeated once a day for 6 successive days to mimic a recurring or chronic stressor.[7,8] During social disruption, residents are attacked by the intruding aggressor and defeated repeatedly. The residents attempt to escape and display the characteristic behavioral signs of fear and submissiveness.

Similar to other models of stress, social disruption activates the HPA axis, resulting in elevated levels of corticotropin and the glucocorticoid hormone, corticosterone.[7,9,10] In many chronic and repeating stress models, activation of the HPA axis results in suppression of multiple immune functions. Thus, it was hypothesized that repeated social defeat would be accompanied by suppression of multiple immune parameters, including both innate and adaptive responses, and that a collateral increased susceptibility to infection would ensue. Unexpectedly, the data showed that despite the high levels of circulating corticosterone, social disruption resulted in splenomegaly, an increase in proinflammatory cytokine responses, and modulation of antimicrobial immunity.[10,11] A further examination of this atypical immune response to the stressor indicated that social disruption decreased the sensitivity of immune cells to glucocorticoids, thus reducing its suppressive influence on inflammation and enhancing proinflammatory cytokine responses.[7,8,10,12–16]

IMMUNOLOGIC EFFECTS OF SOCIAL DISRUPTION

Repeated exposure to social disruption results in the development of a state of glucocorticoid resistance in immune cells taken from the spleens of mice.[7,8] More specifically, social disruption reduces the sensitivity of lipopolysaccharide (LPS)-stimulated splenocytes to the inhibitory effect of corticosterone with regard to cell viability. This effect has been demonstrated in several inbred (C57BL/6, C3H/HeJ, C3H/HeN, BALB/c, and SJL) and outbred (CD-1) mouse strains (Ronit Avistur, PhD, John F. Sheridan, PhD, unpublished data 2005),[7,14] suggesting that this phenomenon does not depend on a specific genetic background.

The development of glucocorticoid resistance is accompanied by splenomegaly,[7] which is characterized by a large increase in the number of splenic CD11b+ myeloid cells.[13,14] Experimental observations suggest that the accumulation of monocytes in the spleen is the result of redistribution from the bone marrow and circulation. After social disruption, LPS-stimulated splenocytes also secrete higher levels of interleukin (IL)-6 and tumor necrosis factor (TNF)-α than do cells from control nonstressed mice.[10,14] The increase in TNF-α secretion was the result of an increase in the number of TNF-α–producing cells and an augmentation in TNF-α secretion per CD11b+ cell.[17]

Although the mechanisms involved in the development of social disruption–induced glucocorticoid resistance are not elucidated fully, glucocorticoid resistance was abolished by depletion of the CD11b+ cell population from splenocyte cultures.[8] Additional studies showed that social disruption–induced glucocorticoid resistance was the result, in part, of the failure of the glucocorticoid receptor to undergo nuclear translocation in the CD11b+ cells after exposure of the cells to corticosterone.[18] Even though the CD11b+ cell seems to be a target cell affected by social disruption, the neuroendocrine mechanism by which social disruption alters the responsiveness of the monocyte to glucocorticoids remains unknown. Several lines of evidence suggest that the development of glucocorticoid resistance might be related to the action of proinflammatory mediators. Molecular studies on the in vitro effects of proinflammatory cytokines on glucocorticoid receptor function have demonstrated that both IL-1 and TNF-α can attenuate glucocorticoid receptor translocation and glucocorticoid receptor–mediated gene transcription in various cell lines. We showed that social disruption attenuated glucocorticoid receptor translocation in vivo.[18] In addition, various types of experimental stressors, including social disruption, have been shown to induce gene expression and protein secretion of IL-1β. Therefore, we examined whether IL-1 was a critical factor in the development of glucocorticoid resistance in socially stressed mice. First, we investigated if repeated social stress altered plasma levels and tissue gene expression of IL-1α and IL-1β. The results revealed that social disruption significantly increased splenic and hepatic mRNA expression, the plasma protein level of IL-1β, and hepatic mRNA expression of IL-1α. Second, we used IL-1 receptor type 1 (IL1R1)–deficient knockout mice to study the role of IL-1 in glucocorticoid resistance. Knockout mice were subjected to social disruption and both the tissue distribution of CD11b+ cells and the glucocorticoid sensitivity of the splenocytes were compared with wild-type mice. Mice lacking the IL1R1 exhibited adrenal hypertrophy and thymic involution in response to stress, but did not show splenic accumulation of CD11b+ cells and failed to develop glucocorticoid resistance. These findings suggest that IL-1 plays a critical role in the development of the social stress–associated glucocorticoid resistance in the murine spleen.[19]

Neuroendocrine mechanisms by which social disruption alters the responsiveness of monocyte populations to glucocorticoids are under investigation and preliminary data indicated that the glucocorticoid receptor is phosphorylated in response to social disruption (Stiner L., unpublished observation, 2008).

Further characterization of the effects of social disruption on the splenic myeloid cell population included the CD11c+, or dendritic cells. Like CD11b+ monocytes, CD11c+ cells from socially disrupted mice were glucocorticoid resistant and displayed an activated phenotype, as indicated by an increase in surface expression of CD80, MHC I, and CD44. In addition, splenic CD11c+ cells from socially disrupted mice produced more cytokines in response to Toll-like receptor stimulation.[20] These social disruption–induced changes in the CD11b+ and CD11c+ myeloid cell populations indicate that social disruption is likely to have a significant impact on the host's response to an infectious challenge, and may provide a mechanism by which social disruption enhances adaptive responses to infection.

SOCIAL DISRUPTION EFFECTS ON THE HOST RESPONSE TO INFECTIOUS DISEASE

Successful resolution of an infection requires termination of microbial replication with little accompanying immunopathology and damage to healthy tissue. Because endocrine hormones broadly influence the immune response, stressors are likely to result in alterations in host susceptibility to infection.[21] In fact, Bailey and colleagues[22] found that social disruption significantly increases the occurrence of gram-positive bacteria in the liver and in inguinal and mesenteric lymph nodes of healthy mice. A closer look suggests that social disruption also induces the translocation of cutaneous and gastrointestinal microflora to secondary lymphoid organs. One could imagine that certain hormonal influences on the immune system could improve host resistance and reduce morbidity and mortality, whereas others might increase susceptibility to disease. Any such changes in host susceptibility would depend upon the effects of a particular stressor on the specific immune mechanisms necessary to terminate microbial replication.

Glucocorticoid hormones serve as a regulatory mechanism to prevent excessive activation of the immune response during an infection.[21] To further clarify the role of glucocorticoid hormones, the authors tested whether or not social disruption–induced changes in glucocorticoid sensitivity of immune cells would have implications for host resistance to a variety of infections. The findings indicate that social disruption did, in fact, alter the course and outcome of several infectious challenges. The effect was different depending on the timing of the stressor and the specific type of microbial challenge. In short, social disruption improved host resistance to a bacterial infection with *Escherichia coli*[23] and increased immunologic memory to an influenza viral challenge (Mays and colleagues, unpublished observation, 2008), but increased susceptibility to a Theiler viral infection.[24]

Enhancement of the immune response to a bacterial infection by social disruption was assessed using an intravenous challenge with *E coli*. When compared with infected control nonstressed mice, infected socially disrupted mice more quickly and effectively cleared *E coli* from the blood and spleen. It was hypothesized that splenocytes from the socially disrupted animals, presumably the CD11b+ monocytes/macrophages, were more adept at killing the bacteria. This hypothesis was supported by the observation that when removed from the spleen and cultured in vitro, adherent CD11b+ splenocytes from mice subjected to social disruption had a greater ability to kill *E coli* than did those cells from control mice.[23]

To further examine the biologic significance of social disruption–induced priming of CD11b+ cells, the activation of specific microbicidal pathways associated with enhanced bacterial killing (mentioned above) were studied. Social disruption–induced increase in bactericidal activity was associated with a significant increase in gene expression for inducible nitric oxide synthase and three subunits of the nicotinamide adenine dinucleotide phosphate oxidase complex. These genes are responsible for bacterial killing by generating reactive nitrogen and oxygen intermediates, respectively. These data indicate that social disruption increases bactericidal activity of CD11b+ splenic macrophages in part by increasing the activity of the pathways responsible for production of reactive nitrogen and oxygen intermediates.[23]

The effect of social disruption on viral infection and immunity has also been examined. In a study of Theiler virus infection, social disruption resulted in higher virus titers and slow viral clearance.[24] In addition, social disruption altered the behavioral signs of illness and motor function associated with the illness. The behavioral changes were accompanied by histologic evidence of inflammation within the central nervous system. The effect of social disruption was dependent on the timing of the stressor relative to infection. Social disruption applied before infection exacerbated behavioral and physiologic responses, whereas social disruption applied concurrent with infection resulted in delayed behavioral responses and a normal inflammatory reaction to the virus.[24]

Studies have been done in the mouse influenza A/PR/8 viral infection model to determine the effects of social disruption on infection and immunity. Mice exposed to social disruption before infection display enhanced immunity to influenza A/PR/8 as evidenced by an increase of cytokine production and clonal expansion of virus-specific memory T cells. In addition to changes in the memory T cell pool, viral replication was terminated earlier in socially disrupted mice (Jacqueline W. Mays, John F. Sheridan, unpublished data 2008). These data show that social stress affects infection and modulates virus-specific immunity, and also highlight the need to consider social factors when designing and implementing experimental models of infectious disease.

The influence of social disruption on the response to a nonreplicating immune challenge also was examined using a laboratory model of endotoxic shock. In this model, bacterial endotoxins (ie, LPS) induce the expression of high levels of the proinflammatory cytokines TNF-α and IL-1. If produced in excessive quantity, these proinflammatory cytokines kick start the production of a myriad of inflammatory mediators that lead to multiple organ failure and possibly death.[25] One of the main mechanisms by which inflammatory responses are regulated is HPA activation. More specifically, the production of glucocorticoid hormones (eg, corticosterone) suppresses excessive TNF-α and IL-1 production, thereby limiting death associated with endotoxin challenge. In this model of endotoxic shock, mice subjected to social disruption were more likely to die than control animals.[26] These data indicate that because social disruption induces a state of glucocorticoid resistance, mice subjected to social disruption were unable to control the excessive LPS-induced proinflammatory cytokine expression. Thus, glucocorticoid insensitivity increased the likelihood of developing endotoxic shock.[26] Although the result of this stress response, glucocorticoid resistance, may not seem to normally provide a competitive advantage for an animal, it may benefit in some situations. Unlike other stress models, social stress in mice likely results in tissue injury because of fighting. Cutaneous wounds may be invaded by bacteria, causing local infection. The repair of these wounds, and clearance of the invading bacteria, may be delayed by high levels of circulating corticosterone secreted in response to social disruption.[27–30] The development of glucocorticoid resistance after social disruption, therefore, may be an adaptive mechanism to enable healing of fight wounds and clearance of bacteria in the presence of high levels of systemic corticosterone.

INDIVIDUAL DIFFERENCES IN THE RESPONSE TO SOCIAL DISRUPTION

An increasing number of reports demonstrate significant individual differences in the response to stress. In fact, although the immunologic influence of social disruption indicates that social disruption has a specific effect on one outcome measure or another, not all animals respond similarly. For example, some animals subjected to social disruption do not develop splenomegaly, some do not accumulate CD11b+ monocytes in their spleens, and some do not develop glucocorticoid resistance.

In humans, studies show that personality and other dispositional traits may play a role in shaping psychologic responses to stressful events. Animal studies show further that stress responses can be modulated by a variety of host- and environment-related factors (for review, see Kemeny and Laudenslager).[5] Individual differences also are demonstrated in various immunologic changes associated with stress. The literature contains many studies showing that stressful life events alter immune activity and increase susceptibility to infection. Together, these studies have examined the effects of a large number of stressors in a wide variety of population study groups. Many of these reports show that the nature, duration, and severity of the stressors play a key role in modulating the immune response to the stressor.

Chronic situations, such as unemployment, bereavement, and caregiving for an ill family member, result in effects different from the more acute, but severe, events, such as earthquakes, hurricanes, or space flights (reviewed by Biondi[4]). Personality traits, coping strategies, and affective state also could account for considerable variability of immune changes in individuals under similar stress conditions. For example, persistent distress and worry, loneliness, and depressed mood are associated with decreased immune function, whereas optimism, social support, and good coping abilities are shown to buffer the negative effects of stress on immune function (reviewed by Biondi).[4] Of particular significance to these studies is the observation that early negative life events are demonstrated to have long-lasting, if not life-long, effects on the behavior and physiology of the organism. These data suggest that individual differences in the immune response to a particular stressor may, in some way, be preprogrammed.[31,32]

Social stress has long been known to affect physical and psychological health. In regard to social disruption, significant individual differences in immunologic and behavioral responses are observed among cohorts of genetically similar inbred animals. As discussed previously, after social disruption, some mice in the cage develop splenic glucocorticoid resistance, whereas others do not.[7] Because genetic differences are not likely to be the cause of the variability, the authors examined possible environmental and behavioral factors. Studies have suggested that these individual differences are mediated by behavioral factors, such as social hierarchy. Social hierarchy within cages of male mice was identified before and after social disruption using a battery of behavioral tests. Results showed that, in the majority of the cages, social order was stable over time.[15] Behavioral observations demonstrate that previous experience of defeat and loss of social status increase the susceptibility of mice to the development of glucocorticoid resistance after social stress.[15] For example, the development of glucocorticoid resistance is more pronounced in mice exhibiting submissive behavior before social disruption.[7,33] In addition, examination of the association between social status and splenic function showed that the splenic response to social disruption in subordinate mice was significantly augmented compared with dominants. This relationship between subordinate social status and the splenic response to social stress was more notable in cages with stable social hierarchies.[33] In sum, the data show a role for socio-behavioral factors in determining the response to social stress. This study further demonstrated the complexity of factors playing a role in mediating the physiologic response to social stress resulting in considerable individual differences.[33]

Age appears to be another factor that influences the response to social stress. We examined whether aging is a factor in social defeat–induced immunoregulatory changes. Proinflammatory cytokine responses were measured in old mice (14 months) and compared with the response of young mice (2 months). The data indicate that repeated social defeat results in a proinflammatory state that is exacerbated in aged mice. The implications of these findings are significant given that inflammation is a contributing factor to many age-related diseases.[34,35]

THE NATURE OF THE STRESSOR AND THE STRESS RESPONSE

The unique endocrine-immunologic response to social disruption provides further support for the notion that the nature of the stressor is important in determining the response to a particular stress. Social disruption elicits an atypical response in that it enhances some aspects of the immune system despite the activation of the HPA axis.[7] A comparison of the response to social disruption with that of other commonly used chronic stress models reveals several significant differences. For example, social disruption induces splenomegaly and an increase in splenocyte viability, whereas restraint stress causes splenic atrophy from cell apoptosis.[21] Additionally, social disruption, but not restraint stress, induces glucocorticoid resistance.[8] To better understand the differences between the response to social disruption and the response to restraint stress, it may be important to examine the nature and characteristics of these two stressors.

The overnight restraint stress paradigm is substantively different from social disruption. For example, mice subjected to restraint experience social isolation, food and water deprivation, and disruption of their normal diurnal rhythm; animals subjected to social disruption do not. From a behavioral perspective, restraint stress may model a naturally occurring event in the life of wild mice. In nature, mice live in underground burrows that may collapse, leaving a mouse trapped. Forced restraint may imitate the collapse of a burrow, triggering a "programmed" response specific for these situations. An appropriate response probably is an attempt to escape by digging a way out. After several fruitless attempts to escape, a mouse might give up and remain in its place, immobile.

Social stress presents a more complicated situation. A mouse threatened by a conspecific may choose between escaping its opponent and fighting back to gain access to territory and other resources. The choice may be based on the evaluation of the situation and the expected outcomes of each response. An attacked mouse probably tries to evaluate its opponent's strength and vigor based on its scent, behavior, and size. Previous experiences in similar situations also would affect behavior. A mouse previously defeated may be more likely to escape future confrontations. Additionally, environmental conditions may affect the response. For example, the likelihood of fighting back may increase if territory or other resources are scarce, putting a greater value on potential gains for risking such a battle. Alternatively, if food and water are plentiful, avoiding a battle may be more of a survival advantage.

In sum, a social stressor, such as social disruption, presents a complex and unique set of circumstances substantively different from those of many other chronic stress models, including repeated cycles of restraint stress. The response to a stressful challenge may be based on an evaluation of the characteristics of the specific situation, the expected outcomes of a particular response to the stressor (ie, fight or flight), and previous experiences in similar situations. In other words, the range of behavioral and environmental factors involved in determining the response to a social stressor may be the basis for some of the individual differences observed in the physiologic response to this stressor.[7]

SUMMARY

This article summarized the endocrine and immune changes induced by an experimental model for social stress characterized by repeated defeat. Furthermore, the article compared and contrasted differences between this stressor and other chronic stress models in mice. Individual differences in the response to social disruption were described and discussed in the context of the unique characteristics of this stressor and the importance of a variety of behavioral and environmental factors in modulating the response to social stress. The data indicate that mice facing a social stressor may use different behavioral coping responses based on the environmental conditions and previous experiences. These different adaptational responses are reflected in their behavioral, endocrine, and immune changes in response to the stressor.[7,8]

In conclusion, although generally it is understood that chronic stressors normally suppress immune function and increase a host's susceptibility to disease, this may not be always true in all cases all the time. For example, under conditions in which individuals face the chance of repeated injury, it may be an adaptive advantage to maintain or even enhance an immune response. The development of glucocorticoid resistance after social disruption may be such a mechanism, allowing animals to heal injuries and clear invading microbes in the presence of the anti-inflammatory stress hormones. Thus, individual differences in response to social disruption are associated with specific behavioral strategies that can have substantive implications for host resistance to infectious disease.

REFERENCES

1. Ramsey JM. Basic pathophysiology: modern stress and the disease process. Menlo Park (CA): Addison-Wesley Publishing; 1982. p. 30–73.
2. Selye H. A syndrome produced by diverse nocuous agents. Nature 1936;138:32.
3. Selye H. The general adaptation syndrome and the diseases of adaptation. J Clin Endocrinol 1946;6:117–230.
4. Biondi M. Effects of stress on immune function: an overview. In: Ader R, Felten DL, Cohen N, editors. Psychoneuroimmunology. San Diego (CA): Academic Press; 2001. p. 189–226.
5. Kemeny ME, Laudenslager ML. Introduction beyond stress: the role of individual difference factors in psychoneuroimmunology. Brain Behav Immun 1999;13:73–5.
6. Ginsburg B, Allee WC. Some effects of conditioning on social dominance and subordination in inbred strains of mice. In: Schein MW, editor. Social hierarchy and dominance. New York: Halsted Press; 1975. p. 282–303.
7. Avitsur R, Stark JL, Sheridan JF. Social stress induces glucocorticoid resistance in subordinate animals. Horm Behav 2001;39:247–57.
8. Stark JL, Avitsur R, Padgett DA, et al. Social stress induces glucocorticoid resistance in macrophages. Am J Physiol Regul Integr Comp Physiol 2001;280: R1799–805.
9. Engler H, Engler A, Bailey MT, et al. Tissue-specific alterations in the glucocorticoid sensitivity of immune cells following repeated social defeat in mice. J Neuroimmunol 2005;163:110–9.
10. Stark JL, Avitsur R, Hunzeker J, et al. Interleukin-6 and the development of social disruption-induced glucocorticoid resistance. J Neuroimmunol 2002;124:9–15.
11. Sheridan JF, Stark JL, Avitsur R, et al. Social disruption, immunity, and susceptibility to viral infection. Role of glucocorticoid insensitivity and NGF. Ann N Y Acad Sci 2000;917:894–905.
12. Avitsur R, Stark JL, Dhabhar FS, et al. Social disruption induced glucocorticoid resistance: kinetics and site specificity. J Neuroimmunol 2002;124:54–61.
13. Avitsur R, Stark JL, Dhabhar FS, et al. Social stress alters splenocyte phenotype and function. J Neuroimmunol 2002;132:66–71.
14. Avitsur R, Padgett DA, Dhabhar FS, et al. Expression of glucocorticoid resistance following social stress requires a second signal. J Leukoc Biol 2003;74:507–13.

15. Avitsur R, Stark JL, Dhabhar FS, et al. Social experience alters the response to social stress in mice. Brain Behav Immun 2003;17:426–37.
16. Bailey MT, Avitsur R, Engler H, et al. Physical defeat reduces the sensitivity of murine splenocytes to the suppressive effects of corticosterone. Brain Behav Immun 2004;18:416–24.
17. Avitsur R, Kavelaars A, Heijnen C, et al. Social stress and the regulation of tumor necrosis factor-alpha secretion. Brain Behav Immun 2005;19:311–7.
18. Quan N, Avitsur R, Stark JL, et al. Molecular mechanisms of glucocorticoid resistance in splenocytes of socially stressed male mice. J Neuroimmunol 2003;137: 51–8.
19. Engler H, Bailey MT, Engler A, et al. Interleukin-1 receptor type 1-deficient mice fail to develop social stress-associated glucocorticoid resistance in the spleen. Psychoneuroendocrinology 2008;33:108–17.
20. Powell ND, Bailey MT, Mays J, et al. Repeated social defeat activates dendritic cells and enhances toll-like receptor dependent cytokine secretion. Brain Behav Immun 2009;23:225–31.
21. Bailey M, Engler H, Hunzeker J, et al. The hypothalamic-pituitary-adrenal axis and viral infection. Viral Immunol 2003;16:141–57.
22. Bailey MT, Engler H, Powell ND, et al. Repeated social defeat increases bactericidal activity of splenic macrophages through a toll-like receptor-dependent pathway. Am J Physiol Regul Integr Comp Physiol 2007;293:R1180–90.
23. Johnson RR, Storts R, Welsh TH, et al. Social stress alters the severity of acute Theiler's virus infection. J Neuroimmunol 2004;148:74–85.
24. Bailey MT, Engler H, Sheridan JF. Stress induces the translocation of cutaneous and gastrointestinal microflora to secondary lymphoid organs of C57BL/6 mice. J Neuroimmunol 2006;171(1–2):29–37.
25. Purvis D, Kirby R. Systemic inflammatory response syndrome: septic shock. Vet Clin North Am Small Anim Pract 1994;24:1225–47.
26. Quan N, Avitsur R, Stark JL, et al. Social stress increases the susceptibility to endotoxic shock. J Neuroimmunol 2001;115:36–45.
27. Almawi WY, Beyhum HN, Rahme AA, et al. Regulation of cytokine and cytokine receptor expression by glucocorticoids. J Leukoc Biol 1996;60:563–72.
28. Cato ACB, Wade E. Molecular mechanisms of anti-inflammatory action of glucocorticoids. Bioessays 1996;18:371–8.
29. Diegelmann RF. Cellular and biochemical aspects of normal and abnormal wound healing: an overview. J Urol 1997;157:298–302.
30. Padgett DA, Sheridan JF, Dorne J, et al. Social stress and the reactivation of latent herpes simplex virus type 1. Proc Natl Acad Sci U S A 1998;95:7231–5.
31. Avitsur R, Hunzeker J, Sheridan JF. Role of early stress in the individual differences in host response to viral infection. Brain Behav Immun 2006;20:339–48.
32. Caldji C, Diorio J, Meaney MJ. Variations in maternal care in infancy regulate the development of stress reactivity. Biol Psychiatry 2000;48:1164–74.
33. Avitsur R, Kinsey S, Bailey MT, et al. Subordinate social stress increases the vulnerability to the immunological effects of social stress. Psychoneuroendocrinology 2007;32:1097–105.
34. Kinsey SG, Bailey MT, Sheridan JF, et al. Repeated social defeat causes increase anxiety-like behavior and alters splenocyte function in C57BL/6 and CD-1 mice. Brain Behav Immun 2007;21:458–66.
35. Kinsey SG, Bailey MT, Sheridan JF, et al. The inflammatory response to social defeat is exaggerated in aged mice. Physiol Behav 2007;93:623–36.

Sleep and Psychoneuroimmunology

Mark R. Opp, PhD[a,b,c,*]

KEYWORDS

- Cytokine • Interleukin-1 • Tumor necrosis factor
- Fever

Historic studies of the impact of infection on the central nervous system provide insight into brain regions involved in the regulation of sleep. Between 1917 and 1928 there was a pandemic of Encephalitis lethargica, an atypical encephalitis characterized by high fever and complex alterations in sleep, among other symptoms. The first case of Encephalitis lethargica seems to have been reported in 1875 by Gayet. This case report was followed by one in 1880 by Wernicke, which led to the designation of this condition as the Gayet-Wernicke syndrome. The general symptoms included fever, agitation or stupor, and sometimes coma. Mauthner[1] localized to the periventricular gray inflammatory lesions that related to symptom complex. Mauthner used these observations to advance the idea that there was a sleep center in brain. The neurologist, Baron Constantin von Economo, working with encephalitic patients in the 1920s and 1930s, advanced the understanding of the impact of this infectious process on sleep. von Economo localized encephalitic lesions to the periventricular gray, the hypothalamus, and the adjacent portions of the mesencephalon. von Economo was the first to suggest that the hypersomnolence or insomnia resulting from this infection were related to lesions of specific regions of the hypothalamus: lesions of the anterior hypothalamus resulted in insomnia whereas lesions of the posterior hypothalamus led to excessive sleep.[2] Thus, neurologic evaluation of effects of encephalitic lesions played a critical role in understanding neuroanatomic substrates critical to the regulation of sleep.

Although the Spanish flu pandemic often has been postulated as the infection associated with subsequent Encephalitis lethargica, recent evidence suggests Encephalitis lethargica likely was a poststreptococcal autoimmune disease.[3,4] A contemporary

This issue is a repurpose of August 2006 issue of the *Neurologic Clinics* (Volume 24, Issue 3). The author was supported by the following grants from the National Institutes of Health during the writing of this article: MH64843, HL080972, and GM067189.

[a] Department of Anesthesiology, University of Michigan, Ann Arbor, MI, USA
[b] Department of Molecular and Integrative Physiology, University of Michigan, Ann Arbor, MI, USA
[c] Neuroscience Graduate Program, University of Michigan, Ann Arbor, MI, USA
* Department of Anesthesiology, 7422 Medical Science Building 1, 1150 West Medical Center Drive, Ann Arbor, MI 48109-0615.
E-mail address: mopp@umich.edu

Immunol Allergy Clin N Am 29 (2009) 295–307
doi:10.1016/j.iac.2009.02.009
0889-8561/09/$ – see front matter © 2009 Elsevier Inc. All rights reserved.

immunology.theclinics.com

disease with a phenotype remarkably similar to that of the historic Encephalitis lethargica now is prevalent. Dale and colleagues[3] report 20 cases in which patients ranging from 2 to 69 years of age had symptoms similar to those reported during the Encephalitis lethargica pandemic. Of these 20 patients, 19 had sleep disturbances: 12 were hypersomnolent, 2 suffered from insomnia, and 5 exhibited sleep inversion (sleepy during the day and wide awake at night). Ten patients had lethargy, which was not associated with any particular sleep phenotype and was in excess of that anticipated due to motor weakness.[3]

Observations of the impact of encephalitic lesions as sequelae of autoimmune disease on central nervous system function, as evidenced by alterations in sleep, underscore the fundamental nature of brain-immune interactions. The brain uses a variety of mechanisms to survey the immune system constantly. Responses of the immune system to invading pathogens are detected by the central nervous system, which responds by orchestrating complex changes in behavior and physiology. Sleep is one of the behaviors altered in response to immune challenge. The role of cytokines as mediators of responses to infectious challenge and regulators and modulators of sleep is the focus of this article.

INFECTION-INDUCED ALTERATIONS IN SLEEP

Although important observations during the early part of the twentieth century of sleep disturbances resulting from postinfection encephalitic lesions contributed much to knowledge of the neuroanatomic basis for sleep, it was not until the 1980s that systematic studies of the impact of infection on sleep were conducted. The impact of infection on sleep of humans and laboratory animals has been evaluated for several classes of pathogens and microorganisms, including viruses, some bacterial strains, fungus, and at least one parasite. There also have been studies of the impact of prion-related diseases on sleep.

Viral Infections

The onset of the AIDS epidemic in the 1980s provided a tragic opportunity to determine the impact of viral infections on sleep of humans. The first reports of HIV effects on sleep[5–8] demonstrated disruptions to nighttime sleep in individuals who were seropositive yet asymptomatic. Many subsequent studies also reported nighttime sleep disturbances and daytime fatigue before onset of AIDS.[8–13] The early reports of Norman and coworkers indicate an increase in non-rapid eye movement (NREM) sleep stages 3 and 4.[12,14] Other studies fail to detect increases in total amounts NREM stages 3 and 4 sleep,[8,15] but demonstrate NREM sleep stages 3 and 4 were distributed more evenly across the night (NREM stages 3 and 4 normally occur primarily in the first half of the night). Such differences among studies may well be the result of variable lengths of time subjects were infected before sleep study and differing rates of disease progression. It is clear, however, that nighttime sleep of HIV-infected individuals is altered long before they become symptomatic for AIDS.

Preclinical studies demonstrate that feline immunodeficiency virus (FIV) alters sleep of cats in conjunction with sequelae that, in many respects, are similar to those of humans infected with HIV. Infection of cats with FIV, a feline retrovirus, induces a gradual change in the normal timing of NREM sleep, increases arousals, and reduces REM sleep.[16] Some aspects of alterations in sleep during HIV infections are mimicked by intracerebroventricular (ICV) administration of the envelope glycoproteins (gp). HIV gp60, gp120, and gp41[17–19] and FIV gp120[16,20] alter sleep of rats. Effects of these HIV gp on sleep may be mediated, in part, by actions of interleukin (IL)-1 or other proinflammatory cytokines, as gp120 and gp160 increase cytokine messenger RNA (mRNA) in rat brain.[19,21] Observations of sleep of HIV-infected humans also supports the hypothesis that HIV infection-induced alterations in sleep are mediated, in part, by actions of cytokines. Darko and colleagues[10] report that the normal coupling of circulating tumor necrosis factor (TNF)-α and the slow frequency components of the electroencephalogram (EEG), known as slow wave sleep delta power, is disrupted in progressive HIV infection. Collectively, clinical studies demonstrate profound alterations in nighttime sleep of individuals infected with HIV that become progressively more severe as the infection progresses to AIDS. Mechanisms contributing to the effects of HIV on sleep are likely to include actions of cytokines in the central nervous system.

Another virus shown to alter sleep is the influenza virus. Influenza/rhinovirus infection of humans variably increases[22] or decreases[23] slow wave sleep time. Brown and colleagues[22] demonstrate reductions in total sleep time during the acute incubation (asymptomatic) period of influenza A and B and rhinovirus colds; total sleep time increased when subjects were symptomatic. In contrast, Drake and colleagues[23] report that rhinovirus type 23 infection of volunteers does not affect sleep during the acute incubation period but reduces total sleep time during the symptomatic period of the infection. The reasons for differences between these studies are not clear, and additional investigation is necessary. In contrast to results from human subjects, multiple studies consistently demonstrate that rabbits[24,25] or mice[26–28] infected with influenza do spend more time in NREM sleep. The increases in NREM sleep of rabbits infected with influenza, although robust, are brief. In contrast, increases in NREM sleep of mice infected with influenza are prolonged, lasting at least 96 hours.[27] Differences in duration of sleep alterations during influenza infections between rabbits and mice may be the result of the degree to which the virus replicates; mouse-adapted strains of influenza undergo complete replication whereas in rabbits the virus undergoes only partial replication. The increases in NREM sleep of mice during influenza infection are most apparent during the dark period of the light-dark cycle, the time when mice are most active and sleep the least. The extent of influenza-induced NREM sleep enhancement in mice likely is the result of the precise interferon response; increased NREM sleep is associated with increased interferon production.[28] The impact of Newcastle disease virus (NDV) on sleep of mice also has been determined: NDV induces a short-lasting increase in NREM sleep.[28] NDV does not replicate in mice, suggesting that viral replication is a critical determinant of the severity of the ensuing infection.

Bacterial Infections

Most studies of the effects of bacterial infections on sleep have been conducted in rabbits. These studies are reviewed extensively elsewhere.[29,30] Briefly, rabbits respond to infections with gram-positive and gram-negative bacterial infections with biphasic changes in NREM sleep; sleep initially is enhanced and subsequently suppressed.[31,32] The duration and magnitude of NREM sleep alterations depend on the specific pathogen, the route of infection, and whether or not the bacteria is viable or has been killed. REM sleep is suppressed for the duration of the infection. The development of fever generally occurs with increases in NREM sleep. The febrile responses of rabbits are protracted and persist during periods when NREM sleep is suppressed, however, indicating that fever and increased NREM sleep may be dissociated. Rabbits also respond to killed bacteria or to isolated bacterial components with increases in NREM sleep, indicating that bacterial replication in the host is not necessary to elicit alterations in sleep. Structure and function studies indicate that particular properties of the pathogen may be responsible for various aspects of alterations in sleep. For example, NREM sleep of rabbits increases more rapidly, but for a shorter duration, in response to gram-negative bacteria than in response to gram-positive bacteria. Lipid A from gram-negative endotoxin elicits increases in NREM sleep of rabbits within an hour of administration, whereas muramyl dipeptide, a synthetic analog of the monomeric muramyl peptide component of bacterial cell wall peptidoglycan, increases NREM sleep after a longer latency.[33,34]

Other Pathogens

Sleep is altered in response to pathogens other than virus and bacteria. For example, the sleep of rabbits is altered by infection with the fungus *Candida albicans* in a manner similar to that of gram-positive bacteria.[32] Prions also disrupt sleep. Scrapie-infected brain homogenates from animals or from human postmortem tissue alter EEG parameters and sleep-wake behavior of rats and cats.[35–37] Mice devoid of the prion protein gene have alterations in circadian rhythms and sleep.[38,39] Human fatal familial insomnia is characterized by profound alterations in sleep secondary to prion-induced degeneration of the thalamus.[40]

"Sleeping sickness," perhaps the most notorious of infection-induced alterations in sleep, is caused by the protozoan *Trypanosoma brucei*. Infection with this parasite induces disruptions to nighttime sleep, there are many short bouts of sleep during daytime, and the normal distribution of sleep and wakefulness across the 24-hour day disappears.[41,42] The impact of trypanosomiasis on sleep-wake behavior has been modeled in rabbits and rats.[43–46] Infection of rabbits induces an increase in NREM sleep after several days that is concurrent with fever and other signs of clinical illness. This initial period of NREM sleep subsides, but there are episodes of increased NREM sleep that occur in association with recrudescence of the parasite.[46] As in humans, rats and rabbits lose the circadian rhythms of sleep and body temperature.

CYTOKINES AND SLEEP REGULATION

During the early period of the Encephalitis lethargica pandemic, two laboratories working independently published studies that resulted eventually in modern research on infection-induced alterations in sleep. The groups of Ishimori in Japan,[47] and Legendre and Piéron in France[48,49] conducted experiments in which dogs were sleep deprived for prolonged periods. Cerebrospinal fluid from these sleep-deprived dogs was injected into rested dogs, which then were observed to fall into a deep sleep that resembled in some ways a narcosis. The results of these studies largely were forgotten until the 1960s, when John Pappenheimer at Harvard University conducted similar experiments. Pappenheimer demonstrated that cerebrospinal fluid from sleep-deprived goats increases sleep and reduced motor activity when injected into rats.[50] This substance in cerebrospinal fluid of sleep-deprived goats, termed factor S,[51] eventually was extracted,[52] purified,[53] characterized,[54] and determined to be muramyl peptide.[55,56]

Because muramyl peptides already were known to induce the synthesis and secretion of lymphocyte activating factor/endogenous pyrogen (now known as IL-1), the first studies to determine the impact of cytokines on sleep followed rapidly. In 1983 and 1984, an abstract and two original papers were published reporting alterations in sleep after administration of IL-1.[57–59] These studies demonstrated that IL-1 injected ICV into rabbits and rats increased the amount of time spend in NREM sleep, suppressed REM sleep, and altered properties of the EEG. In the 2 decades since the initial reports of the effects of IL-1 on sleep-wake behavior, various cytokines, chemokines, and growth factors have been administered to laboratory animals or human volunteers to determine effects on sleep.

Many studies now provide evidence that IL-1 and TNF contribute to the regulation of physiologic, spontaneous NREM sleep. Evidence is accumulating that IL-6 may contribute to alterations in sleep during pathologies in which this cytokine is elevated. The evidence supporting a role for these three cytokines in the regulation and modulation of NREM sleep is the subject of recent reviews.[30,60–62] Data implicating these cytokines in the regulation and modulation of sleep are derived from three types of studies: biochemical, molecular genetic, and electrophysiologic. Biochemical studies use the administration of cytokines, cytokine agonists, or cytokine antagonists in laboratory animals (or, in some cases, human volunteers). A variety of receptor knockout mice are used in molecular genetic studies to determine the impact of deficits in cytokine systems on spontaneous sleep-wake behavior and on responses to challenge. Electrophysiologic studies are conducted in vivo in freely behaving rats and in vitro in slice preparations. In addition, studies of calcium ion imaging evaluate the impact of selected cytokines on calcium flux in primary culture. Data from selected studies representative of each of these aforementioned approaches are reviewed in this section.

Biochemical Studies

The first studies conducted to determine the impact of cytokines on sleep focused on administering cytokine preparations or recombinant cytokine proteins in laboratory animals. Early studies of this type used rats and rabbits as subjects, although cats are the experimental subjects in at least two publications. More recently, cytokines have been administered to mice and the impact on sleep determined. Routes of administration of cytokines include ICV, intraperitoneal, and intravenous. The effects of antagonizing components of selective cytokine systems generally are determined after ICV administration of the antagonist.

The list of cytokines and chemokines administered to laboratory animals or human subjects and demonstrated to alter sleep is extensive and includes IL-1β, IL-1α, IL-2, IL-4, IL-6, IL-8, IL-10, IL-13, IL-15, IL-18, TNF-α, TNF-β, interferon (IFN)-α/β, IFN-γ, and macrophage inflammatory protein-1β (now known as CCL4). Several growth factors have been studied with respect to sleep, including epidermal growth factor, acidic fibroblast growth factor, nerve growth factor, brain-derived neurotrophic factor, glia-derived neurotrophic factor, transforming growth factor-β, granulocyte-macrophage colony-stimulating factor, granulocyte colony-stimulating factor, and insulin-like growth factor. This review focuses on IL-1, TNF, and IL-6; the remainder of these cytokines, chemokines, and growth factors are not discussed further. Interested readers are referred to recent reviews for more details.[30,60–62]

Data derived from biochemical studies that implicate IL-1 and TNF in the regulation of NREM sleep generally are obtained from similar types of studies. For sake of brevity, data concerning multiple aspects of IL-1 and the regulation of sleep are provided. Similar data exist for TNF.[62,63] IL-1, when injected centrally or peripherally into laboratory animals, increases the amount of time spent in NREM sleep.[64–74] Although low doses of IL-1 need not alter REM sleep, the doses of IL-1 used most frequently in laboratory studies (2.5–5.0 ng) consistently reduce REM sleep. Antagonizing the IL-1 system using the IL-1 receptor antagonist,[68] antibodies directed against IL-1,[75,76] or an IL-1 receptor fragment[77] reduces the amount of time laboratory animals spend in NREM sleep. IL-1β mRNA in rodent brain exhibits diurnal rhythms, with peak message expression during the light period,[78,79] the time when laboratory rodents spend the most time in NREM sleep. There also are diurnal rhythms of

IL-1–like activity in cerebrospinal fluid in cat that parallel sleep[80] and IL-1 in human plasma peaks at sleep onset.[81]

In addition to diurnal variation in mRNA and protein, effects of IL-1 depend on the diurnal timing of administration. IL-1 is more effective in increasing NREM sleep and slow frequency components of the EEG of rats when administered before dark onset than when administered before the beginning of the light period.[69,82] This differential responsiveness may be because of the fact that laboratory rodents sleep the most during the early part of the light period, and it may be difficult to increase the amount of sleep further, a so-called "ceiling effect." It is likely, however, that differentially responsiveness of rodents to IL-1 administration is the result primarily of the status at the time IL-1 is administered of feedback mechanisms governing their actions. The hypothalamic-pituitary-adrenal (HPA) axis, via actions of glucocorticoids, is the major regulator of IL-1 synthesis in brain.[83] The diurnal rhythm of HPA axis activity of rodents is out of phase with that of sleep and IL-1 mRNA expression. Manipulating HPA axis activity modulates cytokine mRNA in brain.[84–86] As such, the effects of exogenous IL-1 administration on sleep-wake behavior are greatest when the IL-1 is given at the time when HPA axis activity is lowest (ie, during the dark period).

Molecular Genetic Studies

Many components of cytokine systems in mice have been the target of genetic manipulation. Few of these animals have been the subject of sleep research. To date there are published reports of the impact of genetic ablation (knockout) of the genes for several cytokine receptors. These include the IL-1 receptor type 1,[87] TNF p55 receptor,[88] and TNF p75 receptor.[89] With respect to ligand knockouts, a mouse deficient in both TNF-α and α-lymphotoxin has been studied with respect to sleep.[89] Finally, mice lacking IL-6 also have been investigated in this regard.[90,91] Mice in which the signaling receptors for IL-1 and TNF have been knocked out spend less time in NREM sleep. There are differences in the timing of these reductions in NREM sleep depending on which receptor has been knocked out; mice lacking IL-1R1 spend less time in NREM sleep during the dark period of the light-dark cycle than do control mice,[87] whereas mice lacking the TNF p55 receptor spend less time in NREM sleep during the light period.[88] Double knockout mice lacking TNF and α-lymphotoxin or mice lacking TNF p75 receptors spend less time in REM sleep during the light period,[89] although the mechanisms mediating these effects on REM sleep remain unclear. The timing of NREM and REM sleep is normal in mice lacking IL-6.[90] Mice lacking IL-6 do not differ from control mice in the amount of time spent in NREM sleep, although these animals do spend 30% more time in REM sleep across the 24-hour day.[90]

Mice lacking components of cytokine systems still respond to challenge, although the nature of the response may be modulated. For example, mice lacking the TNF p55 receptor respond to IL-1 with increases in NREM sleep, whereas mice lacking the IL-1R1 spend more time in NREM sleep after administration of TNF.[87,88] IL-6 knockout mice respond to IL-1 with increases in NREM sleep, although the maximal increase in NREM sleep of IL-6 knockout mice is approximately 50% of the increase of C57BL/6J control mice.[92] C57BL/6J mice respond to the immune challenge of intraperitoneal administration of the bacterial cell wall component lipopolysaccharide with increases in NREM sleep and fever, although the magnitude of effect depends on timing of administration.[91] IL-6 knockout mice respond to lipopolysaccharide challenge with increases in NREM sleep that are 50% to 85% less than those of C57BL/6J mice, and develop profound hypothermia instead of fever.[91] IL-6 knockout mice and TNF p75 knockout mice[89] respond to 6-hour sleep deprivation in a manner generally identical to control animals, except in the case of IL-6 knockout mice the recovery process takes longer.[90]

Electrophysiologic Studies

In vivo electrophysiology studies indicate that IL-1 may exert direct effects on neurons in brain regions known to be involved in the regulation of sleep-wake behavior. Brain regions implicated in the regulation of NREM sleep include the hypothalamus and the basal forebrain. The preoptic area of the hypothalamus is a key regulatory region for NREM sleep; the ventrolateral preoptic area and the median preoptic nucleus (MnPN) contain high numbers of c-Fos reactive neurons after spontaneous NREM sleep but not after wakefulness.[93,94] Administration of IL-1 into rats increases the number of c-Fos immunoreactive neurons in the MnPN.[95] In the ventrolateral preoptic area and MnPN are neurons that are sleep active, that is, their discharge rates are higher during sleep than during wakefulness. The adjoining magnocellular basal forebrain contains neurons that are wake active, meaning their spontaneous discharge rats are greater during wakefulness then during NREM sleep. Perfusion of IL-1 by microdialysis into the preoptic area/basal forebrain of unanesthetized, freely behaving rats reduces discharge rates of wake-active neurons.[96] A subset of sleep-active neurons in this brain region increases discharge rates during IL-1 perfusion.

The role of the serotonergic system in the regulation of sleep has been the subject of intense study for more than 40 years. It now is generally accepted that serotonin per se is an arousal-promoting neurotransmitter.[97] The dorsal raphe nucleus of the brainstem is the origin of the major ascending serotonergic pathways to the forebrain. IL-1 receptors are contained in the dorsal raphe nucleus.[98] Microinjection of IL-1 into the dorsal raphe nucleus increases NREM sleep of rats.[99] In vitro studies suggest the effects on NREM sleep of IL-1 microinjected into the dorsal raphe nucleus are mediated by serotonergic neurons. Intracellular recordings from electrophysiologically and pharmacologically defined serotonergic neurons in guinea pig slice preparations indicate that IL-1 reduces discharge rates by 50% in the majority of serotonergic neurons.[99] Because serotonin promotes wakefulness, these results suggest that inhibition of serotonergic neurons in the dorsal raphe nucleus may be one mechanism by which IL-1 promotes NREM sleep.

Additional in vitro evidence supports a role for IL-1 in the regulation of spontaneous NREM sleep. IL-1 in subfemtomolar concentrations suppresses stimulated glutamatergic synapses in hippocampal slice preparations.[100] These effects in slice preparations are receptor mediated as they are attenuated in the presence of the IL-1 receptor antagonist. IL-1 also affects calcium ion flux, as determined in studies using primary culture. Picomolar concentrations of IL-1 increase cytoplasmic calcium ions in primary cultures of rat hypothalamic neurons.[101] The neurons responding to IL-1 under these conditions are primarily γ-aminobutyric acid (GABA)-ergic, suggesting effects on GABAergic neurotransmission. Collectively, data derived from electrophysiologic studies of behaving rats, from slice preparations, and from calcium imaging in primary neuronal cultures indicate direct effects of IL-1 on neurons in brain regions involved in the regulation of sleep.

SUMMARY

Personal experience indicates we sleep differently when sick. Data reviewed demonstrate the extent to which sleep is altered during the course of infection of host organisms by several classes of pathogens. One important unanswered question is whether or not the alterations in sleep during infection are of functional relevance. That is, does the way we sleep when sick facilitate or impede recovery? One retrospective, preclinical study suggests that sleep changes during infection are of functional relevance. Toth and colleagues[102] analyzed sleep responses of rabbits to three different microbial infections. Those rabbits that exhibited robust increases in NREM sleep were more likely to survive than those that exhibited long periods of NREM sleep suppression. These tantalizing data suggest that the precise alterations in sleep through the course of infection are important determinants of morbidity and mortality. Data from healthy subjects demonstrate a role for at least two cytokines in the regulation of spontaneous, physiologic NREM sleep. A second critical yet unanswered question is whether or not cytokines mediate infection-induced alterations in sleep. The hypothesis that cytokines mediate infection-induced alterations in sleep is logical based on observations of the impact of infection on levels of cytokines in the peripheral immune system and in the brain. No attempts have been made to intervene with cytokine systems in brain during the course of infection to determine if there is an impact on infection-induced alterations in sleep. Although substantial progress has been made in elucidating the myriad mechanisms by which cytokines regulate and modulate sleep, much remains to be determined with respect to mechanistic and functional aspects of infection-induced alterations in sleep.

REFERENCES

1. Mauthner L. Zur pathologie und physiologie des schlafes. Wien Klin Wochenschr 1890;3:445–6.
2. von Economo C. Sleep as a problem of localization. J Nerv Ment Dis 1930;71: 249–59.
3. Dale RC, Church AJ, Surtees RAH, et al. Encephalitis lethargica syndrome: 20 new cases and evidence of basal ganglia autoimmunity. Brain 2004;127:21–33.
4. Vincent A. Encephalitis lethargica: part of a spectrum of post-streptococcal autoimmune diseases? Brain 2004;127:2–3.
5. Kubicki S, Henkes H, Terstegge K, et al. AIDS related sleep disturbances— a preliminary report. In: Kubicki S, Henkes H, Bienzle Y, et al, editors. HIV and the nervous system. New York: Gustav Fischer; 1988. p. 97–105.
6. Norman SE, Resnik L, Cohn MA, et al. Sleep disturbances in HIV-seropositive patients. JAMA 1988;260:922.
7. Norman SE, Chediak AD, Kiel M. Sleep disturbances in HIV infected homosexual men. AIDS 1990;4:775–81.
8. Norman SE, Chediak AD, Freeman C, et al. Sleep disturbances in men with asymptomatic human immunodeficiency (HIV) infection. Sleep 1992;15:150–5.
9. Wiegand M, Möller AA, Schreiber W, et al. Nocturnal sleep EEG in patients with HIV infection. Eur Arch Psychiatry Clin Neurosci 1991;240:153–8.
10. Darko DF, Miller JC, Gallen C, et al. Sleep electroencephalogram delta-frequency amplitude, night plasma levels of tumor necrosis factor α, and human immunodeficiency virus infection. Proc Natl Acad Sci U S A 1995;92:12080–4.
11. Ferini-Strambi L, Oldani A, Tirloni G, et al. Slow wave sleep and cyclic alternating pattern (CAP) in HIV-infected asymptomatic men. Sleep 1995;18:446–50.
12. White JL, Darko DF, Brown SJ, et al. Early central nervous system response to HIV infection: sleep distortion and cognitive-motor decrements. AIDS 1995;9: 1043–50.
13. Darko DF, Mitler MM, Miller JC. Growth hormone, fatigue, poor sleep, and disability in HIV infection. Neuroendocrinology 1998;67:317–24.

14. Norman S, Shaukat M, Nay KN, et al. Alterations in sleep architecture in asymptomatic HIV seropositive patients. Sleep Res 1987;16:494.

15. Wiegand M, Moller AA, Schreiber W, et al. Alterations of nocturnal sleep in patients with HIV infection. Acta Neurol Scand 1991;83:141–2.

16. Prospéro-García O, Herold N, Waters AK, et al. Intraventricular administration of a FIV-envelope protein induces sleep architecture changes in rats. Brain Res 1994;659:254–8.

17. Diaz-Ruiz O, Navarro L, Mendez-Diaz M, et al. Inhibition of the ERK pathway prevents HIVgp120-induced REM sleep increase. Brain Res 2001;913:78–81.

18. Gemma C, Opp MR. Human immunodeficiency virus glycoproteins 160 and 41 alter sleep and brain temperature of rats. J Neuroimmunol 1999;97:94–101.

19. Opp MR, Rady PL, Hughes TK Jr, et al. Human immunodeficiency virus envelope glycoprotein 120 alters sleep and induces cytokine mRNA expression in rats. Am J Physiol 1996;270:R963–70.

20. Prospéro-García O, Huitrón-Reséndiz S, Casalman SC, et al. Feline immunodeficiency virus envelope protein (FIVgp120) causes electrophysioloogical alterations in rats. Brain Res 1999;836:203–9.

21. Gemma C, Smith EM, Hughes TK Jr, et al. Human immunodeficiency virus glycoprotein 160 induces cytokine mRNA expression in the rat central nervous system. Cell Mol Neurobiol 2000;20:419–31.

22. Brown R, King MG, Husband AJ. Sleep deprivation-induced hypothermia following antigen challenge due to opioid but not interleukin-1 involvement. Physiol Behav 1992;51:767–70.

23. Drake CL, Roehrs TA, Royer H, et al. Effects of an experimentally induced rhinovirus cold on sleep, performance, and daytime alertness. Physiol Behav 2000;71:75–81.

24. Kimura-Takeuchi M, Majde JA, Toth LA, et al. Influenza virus-induced changes in rabbit sleep and acute phase response. Am J Physiol 1992;263:R1115–21.

25. Kimura-Takeuchi M, Majde JA, Toth LA, et al. The role of double-stranded RNA in induction of the acute phase response in an abortive influenza virus infection model. J Infect Dis 1992;166:1266–75.

26. Fang J, Sanborn CK, Renegar KB, et al. Influenza viral infections enhance sleep in mice. P S E B M 1995;210:242–52.

27. Toth LA, Rehg JE, Webster RG. Strain differences in sleep and other pathophysiological sequelae of influenza virus infection in naive and immunized mice. J Neuroimmunol 1995;58:89–99.

28. Toth LA. Strain differences in the somnogenic effects of interferon inducers in mice. J Interferon Cytokine Res 1996;16:1065–72.

29. Toth LA. Microbial modulation of sleep. In: Lydic R, Baghdoyan HA, editors. Handbook of behavioral state control: cellular and molecular mechanisms. Boca Raton (FL): CRC Press; 1999. p. 641–57.

30. Toth LA, Opp MR. Infection and sleep. In: Lee-Chiong T, Carskadon MA, Sateia M, editors. Sleep medicine. Philadelphia: Hanley & Belfus; 2002. p. 77–84.

31. Toth LA, Krueger JM. Alterations of sleep in rabbits by *Staphylococcus aureus* infection. Infect Immun 1988;56:1785–91.

32. Toth LA, Krueger JM. Effects of microbial challenge on sleep in rabbits. FASEB J 1989;3:2062–6.

33. Krueger JM, Kubillus S, Shoham S, et al. Enhancement of slow-wave sleep by endotoxin and lipid A. Am J Physiol 1986;251:R591–7.

34. Shoham S, Krueger JM. Muramyl dipeptide-induced sleep and fever: effects of ambient temperature and time of injection. Am J Physiol 1988;255:R157–65.

35. Bassant MH, Cathala F, Court L, et al. Experimental scrapie in rats: first electrophysiological observations. Electroencephalogr Clin Neurophysiol 1984;57:541–7.

36. Gourmelon P, Amyx HL, Baron H, et al. Sleep abnormalities with REM disorder in experimental Creutzfeldt-Jakob disease in cats: a new pathological feature. Brain Res 1987;411:391–6.

37. Gourmelon P, Briet D, Clarencon D, et al. Sleep alterations in experimental street rabies virus infection occur in the absence of major EEG abnormalities. Brain Res 1991;554:159–65.

38. Tobler I, Gaus SE, Deboer T, et al. Altered circadian activity rhythms and sleep in mice devoid of prion protein. Nature 1996;380:639–42.

39. Tobler I, Deboer T, Fischer M. Sleep and sleep regulation in normal and prion protein-deficient mice. J Neurosci 1997;17:1869–79.

40. Montagna P, Cortelli P, Gambetti P, et al. Fatal familial insomnia: sleep, neuroendocrine and vegetative alterations. Adv Neuroimmunol 1995;5:13.

41. Buguet A, Bourdon L, Bouteille B, et al. The duality of sleeping sickness: focusing on sleep. Sleep Med Rev 2001;5:139–53.

42. Lundkvist GB, Kristensson K, Bentivoglio M. Why trypanosomes cause sleeping sickness. Physiology (Bethesda) 2004;19:198–206.

43. Berge B, Chevrier C, Blanc A, et al. Disruptions of ultradian and circadian organization of core temperature in a rat model of African trypanosomiasis using periodogram techniques on detrended data. Chronobiol Int 2005;22:237–51.

44. Darsaud A, Bourdon L, Mercier S, et al. Twenty-four-hour disruption of the sleep-wake cycle and sleep-onset REM-like episodes in a rat model of African trypanosomiasis. Sleep 2004;27:42–6.

45. Lundkvist GB, Hill RH, Kristensson K. Disruption of circadian rhythms in synaptic activity of the suprachiasmatic nuclei by African trypanosomes and cytokines. Neurobiol Dis 2002;11:20–7.

46. Toth LA, Tolley EA, Broady R, et al. Sleep during experimental trypanosomiasis in rabbits. Proc Soc Exp Biol Med 1994;205:174–81.

47. Ishimori K. True cause of sleep: a hypnogenic substance as evidenced in the brain of sleep-deprived animals. Tokyo Igakkai Zasshi 1909;23:429–59.

48. Legendre R, Piéron H. Le problème des facteurs du sommeil. Résultats d'injections vasculaires et intracérébrales de liquides insomniques. C R Soc Biol 1910;68:1077–9.

49. Legendre R, Piéron H. Recherches sur le besoin de sommeil consecutif a une vielle prolongee. Z Allg Physiol 1913;14:235–62.

50. Pappenheimer JR, Miller TB, Goodrich CA. Sleep-promoting effects of cerebrospinal fluid from sleep-deprived goats. Proc Natl Acad Sci U S A 1967;58:513–7.

51. Fencl V, Koski G, Pappenheimer JR. Factors in cerebrospinal fluid from goats that affect sleep and activity in rats. J Physiol 1971;216:565–89.

52. Pappenheimer JR, Koski G, Fencl V, et al. Extraction of sleep-promoting factor S from cerebrospinal fluid and from brains of sleep-deprived animals. J Neurophysiol 1975;38:1299–311.

53. Krueger JM, Pappenheimer JR, Karnovsky ML. Sleep-promoting factor S: purification and properties. Proc Natl Acad Sci U S A 1978;75:5235–8.

54. Krueger JM, Pappenheimer JR, Karnovsky ML. The composition of sleep-promoting factor isolated from human urine. J Biol Chem 1982;257:1664.

55. Krueger JM, Pappenheimer JR, Karnovsky ML. Sleep-promoting effects of muramyl peptides. Proc Natl Acad Sci U S A 1982;79:6102–6.

56. Martin SA, Karnovsky ML, Krueger JM, et al. Peptidoglycans as promoters of slow-wave sleep. I. Structure of the sleep-promoting factor isolated from human urine. J Biol Chem 1984;259:12652–8.

57. Krueger JM, Dinarello CA, Chedid L. Promotion of slow-wave sleep (SWS) by a purified interleukin-1 (IL-1) preparation. Fed Proc 1983;42:356.
58. Krueger JM, Walter J, Dinarello CA, et al. Sleep-promoting effects of endogenous pyrogen (interleukin-1). Am J Physiol 1984;246:R994–9.
59. Tobler I, Borbély AA, Schwyzer M, et al. Interleukin-1 derived from astrocytes enhances slow wave activity in sleep EEG of the rat. Eur J Pharmacol 1984;104:191–2.
60. Opp MR. Cytokines and sleep. Sleep Med Rev 2005;9:355–64.
61. Opp MR, Toth LA. Neural-immune interactions in the regulation of sleep. Front Biosci 2003;8:d768–79.
62. Krueger JM, Obal FJ, Fang J, et al. The role of cytokines in physiological sleep regulation. Ann N Y Acad Sci 2001;933:211–21.
63. Krueger JM, Majde JA. Humoral links between sleep and the immune system: research issues. Ann N Y Acad Sci 2003;992:9–20.
64. Opp MR, Krueger JM. Effects of α-MSH on sleep, behavior, and brain temperature: interactions with IL-1. Am J Physiol 1988;255:R914–22.
65. Opp MR, Obál F Jr, Krueger JM. Corticotropin-releasing factor attenuates interleukin-1 induced sleep and fever in rabbits. Am J Physiol 1989;257:R528–35.
66. Obál F Jr, Opp MR, Cady AB, et al. Interleukin 1α and an interleukin 1β fragment are somnogenic. Am J Physiol 1990;259:R439–46.
67. Opp MR, Payne L, Krueger JM. Responsiveness of rats to interleukin-1: effects of monosodium glutamate treatment of neonates. Physiol Behav 1990;48:451–7.
68. Opp MR, Krueger JM. Interleukin 1-receptor antagonist blocks interleukin 1-induced sleep and fever. Am J Physiol 1991;260:R453–7.
69. Opp MR, Obál F, Krueger JM. Interleukin-1 alters rat sleep: temporal and dose-related effects. Am J Physiol 1991;260:R52–8.
70. Opp MR, Postlethwaite AE, Seyer JM, et al. Interleukin 1 receptor antagonist blocks somnogenic and pyrogenic responses to an interleukin 1 fragment. Proc Natl Acad Sci U S A 1992;89:3726–30.
71. Imeri L, Opp MR, Krueger JM. An IL-1 receptor and an IL-1 receptor antagonist attenuate muramyl dipeptide- and IL-1-induced sleep and fever. Am J Physiol 1993;265:R907–13.
72. Opp MR, Toth LA. Somnogenic and pyrogenic effects of interleukin-1β and lipopolysaccharide in intact and vagotomized rats. Life Sci 1998;62:923–36.
73. Imeri L, Mancia M, Opp MR. Blockade of 5-HT$_2$ receptors alters interleukin-1-induced changes in rat sleep. Neuroscience 1999;92:745–9.
74. Opp MR, Imeri L. Rat strains that differ in corticotropin-releasing hormone production exhibit different sleep-wake responses to interleukin 1. Neuroendocrinology 2001;73:272–84.
75. Opp MR, Krueger JM. Interleukin-1 is involved in responses to sleep deprivation in the rabbit. Brain Res 1994;639:57–65.
76. Opp MR, Krueger JM. Anti-interleukin-1β reduces sleep and sleep rebound after sleep deprivation in rats. Am J Physiol 1994;266:R688–95.
77. Takahashi S, Kapás L, Fang J, et al. An interleukin-1 receptor fragment inhibits spontaneous sleep and muramyl dipeptide-induced sleep in rabbits. Am J Physiol 1996;271:R101–8.
78. Taishi P, Bredow S, Guha-Thakurta N, et al. Diurnal variations of interleukin-1β mRNA and β-actin mRNA in rat brain. J Neuroimmunol 1997;75:69–74.
79. Taishi P, Chen Z, Hansen MK, et al. Sleep-associated changes in interleukin-1β mRNA in the brain. J Interferon Cytokine Res 1998;18:793–8.
80. Lue FA, Bail M, Jephthah-Ochola J, et al. Sleep and cerebrospinal fluid interleukin-1-like activity in the cat. Int J Neurosci 1988;42:179–83.

81. Moldofsky H, Lue FA, Eisen J, et al. The relationship of interleukin-1 and immune functions to sleep in humans. Psychosom Med 1986;48:309–18.

82. Lancel M, Mathias S, Faulhaber J, et al. Effect of interleukin-1β on EEG power density during sleep depends on circadian phase. Am J Physiol 1996;270: R830–7.

83. Turnbull AV, Rivier C. Regulation of the hypothalamic-pituitary-adrenal axis by cytokines: actions and mechanisms of action. Physiol Rev 1999;79:1–71.

84. Chang F-C, Opp MR. IL-1 is a mediator of increases in slow-wave sleep induced by CRH receptor blockade. Am J Physiol 2000;279:R793–802.

85. Goujon E, Parnet P, Layé S, et al. Adrenalectomy enhances pro-inflammatory cytokines gene expression, in the spleen, pituitary and brain of mice in response to lipopolysaccharide. Brain Res Mol Brain Res 1996;36:53–62.

86. Mustafa M, Mustafa A, Nyberg F, et al. Hypophysectomy enhances interleukin-1β, tumor necrosis factor-a, and interleukin-10 mRNA expression in the rat brain. J Interferon Cytokine Res 1999;19:583–7.

87. Fang J, Wang Y, Krueger JM. Effects of interleukin-1 beta on sleep are mediated by the type I receptor. Am J Physiol 1998;274(3 Pt 2):R655–60.

88. Fang J, Wang Y, Krueger JM. Mice lacking the TNF 55 kDa receptor fail to sleep more after TNFα treatment. J Neurosci 1997;17:5949–55.

89. Deboer T, Fontana A, Tobler I. Tumor necrosis factor (TNF) ligand and TNF receptor deficiency affects sleep and the sleep EEG. J Neurophysiol 2002;88: 839–46.

90. Morrow JD, Opp MR. Sleep-wake behavior and responses of interleukin-6-deficient mice to sleep deprivation. Brain Behav Immun 2005;19:28–39.

91. Morrow JD, Opp MR. Diurnal variation of lipopolysaccharide-induced alterations in sleep and body temperature of interleukin-6-deficient mice. Brain Behav Immun 2005;19:40–51.

92. Olivadoti M, Opp M. Interleukin-1 (IL-1)-induced changes in sleep and body temperature of IL-6-deficient mice. Sleep 2005;28:A10.

93. Sherin JE, Shiromani PJ, McCarley RW, et al. Activation of ventrolateral preoptic neurons during sleep. Science 1996;271:216–9.

94. Szymusiak R, Alam N, Steininger TL, et al. Sleep-waking discharge patterns of ventrolateral preoptic/anterior hypothalamic neurons in rats. Brain Res 1998;803: 178–88.

95. Baker FC, Shah S, Stewart D, et al. Interleukin 1beta enhances non-rapid eye movement sleep and increases c-Fos protein expression in the median preoptic nucleus of the hypothalamus. Am J Physiol Regul Integr Comp Physiol 2005; 288:R998–R1005.

96. Alam MN, McGinty D, Bashir T, et al. Interleukin-1β modulates state-dependent discharge activity of preoptic area and basal forebrain neurons: role in sleep regulation. Eur J Neurosci 2004;20:207–16.

97. Jouvet M. Sleep and serotonin: an unfinished story. Neuropsychopharmacology 1999;21:24s–7s.

98. Cunningham ET Jr, DeSouza EB. Interleukin 1 receptors in the brain and endocrine tissues. Immunol Today 1993;14:171–6.

99. Manfridi A, Brambilla D, Bianchi S, et al. Interleukin-1β enhances non-rapid eye movement sleep when microinjected into the dorsal raphe nucleus and inhibits serotonergic neurons in vitro. Eur J Neurosci 2003;18:1041–9.

100. Luk WP, Zhang Y, White TD, et al. Adenosine: a mediator of interleukin-1beta-induced hippocampal synaptic inhibition. J Neurosci 1999;19:4238–44.

101. De A, Churchill L, Obal F Jr, et al. GHRH and IL1beta increase cytoplasmic Ca(2+) levels in cultured hypothalamic GABAergic neurons. Brain Res 2002; 949:209–12.
102. Toth LA, Tolley EA, Krueger JM. Sleep as a prognostic indicator during infectious disease in rabbits. Proc Soc Exp Biol Med 1993;203:179–92.

Depression and Immunity: Inflammation and Depressive Symptoms in Multiple Sclerosis

Stefan M. Gold, PhD[a,b,*], Michael R. Irwin, MD[a]

KEYWORDS

- Multiple sclerosis • Neuroimmunology • Cytokine
- Depression • Fatigue • Sickness behavior
- Neurodegeneration

An increasing body of evidence suggests that patients who have major depressive disorder show alterations in immunologic markers including increases in proinflammatory cytokine activity and inflammation. Animal models of a depression-like syndrome called "sickness behavior" have shown clearly that cytokines are implicated in the development of these symptoms. Inflammation of the central nervous system (CNS) is a pathologic hallmark of multiple sclerosis (MS). Patients affected by this disease also show a high incidence of depression. Accumulating evidence for cytokine-mediated sickness behavior from animal studies suggests that some aspects of depression and fatigue in MS may be linked to inflammatory markers. This article reviews the current knowledge in the field and illustrates how the sickness behavior model may be applied to investigate depressive symptoms in inflammatory neurologic diseases such as MS.

MAJOR DEPRESSION AND MEDICAL COMORBIDITY

Neuropsychiatric disorders, especially major depressive disorder, are now one of the leading causes of disability.[1] Major depressive disorder, with a lifetime incidence of

This issue is a repurpose of August 2006 issue of the *Neurologic Clinics* (Volume 24, Issue 3).
This work was supported by MH55253, AG18367, T32-MH19925, M01 RR00827, General Clinical Research Centers Program, the Cousins Center for Psychoneuroimmunology, and the Deutsche Forschungsgemeinschaft (GO-1357/1-1).
[a] Cousins Center for Psychoneuroimmunology, Semel Institute for Neuroscience, 300 Medical Plaza, Suite 3109, Los Angeles, CA 90095
[b] Multiple Sclerosis Program, Department of Neurology, Geffen School of Medicine, University of California-Los Angeles, 635 Charles E. Young Drive South, Los Angeles, CA 90095, USA
* Corresponding author. Multiple Sclerosis Program, Department of Neurology, Geffen School of Medicine, University of California-Los Angeles, 635 Charles E. Young Drive South, Los Angeles, CA 90095.
E-mail address: sgold@mednet.ucla.edu (S.M. Gold).

more than 10%,[2,3] is a potent risk factor for disease morbidity, with depressed persons showing a mortality rate twice that found in nondepressed persons.[4–7] Altered functioning of the immune system is a mechanism that might contribute to medical morbidity of major depression including risk of infectious disease[8] as well as inflammatory disorders.[9] Depressed persons show reductions of cellular and innate immune responses that are associated with susceptibility to infectious disease,[10,11] whereas other studies have found that depression is linked to immune activation in patients who have inflammatory disorders such as rheumatoid arthritis[9] or cardiovascular disease[12,13] or who are undergoing cytokine therapy.[14]

Association of Depression with Enumerative and Functional Immune Measures

Increases in the total number of white blood cells and in the numbers and percentages of neutrophils and lymphocytes were among the first immunologic changes identified in depressed persons.[15] Further evaluation of lymphocyte subpopulations found that depression is related negatively to the number and percentage of lymphocytes (B cells, T cells, T-helper [Th] cells, and T-suppressor/cytotoxic cells) as well the natural killer (NK) cell phenotype, although such differences have not been replicated consistently.[16]

To evaluate the function of the immune system in depressed patients, most studies have relied on results from assays of nonspecific mitogen-induced lymphocyte proliferation, mitogen-stimulated cytokine production, and NK cytotoxicity. More than a dozen studies have been conducted on lymphocyte proliferation in depression, and there is a reliable association between major depression and lower proliferative responses to the three nonspecific mitogens, phytohaemaglutinin, concanavalin-A, and pokeweed.[16] In addition, a number of independent laboratories have confirmed reduced NK activity in major depression.[16]

Cytokines and Depression

Animal models that use chronic mild stress to induce depression-like syndromes report alterations in immune parameters including increased interleukin (IL)-1 production.[17] Studies of stimulated cytokine production in humans have not yielded consistent findings, however. For example, in whole-blood assays, Kronfol and colleagues[18] found increased lipopolysaccharide-stimulated production of IL-1 and IL-6 but no change in the expression of tumor necrosis factor (TNF)-α. Other studies have suggested a shift in the relative balance of Th1 versus Th2 cytokine production with increases in the capacity of lymphocytes to produce interferon (IFN) in depression,[19] but no difference in the stimulated production of IL-2 has been found.[19,20] These negative findings cannot be ascribed to differences in depressed samples, because reduced NK activity has been found in depressed patients whose IL-2 production was normal.[20]

Recent attention has focused on evaluating different patterns of cytokine activation in subtypes of depression. Whereas one study found no differences in the capacity of lymphocytes to produce IL-2 in melancholic and non-melancholic depression,[21] another study suggested that peripheral blood mononuclear cells of non-melancholic depressed patients showed a greater stimulated capacity to produce IL-1 β and IL-1 receptor antagonist as compared with responses from controls and melancholic depressed patients,[22] although earlier work by this group of investigators did not identify such increases in IL-1 production.[23] Nevertheless, further observations suggest that the melancholic, but not non-melancholic, depressed patients showed evidence of activation of the hypothalamic-pituitary-adrenal (HPA) axis, which is thought to inhibit immune activation and the expression of inflammatory markers and might account for the reported differences in the melancholic and non-melancholic groups.[22]

In contrast to the inconsistent findings regarding association between depression and production of inflammatory cytokines, meta-analyses indicate that depression is associated with an increase in circulating levels of the proinflammatory cytokine IL-6.[16] As compared with controls, elevated levels of IL-6 have been found in adults who have major depression,[24–26] in depressed elderly populations[27] and in persons who have chronic medical disorders such as rheumatoid arthritis,[9] cancer,[28] and cardiovascular disease.[29] It is hypothesized that increases in circulating levels of proinflammatory cytokine are caused by activation of monocyte populations. Increases in circulating levels of other proinflammatory cytokines such as tumor TNF-α and IL-1β have been reported in depressed patients[30,31] including patients who have late-life depressive disorder.[32] The number of studies that have examined these additional cytokines is too few to make firm conclusions, however. One study also reported increased plasma levels of IL-12 in a large cohort of depressed patients.[33]

Behavioral Effects of Proinflammatory Cytokines

Abundant evidence indicates that peripheral and central administration of cytokines is associated with the development of so-called "sickness behavior." For example, in animal models, proinflammatory cytokine induction or administration yields a set of behavior changes characterized by decreased appetite, weight loss, sleep disturbances, retardation of motor activity, reduced interest in the physical and social environment, and loss of libido.[34] In healthy human volunteers, endotoxin-induced endogenous cytokine production is associated with the transient development of depressed mood, anxiety, and memory impairments.[35]

The therapeutic administration of cytokines (eg, in antiviral or cancer therapy) provides another paradigm to study the effects of cytokines on behavioral and cognitive measures in humans. Several studies have reported that IFN-α administration in patients who have cancer or hepatitis C is accompanied by behavioral side effects that are similar to the sickness behaviors observed in animals. A few studies have reported similar observations for IFN-β (MS therapy), IL-1, IL-2, and TNF-α (cancer treatment). The most common side effects of these treatments are flulike symptoms such as fever, malaise, headache, and myalgia, which typically occur early (approximately 2 weeks) after the start of treatment but tend to attenuate as treatment continues. In contrast, neuropsychiatric symptoms, including anxiety, dysphoria, anhedonia, fatigue, anorexia, and cognitive and psychomotor slowing, generally occur after 1 to 3 months of therapy; these depressive symptoms persist unless treatment is terminated or supplemented by antidepressant medications.[36] Administration of IL-2 or IFN-α can activate the proinflammatory cytokine network and cause the subsequent elevation of IFN-γ, IL-6, IL-8, and other cytokines. It therefore is conceivable that the comparatively late onset of neuropsychiatric symptoms reflects an epiphenomenon to the induction of endogenous cytokines.

Brain Signaling by Cytokines

Cytokines are relatively large, hydrophilic molecules that under physiologic conditions do not readily cross the blood–brain barrier. There are, however, several ways by which peripheral cytokines may enter the brain. For example, passive diffusion may allow entry of cytokines in certain brain regions (eg, the circumventricular regions) where the blood–brain barrier is less restricted or absent. Furthermore, active transport mechanisms have been identified for some cytokines such as IL-1α, IL-1β, and TNF-α.[37] Other mechanisms by which peripheral cytokines may influence the brain include second-messenger induction through receptor binding on cerebral vascular endothelial cells and signaling through the vagus nerve.[38]

Of particular relevance to this article, cytokines themselves have been found to promote degeneration of the blood–brain barrier in inflammatory conditions.[39] In MS a pronounced breakdown of the blood–brain barrier, entry of inflammatory cells into the CNS, and local production of cytokines within the brain are at the core of presumed pathogenesis. Thus in MS, the effect of cytokines on the brain, in addition to their contribution to neuronal and oligodentroglial damage, may be important for behavioral symptoms. This possibility is discussed in detail later.

Effects of Cytokines on Neuroendocrine Function and Neurotransmitters

Several biologic mechanisms have been proposed to explain the association between depression and inflammation. The effects of cytokines on neurotransmitters in the CNS, most notably serotonin and norepinephrine, are explained by a prevailing biologic hypothesis of depression, which states that serotonin deficiency plays a crucial role in the pathogenesis of this disorder. This hypothesis is based largely on the observation that pharmacologic enhancers of serotonergic neurotransmission (eg, selective serotonin re-uptake inhibitors) are effective antidepressants. Evidence suggests that some cytokines may be involved in serotonergic depletion in the CNS. For example, IFN-α has been shown to interfere with serotonin metabolism and reduce serotonergic availability.[40] Similarly, cytokines may affect the noradrenergic system, which also is thought to play an important role in depression. Pronounced and sustained hypersecretion of brain norepinephrine has been reported in patients who have major depression.[41] A number of studies have shown that IL-1 administration can activate the central noradrenergic system in animals markedly,[40] thus providing another potential pathway related to cytokine-induced depression.

Another important mechanism involves the activation of the neuroendocrine system by cytokines. Patients who are depressed show elevated levels of corticotropin-releasing hormone (CRH),[42] and this key peptide is involved in integrating neural neuroendocrine as well as immune responses to stress. Release of this peptide in the brain alters a variety of immune processes, including aspects of innate immunity, cellular immunity, and in vivo measures of antibody production.[43,44] Peripheral immune measures also change after lesioning of the brain (eg, hypothalamus) or in response to the stimulation of certain brain regions that ultimately impact CRH systems. The brain controls immune cells in lymphoid tissue in the same way it controls other visceral organs, namely by coordinating autonomic and neuroendocrine pathways. When these pathways are blocked by specific factors that bind to sympathetic or hormone receptors, the effects of CRH on immune function are blocked also.[45,46]

CLINICAL APPLICATION: DEPRESSION IN MULTIPLE SCLEROSIS

Immune infiltration and inflammation of the central nervous system are pathologic hallmarks of MS,[47] and cytokines are secreted in the brain by invading cells as well as by resident microglia and astrocytes.[48] Depression is one of the most common symptoms in MS: numerous clinical studies have reported that patients who have MS have a lifetime risk of major depression of 25% to 50%.[49] A recent large-scale community-based study[50] showed that 40% of patients who had MS had clinical depressive symptoms. Based on the sickness behavior literature reviewed previously, it is possible that inflammatory markers may be linked causally to the high prevalence of depression in patients who have MS. Depressive disorders within neuromedical illnesses such as MS present special challenges for detection and treatment. In particular, the understanding of the pathogenesis of depressive symptoms in MS is crucial for the development of novel treatment strategies.

Although the presence of depression in MS does not seem to be related to the severity of neurologic impairment[51] and also can occur in early stages of the disease,[52] it has a strong impact on the patient's functional status. Patients who have MS and comorbid depression perform more poorly on tests of cognitive function.[53,54] It also has been shown that depression adversely affects quality of life in patients who have MS,[55] contributes to disruptions of social support,[56] and interferes with work attendance.[57] Because depression is linked to poorer treatment compliance,[58] it potentially can affect long-term health outcomes. Finally, it is reported that depression is the most powerful determinant of suicidal intent in patients who have MS.[59]

Despite evidence that depression is a major complication of MS with implications for the health status of these patients, this condition remains underdiagnosed and undertreated.[59] It is therefore important to understand better the pathogenesis of depression and its potential interactions with MS disease processes to develop novel treatment options.

Pathogenetic Models of Depression in Multiple Sclerosis

To date, little is known about the pathogenetic factors that account for the development of depressive symptoms in MS. Several models have been proposed to explain the strong association of depression and MS. A recent consensus statement issued by experts assembled by the National Multiple Sclerosis Society[60] stated that the pathogenesis is most likely multifactorial, including psychologic, social, neurobiologic, immunologic, and genetic factors. Some of the pathogenetic models proposed are reviewed briefly here.

Psychosocial factors

A simple explanation for the occurrence of depression in MS is that it is primarily reactive in nature, that is, a response to facing a chronic illness characterized by an uncertain prognosis and with no therapeutic cure available. There is no direct correlation between disease severity and depression in MS.[51] Whether or not depression develops in response to the illness, psychosocial factors such as coping strategies or social support may play a role. For example, coping and social support seem to mediate the relationship between disease and depression in MS,[61,62] although depression is not simply a failure of patients to cope with the psychosocial challenges.[60] Interventions designed to provide social support (eg, peer groups) have failed to show an effect on mood.[63] Furthermore, psychosocial factors alone cannot account for the higher frequency of depression seen in MS than in other chronic progressive diseases.[64] It therefore has been proposed that depression may be related to disease-specific processes such as CNS damage or changes in immune parameters, as hypothesized previously in this article.

Damage to the central nervous system

Another plausible explanation for the higher incidence of depression in MS may involve disease-specific and damage to particular locations in the CNS. Pujol and colleagues[65] reported a specific association of lesions in the left suprainsular white matter and depressive symptoms, accounting for a significant 17% of the depression variance. More recently, black holes as detected on T1-weighted images (which are thought to reflect severe tissue damage) in superior frontal and superior parietal regions have been found to predict depression.[66] Feinstein and colleagues[67] found greater volume of left medial inferior prefrontal lesions detected on T2-weighted images. One other study has shown more frontal atrophy in patients who have MS and depression than in nondepressed patients who have MS.[68] Although these studies suggest that the location and severity of MS lesions may be associated with certain depressive features in MS, no clear anatomic pattern has been established so far.

Experimental Autoimmune Encephalomyelitis is Associated with Depression-Like Behavioral Symptoms

A limited number of studies have investigated sickness behavior in experimental auto-immune encephalomyelitis (EAE), the animal model of MS. Behavioral signs including anorexia, weight loss, and reduced social exploration characterize EAE,[69] and these behavioral alterations occur after immunization but before the onset of neurologic signs of disease. Hence it is thought that these symptoms reflect motivational defects rather than impairments in motor function. For example, EAE is accompanied by decreased sucrose consumption (but no change in water consumption), which can be interpreted as a sign of anhedonia. Furthermore, in accordance with a cytokine-mediated pathogenesis of these symptoms, a later study showed that the onset of sickness behavior coincided with inflammatory cell infiltration of the brain as well as mRNA expression of IL-1, TNF-α, and prostaglandin E2 in brain tissue.[70] Anti-inflammatory treatment ameliorated the behavioral effects.[71]

Aspects of Depression and Fatigue in Multiple Sclerosis Resemble Sickness Behavior Seen in Animal Models

One intriguing aspect of depression in MS is its relation to fatigue. Fatigue is a common symptom in depression and in MS. Mohr and colleagues[72] noted "a relationship between fatigue and depression has long been suspected in MS," but "why and how this relationship might exist has remained generally unarticulated." Although earlier studies have not found evidence for an association of depression and fatigue in MS,[73,74] later reports usually have confirmed a moderate correlation.[75–79] The relationship seems to differ in the different dimensions of fatigue (the association was stronger with mental fatigue than with physical fatigue),[76] thus suggesting that different mechanisms may contribute to fatigue in MS. A cytokine-mediated pathogenesis of depression and mental fatigue (but not physical fatigue) could explain these differential associations.

Clinical Evidence for the Role of Inflammation in Multiple Sclerosis Sickness Behavior

Depression is a suspected side effect of MS treatment with IFNβ-1a. It has been suggested that IFN treatment in MS may induce depression or worsen existing depressive symptomatology. Although several studies have investigated this hypotheses using datasets from phase III clinical trials, it seems that anecdotal evidence of increased depression during IFN treatment is explained better by prior history of depression.[80]

Some recent studies have investigated the inflammation hypothesis of depression in MS by correlating endogenous inflammatory markers and depressive symptoms. The first study published by Fassbender and colleagues[81] showed that during relapse MS patients who had higher depression scores had significantly increased white blood cell counts in the cerebrospinal fluid. Depression scores also were higher in patients who had MRI evidence for CNS inflammation as indicated by gadolinium-enhancing lesions on T1-weighted MRI. Depression scores in this study also correlated with activation of the HPA axis. In another study assessing MS patients during relapse, Kahl and colleagues[82] reported that mRNA levels of TNF-α and IFN-γ obtained from whole-blood samples were increased, and both cytokines significantly correlated with scores on the Beck Depression Inventory (BDI). Th2-type cytokines such as IL-10 and IL-4 were not correlated with BDI scores. During remission in a subgroup of patients (with follow-up at 3 and 6 months and 1 year), only TNF levels showed a significant correlation with BDI scores. In line with these findings, Mohr and colleagues[83] also showed a positive correlation of depression and in vitro IFN-γ production. In this small study, amelioration of depression after psychotherapy or antidepressant medication treatment was paralleled by decreases in the capacity to produce IFN-γ. In another study, treatment of MS depression with lofepramine, a derivative of the antidepressant medication imipramine, was associated with decreases of gadolinium-enhancing lesion load on T1-weighted scans.[84]

A few studies have investigated the association of inflammatory markers and fatigue in MS. An early study could not find correlations of fatigue and urinary neopterin, C-reactive protein, and soluble intercellular adhesion molecule 1 in a sample of 38 patients who had MS.[85] More recently, however, cytokines typically associated with sickness behavior have been found to be associated with MS fatigue. For example, Flachenecker and colleagues[86] showed a positive correlation with TNF-α mRNA levels. Heesen and colleagues[87] reported correlations of TNF-α and IFN-γ in vitro production and fatigue severity. TNF-α levels also were associated with self-report measures of daytime sleepiness.

In summary, these findings are in accordance with the cytokine hypothesis of MS depression and fatigue. It is not known, however, whether depression is secondary, primary, or coincidental with inflammation in this population, even though treatment with antidepressant medication has been shown to decrease inflammatory markers in MS.

SUMMARY

There is strong evidence that depression involves alterations in multiple aspects of immunity that may contribute to the development or exacerbation of a number of medical disorders and also may play a role in the pathophysiology of depressive symptoms. Accordingly, aggressive management of depressive disorders in medically ill populations or individuals at risk for disease may improve disease outcome or prevent disease development. On the other hand, in light of data suggesting that immune processes may interact with the pathophysiologic pathways known to contribute to depression, novel approaches to the treatment of depression may target relevant aspects of the immune response. Taken together, the data provide compelling evidence that a psychoimmunologic frame of reference may have profound implications regarding the consequences and treatment of depression.

In addition, this approach may be used to investigate the possibility that peripheral and central production of cytokines may account for neuropsychiatric symptoms in inflammatory diseases. This article summarizes evidence for a cytokine-mediated pathogenesis of depression and fatigue in MS. The effects of central inflammatory processes may account for some of the behavioral symptoms seen in patients who have MS that cannot be explained by psychosocial factors or CNS damage. This immune-mediated hypothesis is supported by indirect evidence from experimental and clinical studies of the effect of cytokines on behavior, which have found that both peripheral and central cytokines may cause depressive symptoms. Emerging clinical data from patients who have MS support an association of central inflammation (as measured by MRI) and inflammatory markers with depressive symptoms and fatigue.

Based on the literature reviewed in this article, subtypes of MS fatigue and depression may exist that are caused by different pathogenetic mechanisms, including inflammation and CNS damage as well as psychosocial factors or predisposition. The existence of these subtypes could have important clinical implications. For example, an inflammatory depression may require different therapeutic approaches than a reactive depression in MS. Future research should aim to characterize these subtypes better with the goal of optimizing treatment.

REFERENCES

1. Mental health: new understanding, new hope. World Health Report. Geneva (Switzerland): World Health Organization; 2001. p. 20–45.
2. Michaud CM, Murray CJ, Bloom BR. Burden of disease—implications for future research. JAMA 2001;285(5):535–9.
3. Irwin M. Psychoneuroimmunology of depression: clinical implications. [presidential address]. Brain Behav Immun 2002;16:1–16.
4. Penninx BW, Geerlings SW, Deeg DJ, et al. Minor and major depression and the risk of death in older persons. Arch Gen Psychiatry 1999;56(10):889–95.
5. Cuijpers P, Smit F. Excess mortality in depression: a meta-analysis of community studies. J Affect Disord 2002;72(3):227–36.
6. Wulsin LR, Vailant GE, Wells VE. A systematic review of the mortality of depression. Psychosom Med 1999;61:6–17.
7. Rudisch B, Nemeroff CB. Epidemiology of comorbid coronary artery disease and depression. Biol Psychiatry 2003;54(3):227–40.
8. Evans DL, Ten Have TR, Douglas SD, et al. Association of depression with viral load, CD8 T lymphocytes, and natural killer cells in women with HIV infection. Am J Psychiatry 2002;159(10):1752–9.
9. Zautra AJ, Yocum DC, Villanueva I, et al. Immune activation and depression in women with rheumatoid arthritis. J Rheumatol 2004;31:457–63.
10. Leserman J. HIV disease progression: depression, stress, and possible mechanisms. Biol Psychiatry 2003;54(3):295–306.
11. Cohen S, Miller G. Stress, immunity and susceptibility to upper respiratory infection. Psychoneuroimmunology 2000;25:499–509.
12. Lesperance F, Frasure-Smith N, Theroux P, et al. The association between major depression and levels of soluble intercellular adhesion molecule 1, interleukin-6, and C-reactive protein in patients with recent acute coronary syndromes. Am J Psychiatry 2004;161(2):271–7.
13. Miller GE, Stetler CA, Carney RM, et al. Clinical depression and inflammatory risk markers for coronary heart disease. Am J Cardiol 2002;90(12):1279–83.
14. Capuron L, Miller AH. Cytokines and psychopathology: lessons from interferon-alpha. Biol Psychiatry 2004;56(11):819–24.
15. Kronfol Z, Turner R, Nasrallah H, et al. Leukocyte regulation in depression and schizophrenia. Psychiatry Res 1984;13(1):13–8.
16. Zorrilla EP, Luborsky L, McKay JR, et al. The relationship of depression and stressors to immunological assays: a meta-analytic review. Brain Behav Immun 2001;15(3):199–226.
17. Kubera M, Symbirtsev A, Basta-Kaim A, et al. Effect of chronic treatment with imipramine on interleukin 1 and interleukin 2 production by splenocytes obtained from rats subjected to a chronic mild stress model of depression. Pol J Pharmacol 1996;48(5):503–6.

18. Kronfol Z. Cytokine regulation in major depression. In: Kronfol Z, editor. Cytokines and mental health. Boston: Kluwer Academic Publishers; 2003. p. 259–80.
19. Seidel A, Arolt V, Hunstiger M, et al. Cytokine production and serum proteins in depression. Scand J Immunol 1995;41:534–8.
20. Irwin M, Clark C, Kennedy B, et al. Nocturnal catecholamines and immune function in insomniacs, depressed patients, and control subjects. Brain Behav Immun 2003;17:365–72.
21. Schlatter J, Ortuno F, Cervera-Enguix S. Lymphocyte subsets and lymphokine production in patients with melancholic versus nonmelancholic depression. Psychiatry Res 2004;128(3):259–65.
22. Kaestner F, Hettich M, Peters M, et al. Different activation patterns of proinflammatory cytokines in melancholic and non-melancholic major depression are associated with HPA axis activity. J Affect Disord 2005;87(2–3):305–11.
23. Rothermundt M, Arolt V, Peters M, et al. Inflammatory markers in major depression and melancholia. J Affect Disord 2001;63(1–3):93–102.
24. Frommberger UH, Bauer J, Haselbauer P, et al. Interleukin-6 (IL-6) plasma levels in depression and schizophrenia: comparison between the acute state and after remission. Eur Arch Psychiatry Clin Neurosci 1997;247(4):228–33.
25. Pike JL, Irwin MR. Dissociation between natural killer cell activity and inflammatory markers in major depression. Brain Behav Immun 2006;20(2):169–74.
26. Motivala SJ, Sarfatti A, Olmos L, et al. Inflammatory markers and sleep disturbance in major depression. Psychosom Med 2005;67(2):187–94.
27. Penninx BW, Kritchevsky SB, Yaffe K, et al. Inflammatory markers and depressed mood in older persons: results from the Health, Aging and Body Composition study. Biol Psychiatry 2003;54(5):566–72.
28. Musselman DL, Miller AH, Porter MR, et al. Higher than normal plasma interleukin-6 concentrations in cancer patients with depression: preliminary findings. Am J Psychiatry 2001;158:1252–7.
29. Empana JP, Sykes DH, Luc G, et al. Contributions of depressive mood and circulating inflammatory markers to coronary heart disease in healthy European men: the Prospective Epidemiological Study of Myocardial Infarction (PRIME). Circulation 2005;111(18):2299–305.
30. Maes M, Scharpe S, Meltzer HY, et al. Relationships between interleukin-6 activity, acute phase proteins, and function of the hypothalamic-pituitary-adrenal axis in severe depression. Psychiatry Res 1993;49(1):11–27.
31. Anisman H, Ravindran AV, Griffiths J, et al. Endocrine and cytokine correlates of major depression and dysthymia with typical or atypical features. Mol Psychiatry 1999;4:182–8.
32. Thomas AJ, Davis S, Morris C, et al. Increase in interleukin-1beta in late-life depression. Am J Psychiatry 2005;162(1):175–7.
33. Kim YK, Suh IB, Kim H, et al. The plasma levels of interleukin-12 in schizophrenia, major depression, and bipolar mania: effects of psychotropic drugs. Mol Psychiatry 2002;7(10):1107–14.
34. Kelley KW, Bluthe RM, Dantzer R, et al. Cytokine-induced sickness behavior. Brain Behav Immun 2003;17(Suppl 1):S112–8.
35. Reichenberg A, Yirmiya R, Schuld A, et al. Cytokine-associated emotional and cognitive disturbances in humans. Arch Gen Psychiatry 2001;58(5):445–52.
36. Capuron L, Gumnick JF, Musselman DL, et al. Neurobehavioral effects of interferon-alpha in cancer patients: phenomenology and paroxetine responsiveness of symptom dimensions. Neuropsychopharmacology 2002;26(5):643–52.

37. Banks WA, Kastin AJ, Broadwell RD. Passage of cytokines across the blood-brain barrier. Neuroimmunomodulation 1995;2(4):241–8.

38. Watkins LR, Maier SF, Goehler LE. Cytokine-to-brain communication: a review and analysis of alternative mechanisms. Life Sci 1995;57(11):1011–26.

39. Chandler S, Miller KM, Clements JM, et al. Matrix metalloproteinases, tumor necrosis factor and multiple sclerosis: an overview. J Neuroimmunol 1997; 72(2):155–61.

40. Dunn AJ, Swiergiel AH, de Beaurepaire R. Cytokines as mediators of depression: what can we learn from animal studies? Neurosci Biobehav Rev 2005;29(4–5):891–909.

41. Wong ML, Kling MA, Munson PJ, et al. Pronounced and sustained central hyper-noradrenergic function in major depression with melancholic features: relation to hypercortisolism and corticotropin-releasing hormone. Proc Natl Acad Sci U S A 2000;97(1):325–30.

42. Owens MJ, Nemeroff CB. Physiology and pharmacology of corticotropin-releasing factor. Pharmacol Rev 1991;91:425–73.

43. Friedman EM, Irwin M. A role for CRH and the sympathetic nervous system in stress-induced immunosuppression. Ann N Y Acad Sci 1995;771:396–418.

44. Friedman EM, Irwin MR. Modulation of immune cell function by the autonomic nervous system. Pharmacol Ther 1997;74:27–38.

45. Irwin M, Hauger RL, Jones L, et al. Sympathetic nervous system mediates central corticotropin-releasing factor induced suppression of natural killer cytotoxicity. J Pharmacol Exp Ther 1990;255(1):101–7.

46. Irwin M, Vale W, Rivier C. Central corticotropin-releasing factor mediates the suppressive effect of stress on natural killer cytotoxicity. Endocrinology 1990; 126:2837–44.

47. Noseworthy JH, Lucchinetti C, Rodriguez M, et al. Multiple sclerosis. N Engl J Med 2000;343(13):938–52.

48. Link H. The cytokine storm in multiple sclerosis. Mult Scler 1998;4(1):12–5.

49. Siegert RJ, Abernethy DA. Depression in multiple sclerosis: a review. J Neurol Neurosurg Psychiatry 2005;76(4):469–75.

50. Chwastiak L, Ehde DM, Gibbons LE, et al. Depressive symptoms and severity of illness in multiple sclerosis: epidemiologic study of a large community sample. Am J Psychiatry 2002;159(11):1862–8.

51. Moller A, Wiedemann G, Rohde U, et al. Correlates of cognitive impairment and depressive mood disorder in multiple sclerosis. Acta Psychiatr Scand 1994; 89(2):117–21.

52. Sullivan MJ, Weinshenker B, Mikail S, et al. Depression before and after diagnosis of multiple sclerosis. Mult Scler 1995;1(2):104–8.

53. Arnett PA, Higginson CI, Voss WD, et al. Depression in multiple sclerosis: relationship to working memory capacity. Neuropsychology 1999;13(4):546–56.

54. Arnett PA, Higginson CI, Voss WD, et al. Depressed mood in multiple sclerosis: relationship to capacity-demanding memory and attentional functioning. Neuropsychology 1999;13(3):434–46.

55. Jonsson A, Dock J, Ravnborg MH. Quality of life as a measure of rehabilitation outcome in patients with multiple sclerosis. Acta Neurol Scand 1996;93(4):229–35.

56. McIvor GP, Riklan M, Reznikoff M. Depression in multiple sclerosis as a function of length and severity of illness, age, remissions, and perceived social support. J Clin Psychol 1984;40(4):1028–33.

57. Vickrey BG, Hays RD, Harooni R, et al. A health-related quality of life measure for multiple sclerosis. Qual Life Res 1995;4(3):187–206.

58. Mohr DC, Goodkin DE, Likosky W, et al. Treatment of depression improves adherence to interferon beta-1b therapy for multiple sclerosis. Arch Neurol 1997;54(5): 531–3.
59. Feinstein A. An examination of suicidal intent in patients with multiple sclerosis. Neurology 2002;59(5):674–8.
60. Goldman Consensus Group. The Goldman Consensus statement on depression in multiple sclerosis. Mult Scler 2005;11(3):328–37.
61. Pakenham KI. Adjustment to multiple sclerosis: application of a stress and coping model. Health Psychol 1999;18(4):383–92.
62. McCabe MP, McKern S, McDonald E. Coping and psychological adjustment among people with multiple sclerosis. J Psychosom Res 2004;56(3):355–61.
63. Messmer Uccelli M, Mancuso Mohr L, Battaglia MA, et al. Peer support groups in multiple sclerosis: current effectiveness and future directions. Mult Scler 2004; 10(1):80–4.
64. Patten SB, Beck CA, Williams JV, et al. Major depression in multiple sclerosis: a population-based perspective. Neurology 2003;61(11):1524–7.
65. Pujol J, Bello J, Deus J, et al. Lesions in the left arcuate fasciculus region and depressive symptoms in multiple sclerosis. Neurology 1997;49(4):1105–10.
66. Bakshi R, Czarnecki D, Shaikh ZA, et al. Brain MRI lesions and atrophy are related to depression in multiple sclerosis. Neuroreport 2000;11(6):1153–8.
67. Feinstein A, Roy P, Lobaugh N, et al. Structural brain abnormalities in multiple sclerosis patients with major depression. Neurology 2004;62(4):586–90.
68. Zorzon M, Zivadinov R, Nasuelli D, et al. Depressive symptoms and MRI changes in multiple sclerosis. Eur J Neurol 2002;9(5):491–6.
69. Pollak Y, Ovadia H, Goshen I, et al. Behavioral aspects of experimental autoimmune encephalomyelitis. J Neuroimmunol 2000;104(1):31–6.
70. Pollak Y, Ovadia H, Orion E, et al. The EAE-associated behavioral syndrome: I. Temporal correlation with inflammatory mediators. J Neuroimmunol 2003; 137(1–2):94–9.
71. Pollak Y, Ovadia H, Orion E, et al. The EAE-associated behavioral syndrome: II. Modulation by anti-inflammatory treatments. J Neuroimmunol 2003;137(1–2): 100–8.
72. Mohr DC, Hart SL, Goldberg A. Effects of treatment for depression on fatigue in multiple sclerosis. Psychosom Med 2003;65(4):542–7.
73. Krupp LB, Alvarez LA, LaRocca NG, et al. Fatigue in multiple sclerosis. Arch Neurol 1988;45(4):435–7.
74. Vercoulen JH, Hommes OR, Swanink CM, et al. The measurement of fatigue in patients with multiple sclerosis. A multidimensional comparison with patients with chronic fatigue syndrome and healthy subjects. Arch Neurol 1996;53(7): 642–9.
75. Schwartz CE, Coulthard-Morris L, Zeng Q. Psychosocial correlates of fatigue in multiple sclerosis. Arch Phys Med Rehabil 1996;77(2):165–70.
76. Ford H, Trigwell P, Johnson M. The nature of fatigue in multiple sclerosis. J Psychosom Res 1998;45:33–8.
77. Bakshi R, Shaikh ZA, Miletich RS, et al. Fatigue in multiple sclerosis and its relationship to depression and neurologic disability. Mult Scler 2000;6(3):181–5.
78. van der Werf SP, Evers A, Jongen PJ, et al. The role of helplessness as mediator between neurological disability, emotional instability, experienced fatigue and depression in patients with multiple sclerosis. Mult Scler 2003;9(1):89–94.
79. Voss WD, Arnett PA, Higginson CI, et al. Contributing factors to depressed mood in multiple sclerosis. Arch Clin Neuropsychol 2002;17(2):103–15.

80. Feinstein A, O'Connor P, Feinstein K. Multiple sclerosis, interferon beta-1b and depression. A prospective investigation. J Neurol 2002;249(7):815–20.
81. Fassbender K, Schmidt R, Mossner R, et al. Mood disorders and dysfunction of the hypothalamic-pituitary-adrenal axis in multiple sclerosis: association with cerebral inflammation. Arch Neurol 1998;55(1):66–72.
82. Kahl KG, Kruse N, Faller H, et al. Expression of tumor necrosis factor-alpha and interferon-gamma mRNA in blood cells correlates with depression scores during an acute attack in patients with multiple sclerosis. Psychoneuroendocrinology 2002;27(6):671–81.
83. Mohr DC, Goodkin DE, Islar J, et al. Treatment of depression is associated with suppression of nonspecific and antigen-specific T(h)1 responses in multiple sclerosis. Arch Neurol 2001;58(7):1081–6.
84. Puri BK, Bydder GM, Chaudhuri KR, et al. MRI changes in multiple sclerosis following treatment with lofepramine and L-phenylalanine. Neuroreport 2001; 12(9):1821–4.
85. Giovannoni G, Thompson AJ, Miller DH, et al. Fatigue is not associated with raised inflammatory markers in multiple sclerosis. Neurology 2001;57(4):676–81.
86. Flachenecker P, Bihler I, Weber F, et al. Cytokine mRNA expression in patients with multiple sclerosis and fatigue. Mult Scler 2004;10(2):165–9.
87. Heesen C, Nawrath L, Reich C, et al. Fatigue in multiple sclerosis: an example for cytokine-mediated sickness behavior. J Neurol Neurosurg Psychiatry 2006;77(1): 34–9.

Age and Neuroinflammation: A Lifetime of Psychoneuroimmune Consequences

Jonathan P. Godbout, PhD[a,b,*], Rodney W. Johnson, PhD[c]

KEYWORDS

• Aging • Microglia • Brain • Cytokines • Inflammation

Aging is a process of intrinsic, progressive, and generalized physical deterioration that occurs over time, beginning at about the age of reproductive maturity. Aging steadily reduces an organism's ability to cope with intrinsic and extrinsic factors that cause stress, and thus it increases the probability of morbidity and mortality. It is well established that one of the intrinsic factors associated with aging is attenuated immune function or immunosenescence.[1] This age-dependent impairment of immune function results from weakened defenses by cells involved in innate[2] and adaptive immunity.[3] Specifically there is a reduction in naive T cells, which are critical for mounting both cell-mediated (T-cell) and humoral-mediated (B-cell) adaptive immune responses to novel antigens.[4] Immune dysfunction in the elderly is confounded further by a decrease in the production of anti-inflammatory hormones.[5] A consequence of these age-related impairments in the immune and endocrine systems is a heightened proinflammatory profile in the aged brain.[6] For example, increased innate immune activity and inflammation in the brain of the aged are involved in the pathophysiology of several neurodegenerative diseases including Alzheimer's disease and Parkinson's disease.[7] Furthermore, even in the absence of neurologic disease, an elevated inflammatory profile has been detected in aging brain[8] with innate immune glia (astrocytes and

This issue is a repurpose of August 2006 issue of the *Neurologic Clinics* (NCL Volume 24, Issue 3).

[a] Institute for Behavioral Medicine Research, the Ohio State University, Columbus, OH 43210, USA

[b] Department of Molecular Virology, Immunology, and Medical Genetics, the Ohio State University, Columbus, OH 43210, USA

[c] Integrative Immunology and Behavior, Department of Animal Sciences, University of Illinois, Urbana, IL 61801, USA

* Corresponding author. 2166B Graves Hall, 333 West 10th Avenue, The Ohio State University, Columbus, OH 43210.

E-mail address: godbout.2@osu.edu (J.P. Godbout).

microglia) displaying a more reactive phenotype.[9–12] Recent findings indicate that a reactive glia population sets the stage for an exaggerated neuroinflammatory cytokine response after peripheral innate immune activation.[10,13,14]

The potential for reactive glia to mount an exaggerated response to a secondary stimulus from the peripheral innate immune system is important for several reasons. First, inflammatory cytokines in the brain including interleukin (IL)-1β, IL-6, and tumor necrosis factor alpha (TNF-α) are key mediators of the sickness behavior syndrome.[15] Although transient brain exposure to inflammatory cytokines is beneficial in the host's innate immune response,[16] excessive or prolonged exposure is associated with a myriad of neurobehavioral complications including cognitive dysfunction,[17] anorexia,[18] and mood and depressive disorders.[19–21] Second, inflammatory cytokines are involved in chronic neurodegenerative diseases such as multiple sclerosis and Alzheimer's disease.[22] Finally, excessive or prolonged exposure to inflammatory cytokines in the brain abrogates neuronal plasticity, resulting in behavioral and cognitive impairments.[23–25] Therefore it is hypothesized that an exacerbated neuroinflammatory cytokine response in the aged disrupts neuronal synaptic plasticity, creating a brain environment that is permissive to severe long-lasting mental health complications (**Fig. 1**).

This hypothesis is clinically relevant, because cognitive and behavioral disorders are more frequent in older patients during an illness and are positively correlated with increased morbidity and mortality.[26–28] For example, it is estimated that 15% to 30% of the elderly suffer from a depressive disorder associated with disease or illness.[27] Furthermore, acute cognitive impairment (ie, delirium) is the most common psychiatric condition experienced by the elderly admitted to emergency department with a chronic disease or infection.[28] The overall occurrence of neurobehavioral complications in the elderly is expected to increase dramatically because, based on 2001 Census Bureau projections, by the year 2025 20% of the U.S. population will be over the age of 65 years.[29] In fact, in the last century the average life span increased

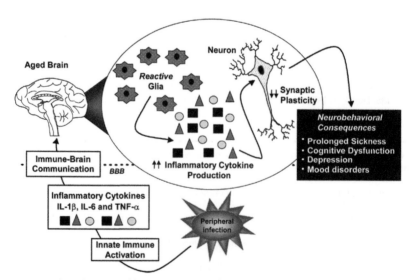

Fig. 1. Proposed mechanism of how aging exacerbates neuroninflammation and neurobehavioral deficits when the peripheral innate immune system is activated. BBB, blood–brain barrier; IL, interleukin; TNF, tumor necrosis factor.

from 47 to 78 years, and the elderly population tripled, from 4% to 13%. Unfortunately it is predicted that this greater life expectancy will result in only a modest increase in health span, with significant increase in years of poor or compromised physical and mental health. Thus, a better understanding of how the interaction between the brain and immune system is dysregulated with age is needed to improve the likelihood of successful aging.

THE RELATIONSHIP BETWEEN THE BRAIN AND THE INNATE IMMUNE SYSTEM

The bidirectional communication between the immune system and brain is critical for mounting the appropriate immunologic, physiologic, and behavioral responses to immune activation by infectious pathogens. The host's first line of defense is the innate immune system. Innate immune cells are armed with pathogen-associated molecular pattern receptors, such as the family of Toll-like receptors, which recognize specific pathogenic elements and elicit an immune response.[30] This innate immune stimulation results in the production of inflammatory cytokines including IL-1β, IL-6, and TNF-α by active peripheral macrophages or monocytes. These cytokines utilize both neural (by the afferent vagus nerve)[31,32] and humoral (by circumventricular organs[33,34] and direct transport[35]) pathways to communicate this innate immune challenge to the brain. This cytokine-mediated immune system–brain communication activates microglia, the resident innate immune cells of the brain, which induce and propagate these same cytokine signals throughout the central nervous system (CNS).[16] Inflammatory cytokines produced within the CNS target neuronal substrates and elicit the behavioral symptoms of sickness, including fever, increased sleep, reduced appetite, lethargy, and decreased social behavior.[15] Collectively these behavioral symptoms of sickness are evolutionarily conserved and function to increase the metabolic demand for clearance of pathogens as well as limit the spread of infection to others.[36] Moreover, the neuroinflammatory-modulated response associated with sickness behavior is a beneficial and transient response.[37] Thus, it is important to distinguish this neuroinflammatory process from that caused by encephalitis, which is associated with infiltration of T cells into the brain, neurodegeneration, and a break down of the blood–brain barrier.

Critical for this immune system–CNS interaction and the modulation of sickness behavior are the resident innate immune cells of the brain. Aside from neurons, macroglia and microglia are the two primary cell types located throughout the CNS. The macroglia are derived from a nerve cell lineage and are classified into three distinct subtypes: astrocytes, oligodendrocytes, and Schwann cells. These macroglia are the most populous cells of the CNS and support and maintain neuronal plasticity throughout the CNS. Microglia also are interspersed throughout the brain and represent approximately 10% of the CNS population. Microglia differ from the macroglia because they are derived from a monocyte/macrophage cell lineage. Microglia are pivotal in innate immune activation and function to modulate neuroinflammatory signals throughout the brain. In the absence of stimulus, microglia are quiescent and have a ramified morphology.[38] During an innate immune response microglia are activated and become deramified. Active microglia show macrophage-like activities including scavenging, phagocytosis, antigen presentation, complement activation, and inflammatory cytokine production. Moreover microglia recruit and activate astrocytes to propagate these inflammatory signals further.[7] Normally these neuroinflammatory changes are transient, with microglia returning to a quiescent state after the resolution of the immune challenge. Aging, however, may provide a brain environment in which microglia activation is not resolved, leading to a heightened sensitivity to immune activation; this lack of resolution may contribute to the pathogenesis of neurologic disease.

Evidence of an Altered Glia Population in the Aged Brain

Age-associated alterations in immunity are apparent in the innate immune cells of the brain. Recent evidence indicates there is an elevated inflammatory profile in the aging brain consisting of an increased population of reactive or primed glia. Glial phenotypes of reactivity include increased microglia expression of major histocompatibility complexes (MHC), scavenger receptors, and complement receptors and increased astrocyte expression of glial fibrillary protein (GFAP). For example, increased microglial expression of MHC class II was detected in brains of aged but otherwise healthy humans, nonhuman primates, and rodents using either immunohistochemical or mRNA measurements.[9–12,39–43] Microglial expression of complement receptor-3[12] and the macrosialin (CD68) scavenger receptor[10,44] also were elevated in the brain of aged rodents. Furthermore, the expression of GFAP, a marker of astrogliosis, was increased in several of these same rodent models of aging.[8,10,11] It is noteworthy that the actual number of resident astrocytes and microglia did not increase in the brain with age.[11,45] Therefore the expression of markers indicative of glial reactivity seems to be increased in existing astrocytes and microglia populations. There is, however, evidence of sex-dependent and region-specific glia increases with age.[46] Also, although active and reactive glia have a similar morphology (ie, deramified), reactive glia do not produce appreciable levels of proinflammatory cytokines in this state.[36] In fact, in rodent models of prion and Parkinson's disease reactive microglia have an anti-inflammatory or atypical cytokine profile in the absence of immune stimulation.[47,48]

In humans, alterations in microglia phenotype are especially prevalent in patients who have inflammatory disease or injury. For example the MHC class II marker in humans, HLA-DR, was detected in patients who have Alzheimer's disease[49] and in older patients who have coronary artery disease[43] or spinal cord tract degeneration.[50] These alterations in the glia population were detected in healthy, cognitively normal (ie, nondemented) subjects as well, however. For instance, older individuals had increased IL-1α–positive microglia with morphologic changes indicative of enlarged or phagocytic microglia in the hippocampus.[51] Increased HLA-DR expression on the surface of microglia also was found in the hippocampus of older individuals.[43] A subsequent study using a cognitively normal elderly donor revealed increased HLA-DR–positive microglia in the cortex and morphologic alterations in microglia including deramification, spheroid formation, and fragmentation of processes. These morphologic alterations were interpreted as indicating microglial senescence. These changes, however, were predicted to result in functional defects that trigger an intracerebral inflammatory response that supports the development of age-associated neurodegenerative diseases such as Alzheimer's disease.[7,2] Taken together, these findings suggest that even in the absence of detectable disease, the glia population undergoes an age-related transformation that creates a more sensitive brain environment (**Table 1**).

Immune Consequences of Reactive Glia in the Aged Brain

A potential consequence of a reactive glial cell population in the brain is an exaggerated inflammatory response to innate immune activation. Perry and colleagues[36] at the University of Southampton, United Kingdom, have proposed that systemic infection exacerbates the progression of neurodegenerative disease. In this circumstance the brain environment created by the neurologic disease provides a primary trigger for

Table 1
Evidence for an age-related increase in reactive glia

Author	Principal Finding	Detection	Model	Brain Region
Perry et al (1993)	MHC class II (Ox-6) and Complement type-3 receptor (Ox-42)	IHC	Rat	Multiple
Ogura et al (1994)	MHC class II (Ox-6)	IHC	Rat	Multiple
Sheffield et al (1997)	MHC class II (LN-3)	IHC	Monkey	Hippocampus
Streit et al (1997)	HLA-DR (LN-3)	IHC	Human	Hippocampus
Sheng et al (1998)	IL-1alpha	IHC/morphology	Human	Hippocampus
Morgan et al (1999)	MHC class II (Ox-6) and GFAP	IHC	Rat	Hippocampus
Lee et al (2000)	GFAP	mRNA/microarray	Mouse	Cortex and cerebellum
Nicolle et al (2001)	MHC class II (Ox-6)	IHC	Rat	Hippocampus
Streit et al (2004)	HLA-DR (LN-3)	IHC/morphology	Human	Cortex
Godbout et al (2005)	MHC class II, CD68, GFAP	mRNA/microarray	Mouse	Whole brain
Frank et al (2005)	MHC class II and CD86	mRNA/qPCR	Rat	Hippocampus
Wong et al (2005)	CD68	IHC/qPCR	Mouse	Corpus callosum

Abbreviations: GFAP, glial fibrillary protein; IHC, immunohistochemistry; IL, interleukin; MHC, major histocompatibility class; PCR, polymerase chain reaction.

microglia reactivity, and peripheral infection provides the secondary stimulus.[52] In the ME-7 murine model of prion disease, microglia are activated throughout the limbic system, including the hippocampus where neuron loss occurs.[53] In mice with preclinical ME-7–induced prion disease, peripheral lipopolysaccharide (LPS) challenge, a potent activator of the innate immune system, induced an exaggerated depression in locomotor behavior and body temperature and increased brain IL-1β compared with controls.[14] In a transgenic murine model of amyotrophic lateral sclerosis, disease progression was exacerbated in presymptomatic mice given repeated intraperitoneal injections of LPS.[54] The expression of Toll-like receptor 2 and TNF-α was increased in discrete brain and spinal cord regions where degeneration occurred,[54] and the average life span of amyotrophic lateral sclerosis mice given LPS was decreased by 3 weeks. These experimental findings have clinical relevance, because systemic infection in humans exacerbates disease progression of Alzheimer's disease and multiple sclerosis.[52] For instance, peripheral infection precipitated relapse in patients who had multiple sclerosis[55] and enhanced the progression into dementia in patients who had Alzheimer's disease.[56] Furthermore, deposition of β amyloid within senile plaques is a classic feature of Alzheimer's disease, and conditions leading to the expression of inflammatory cytokines in brain are associated with the induction of β amyloid precursor protein.[57] In the Tg2576 murine model of Alzheimer's disease, intravenous injection of LPS caused age-dependent increases in brain IL-1β and TNF-α levels and increased β amyloid deposition.[58] This deposition may promote neuroinflammation further, because β amyloid activates microglia.[59] Collectively these data indicate that innate immune activation contributes both to the pathogenesis of neurodegenerative disease and to the severity of the associated neurobehavioral complications.

Hypersensitivity to innate immune activation in the brain also is evident in several animal models of aging. For instance, primary mixed glia cultures and coronal brain sections established from the brain of aged rodents were hyper-responsive to LPS stimulation and produced more inflammatory cytokines (IL-1β and IL-6) than cultures established from adult brains.[60,61] In a murine model of aging, older mice were more sensitive to septic shock induced by intracerebroventricular (ICV) administration of LPS. Older mice had elevated TNF-α production in the brain and plasma after LPS challenge compared with adult controls.[62] In another murine model of aging, microarray analysis revealed that peripheral injection of LPS induced a higher expression of IL-1β and TNF-α in the hippocampus of aged mice than in adults.[63] Moreover, a recent study using microarray analysis showed increased markers of glia reactivity, including MHC class II, CD68, and GFAP, in the brain of aged mice.[10] In this model peripheral stimulation of the innate immune system with LPS caused an exaggerated inflammatory cytokine response in the aged brain with increased production of IL-6 and IL-1β. Furthermore, aged mice that experienced a LPS-induced amplified and prolonged neuroinflammatory response showed a delayed recovery from sickness behavior.[10] Finally, in a rat model of aging, in which increased reactive glia with MHC class II expression were detected,[9] peripheral injection of Escherichia coli promoted higher levels of IL-1β in the hippocampus of aged rats than in adults.[13] This increased IL-1β production in the hippocampus of aged rats after E coli challenge was associated with impaired long-term hippocampal-dependent memory.[13] Neither of these studies[10,13] found peripheral inflammatory cytokines to be a reliable indicator of the exaggerated neuroinflammatory response. Taken together these results suggest that the presence of reactive glia in the aged or diseased brain is permissive to an amplified and prolonged neuroinflammatory response, which may lead to subsequent behavioral and cognitive complications.

ARE NEUROBEHAVIORAL COMPLICATIONS A CONSEQUENCE OF PROLONGED EXPOSURE TO PROINFLAMMATORY CYTOKINES?

Recent experimental evidence suggests that an amplified and prolonged inflammatory response in the aged brain promotes protracted behavioral and cognitive impairments.[10,13] These findings seem to be supported by clinical evidence indicating that many of the behavioral consequences of illness and infection in the elderly, if prolonged, can have deleterious affects on mental health. For example, there is an increased prevalence of delirium in elderly emergency department patients[64] as a result of infections unrelated to the CNS.[28,65] The most striking characteristic of pneumonia (either viral or bacterial) in the aged is that it frequently presents clinically as delirium, even in the absence of classic pneumonia symptoms.[66] A clinical study showed that 34% of elderly patients diagnosed with delirium had an infection. A follow-up of these patients 1 year later revealed increased rates of mortality, institutionalization, and hospital readmittance.[67] Furthermore, delirium is a risk factor for progression into dementia. For example, a recent clinical trial of 203 subjects over the age of 65 years found that those initially diagnosed as having delirium had an 18% probability of developing dementia within 1 year and had a significantly higher mortality rate within a 3-year period.[68] Moreover, peripheral infection increased the risk of dementia in otherwise healthy individuals over the age of 84 years.[69] Acute cognitive impairment or dementia often results in a failure of self-care and is associated with delayed recovery from illness, resulting in increased rates of hospitalization,[64,70] institutionalization,[67] and mortality.[71] Taken together these data indicate that age is a risk factor for delirium and dementia following a peripheral infection and suggest that inflammatory cytokines play a role in the origin of these deficits.[56]

Mood and depressive symptoms also are common in elderly patients who are ill and are associated with increased morbidity and mortality.[26] A number of clinical and laboratory studies of depression support the premise that there is a causative relationship between inflammatory cytokines and depressive disorders. For example, the chronic stress associated with care-giving for a patient who had Alzheimer's disease was associated with increased peripheral IL-6 and depressive symptoms.[72] Elderly patients who experienced a prolonged inflammatory response to an influenza vaccination also had a higher incidence of mild depressive symptoms.[73] Moreover, increased inflammatory cytokines have been associated with major depression in chronically infected patients,[20,74] in patients who have chronic inflammatory diseases (eg, coronary heart disease and rheumatoid arthritis),[75] and in patients who have cancer and are undergoing cytokine immunotherapy.[76] Several studies have found evidence of increased cytokines, including IL-6 and IL-1β, in the plasma or in the cerebrospinal fluid of depressed patients.[73,77–80] Furthermore, the heightened levels of cytokines were associated with the severity of the depressive symptoms.[76–78,81] Collectively these findings suggest that a prolonged neuroinflammatory response in the elderly has a profound effect on mental health and lifespan (**Fig. 2**).

DOES HEIGHTENED INFLAMMATORY CYTOKINE EXPOSURE IMPAIR NEURONAL PLASTICITY AND CAUSE NEUROBEHAVIORAL COMPLICATIONS?

Inflammatory cytokines provoke behavioral responses, in part, by modulating neuronal activity. Synaptic plasticity encompasses a number of important brain functions that maintain cognitive and behavioral homeostasis including long-term potentiation (LTP), neurogenesis, and neurite outgrowth. This effect is clinically relevant because impaired neuronal plasticity may underlie several complications in mood and behavior.[82,83] Neuronal plasticity is essential in brain areas associated with modulating cognition and behavior, such as the hippocampus. In fact, the hippocampus and the hypothalamus have the highest expression of inflammatory cytokine receptors for IL-1β[84] and IL-6.[85] In some instances inflammatory cytokine exposure leads to neuronal cell death,[86] especially in neurologic disease, endotoxic shock, or chronic inflammatory conditions, but normal neuroinflammatory responses that mediate sickness behavior do not.[16] In fact, in primary or transformed cultures cytokines such as IL-6 and IL-1β have growth-promoting effects on neurons[87] and may play a role in early brain development. Several experimental examples, however, indicate that

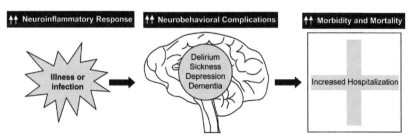

Fig. 2. The elderly population is more susceptible to peripheral infection and has a higher incidence of mental health complications that affect health and lifespan.

excessive and prolonged exposure to inflammatory cytokines impairs synaptic plasticity and may underlie cognitive and behavioral complications seen with age and infection.

Several studies have demonstrated that inflammatory cytokines impair the ability to maintain LTP in the hippocampus, a critical physiologic process involved in memory consolidation. For example, IL-6 exposure abrogated LTP in rat hippocampal brain slices.[88] Lynch and colleagues[89] at Trinity College, Ireland, demonstrated that peripheral LPS injection impaired LTP in the hippocampus of rats through a pathway involving IL-1β production.[89] Moreover, ICV infusion of recombinant IL-1β alone attenuated LTP in the hippocampus.[25] The inflammatory-dependent impairment of LTP was associated with increased oxidative stress, decreased glutamate release, and neuronal apoptosis.[25,89] Moreover, activation of p38 stress kinase and nuclear factor κB (NFκB) transcription factor also were involved in this inflammatory cytokine-dependent disruption of LTP.[90] Finally, in this model inhibition of LTP was reversed by ICV infusion of the anti-inflammatory cytokine IL-10.[91]

Inflammatory cytokines also can impair neurite outgrowth, a critical process involved in modifying existing synaptic connections. For example, in primary hippocampal neurons cultured on astrocytes, IL-1β stimulated astrocytes to produce TNF-α, which inhibited the neurite outgrowth and branching.[92] Furthermore neurite outgrowth and branching was unaffected by TNF-α in primary neurons established from TNF receptor I- and II–deficient mice.[92] Astrocytes with a more reactive phenotype, even in the absence of immune stimulus, may impair neuronal plasticity in the aged brain. For instance, neurite outgrowth of embryonic neurons was reduced when co-cultured with reactive astrocytes derived from aged brains compared with results in adults. Decreasing astrocyte reactivity through the attenuation of GFAP expression by RNA interference restored neurite outgrowth in this culture system.[93]

Several studies have shown that inflammatory cytokines reduce hippocampal neurogenesis, a process that is critical for memory and learning.[94] Neurogenesis is significant because it allows new neurons with a high degree of plasticity to become incorporated into the hippocampal circuitry.[95] For instance, neuroinflammation induced by ICV or intraperitoneal injection of LPS reduced neurogenesis in the hippocampal dentate gyrus.[23,96] Resident microglia activated to produce cytokines were implicated, because two anti-inflammatory drugs known to attenuate microglia activity, idomethacin (a nonsteroidal anti-inflammatory drug) and minocycline, restored neurogenesis. Finally, inflammatory cytokine exposure in the brain can also diminish neurogenesis. In transgenic mice whose astrocytes chronically overproduce IL-6, hippocampal neurogenesis was decreased by 63%.[24] Collectively, inflammatory cytokine exposure disrupts synaptic plasticity, which may underlie mental health complications associated with age and inflammation.

HOW DO GLIA BECOME MORE REACTIVE WITH AGE?

There are several plausible explanations for increased glia sensitivity with age (**Fig. 3**). One explanation is that inflammatory cytokine exposure over a course of a lifespan increases the number of reactive glia in the brain. A recent longitudinal study from Sweden demonstrated that young individuals exposed to inflammatory events early in life had a higher morbidity and mortality rate as they aged.[97] Therefore inflammatory exposure, especially early in life, may predict inflammatory associated complications later in life. Several experimental rodent studies have demonstrated that neonatal exposure to inflammatory stimulus interferes with brain–immune system coordination and may predispose these animals to inflammatory processes later in life.[98–100]

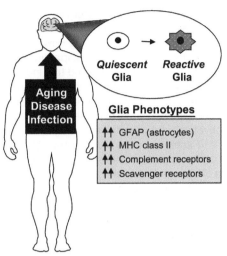

Fig. 3. Inflammatory exposure over the course of a lifespan may influence thenuber of reative glia in the brain. GFAP, glial fibrillary protein; MHC, major histocompatibility class.

Although neonatal exposure to a pathogen may interfere with the development of the immune system, this model system also may provide insight into why reactive glia populations are more prevalent with age. In a recent study, neonatal rats were challenged with live replicating *E coli* and then in adulthood were given a secondary challenge with LPS. The secondary challenge with LPS caused a significant increase in astrocyte expression of GFAP in the CA3 region of the hippocampus in rats infected as neonates.[101] Moreover, astrocyte reactivity to secondary challenge of LPS in adulthood was associated with a severe deficit in hippocampal-dependent memory.[101] Although the IL-1β cytokine response was unchanged in the hippocampus, increased astrocyte expression of GFAP was interpreted as suggesting an exaggerated neuro-inflammatory response. Reactive glia also may be derived by inflammatory process later in life. For example, inflammatory cytokines such as IL-6 and IL-1β have been detected in the aged brain, even in the absence of inflammatory stimulus or neurologic disease.[102–104] A potential outcome of increased IL-6 exposure with age is a more reactive or abundant glia population. Support for this notion comes from studies in which heightened expression of IL-6 in neurons of transgenic mice increased the number and size of astrocytes and the number of ramified microglial cells.[105] Furthermore, IL-6 also stimulated embryonic cerebral precursor cells to differentiate into astrocytes.[106] Thus, IL-6 may also increase the number of astrocytes in the brain by redirecting progenitor cells toward a glial cell lineage. Taken together these data suggest that inflammatory exposure may prime the glia of the brain to secondary insult and predispose individuals for inflammatory complications.

Another possible explanation for reactive glia in the aged brain is increased oxidative stress and damage. According to the free radical hypothesis of aging, oxidative damage to cell membranes and intracellular proteins increases because of an increase in oxygen free radicals (ie, reactive oxygen species), a decrease in the capacity of the antioxidant defense mechanisms to scavenge reactive oxygen species, or some combination of these two.[107] For example oxidative stress contributes to the inflammatory milieu of the aging brain and is associated with the age-related decline in cognitive and motor function.[108,109] An age-related decline in cognition was associated with increased MHC class II–positive microglia in the hippocampus.[39] Supporting evidence for this premise is derived from recent rodent studies of aging using the caloric restriction model. In the calorie restriction model, total calories are restricted by 40% from weaning onwards, while dietary intake of essential nutrients is maintained. One of the principal findings of this model is that life span is extended by 30% to 50%. It is proposed that increased lifespan is caused by increased DNA repair, increased metabolic efficiency, and reduced reactive by-products.[110] Global evaluations of the inflammatory state of the aged brain using microarray analysis have revealed a gene-expression profile indicative of oxidative stress, complement activation, and glial cell reactivity in the neocortex, cerebellum, and hippocampus.[8,10,111] Restricting caloric intake reversed the age-related expression of the oxidative and inflammatory markers.[8] In fact, calorie restriction both limited the inflammatory profile of the aged brain and enhanced the expression of growth and trophic factors.[8] In several other models, calorie restriction also reduced other inflammatory markers in the aged rodent brain, including GFAP and CD68 scavenger receptor.[11,44] Thus, an inflammatory brain profile is detrimental to successful aging, potentially through the reduction of important neurotrophic factors involved in the maintenance of neuronal plasticity.

LIMITING INFLAMMATORY EXPOSURE WITH ANTIOXIDANTS

The induction of sickness behavior is a necessary and important response to systemic infection.[37] Instances when sickness behavior is too severe or prolonged, however, may cause long-lasting behavioral and cognitive impairments.[10,13] Therefore developing interventions that limit this neuroinflammatory process without affecting induction of the response is of particular interest. One potential cytokine target could be IL-6. Although IL-6 exposure alone does not induce sickness behavior,[112] in combination with other cytokines it has an important role in the maintenance of sickness behavior. This notion is supported by evidence that IL-6 knockout mice recovered faster from LPS-induced sickness,[113] and protracted IL-6 expression in the brain of aged mice was positively correlated with prolonged sickness behavior.[10] Moreover, the antioxidant α-tocopherol (vitamin E) attenuates the inflammatory response induced by LPS by reducing lipid peroxidation and IL-6 cytokine production in the brain and primary microglia.[114] This immunomodulary action of α-tocopherol facilitated the recovery from LPS-induced sickness behavior in adult[115] and aged mice.[116] Furthermore, attenuation of NFκB in the brain with α-tocopherol or central injection of NFκB decoy also improved the recovery from LPS-induced sickness behavior.[117,118] Thus, attenuating neuroinflammation with antioxidants facilitates recovery from the behavioral symptoms of sickness and may prevent the onset of neurobehavioral impairments. Therefore it may be worthwhile to investigate whether antioxidant therapy decreases the incidence of peripheral infections in a susceptible elderly population[119] and whether it aids in the recovery from infection in this same population.

SUMMARY

This article reviews the literature indicating that the innate immune cells of the brain become more reactive with age. Although it is unclear how glia reactivity increases, emerging evidence suggests these alterations allow exacerbated neuroinflammation and sickness behavior following peripheral immune activation. This amplified or prolonged exposure to inflammatory cytokines in the brain may impair neuronal plasticity and underlie a heightened neuroinflammatory response in the aged that also may lead to other neurobehavioral impairments such as delirium, depression, and, potentially, the onset of neurologic disease. Therefore pharmacologic strategies to decrease neuroinflammation associated with infection may be important for improving recovery from sickness and reducing neurobehavioral deficits in the elderly.

REFERENCES

1. Castle SC. Clinical relevance of age-related immune dysfunction. Clin Infect Dis 2000;31(2):578–85.
2. Plowden J, Renshaw-Hoelscher M, Engleman C, et al. Innate immunity in aging: impact on macrophage function. Aging Cell 2004;3(4):161–7.
3. Miller RA. The aging immune system: primer and prospectus. Science 1996; 273(5271):70–4.
4. Ginaldi L, Loreto MF, Corsi MP, et al. Immunosenescence and infectious diseases. Microbes Infect 2001;3(10):851–7.
5. Straub RH, Miller LE, Scholmerich J, et al. Cytokines and hormones as possible links between endocrinosenescence and immunosenescence. J Neuroimmunol 2000;109(1):10–5.
6. Godbout JP, Johnson RW. Interleukin-6 in the aging brain. J Neuroimmunol 2004; 147(1-2):141–4.
7. Blasko I, Stampfer-Kountchev M, Robatscher P, et al. How chronic inflammation can affect the brain and support the development of Alzheimer's disease in old age: the role of microglia and astrocytes. Aging Cell 2004;3(4):169–76.
8. Lee CK, Weindruch R, Prolla TA. Gene-expression profile of the ageing brain in mice. Nat Genet 2000;25(3):294–7.
9. Frank MG, Barrientos RM, Biedenkapp JC, et al. mRNA up-regulation of MHC II and pivotal pro-inflammatory genes in normal brain aging. Neurobiol Aging 2005.
10. Godbout JP, Chen J, Abraham J, et al. Exaggerated neuroinflammation and sickness behavior in aged mice following activation of the peripheral innate immune system. FASEB J 2005;19(10):1329–31.
11. Morgan TE, Xie Z, Goldsmith S, et al. The mosaic of brain glial hyperactivity during normal ageing and its attenuation by food restriction. Neuroscience 1999;89(3):687–99.
12. Perry VH, Matyszak MK, Fearn S. Altered antigen expression of microglia in the aged rodent CNS. Glia 1993;7(1):60–7.
13. Barrientos RM, Higgins EA, Biedenkapp JC, et al. Peripheral infection and aging interact to impair hippocampal memory consolidation. Neurobiol Aging 2005.
14. Combrinck MI, Perry VH, Cunningham C. Peripheral infection evokes exaggerated sickness behaviour in pre-clinical murine prion disease. Neuroscience 2002;112(1):7–11.
15. Konsman JP, Parnet P, Dantzer R. Cytokine-induced sickness behaviour: mechanisms and implications. Trends Neurosci 2002;25(3):154–9.
16. Rivest S. Molecular insights on the cerebral innate immune system. Brain Behav Immun 2003;17(1):13–9.
17. Heyser CJ, Masliah E, Samimi A, et al. Progressive decline in avoidance learning paralleled by inflammatory neurodegeneration in transgenic mice expressing interleukin 6 in the brain. Proc Natl Acad Sci U S A 1997;94(4):1500–5.
18. Finck BN, Johnson RW. Anorexia, weight loss and increased plasma interleukin-6 caused by chronic intracerebroventricular infusion of interleukin-1beta in the rat. Brain Res 1997;761(2):333–7.
19. Musselman DL, Lawson DH, Gumnick JF, et al. Paroxetine for the prevention of depression induced by high-dose interferon alfa. N Engl J Med 2001;344(13): 961–6.

20. Pollmacher T, Haack M, Schuld A, et al. Low levels of circulating inflammatory cytokines—do they affect human brain functions? Brain Behav Immun 2002; 16(5):525–32.
21. Capuron L, Neurauter G, Musselman DL, et al. Interferon-alpha-induced changes in tryptophan metabolism. Relationship to depression and paroxetine treatment. Biol Psychiatry 2003;54(9):906–14.
22. Wilson CJ, Finch CE, Cohen HJ. Cytokines and cognition—the case for a head-to-toe inflammatory paradigm. J Am Geriatr Soc 2002;50(12):2041–56.
23. Monje ML, Toda H, Palmer TD. Inflammatory blockade restores adult hippo-campal neurogenesis. Science 2003;302(5651):1760–5.
24. Vallieres L, Campbell IL, Gage FH, et al. Reduced hippocampal neurogenesis in adult transgenic mice with chronic astrocytic production of interleukin-6. J Neurosci 2002;22(2):486–92.
25. Vereker E, O'Donnell E, Lynch MA. The inhibitory effect of interleukin-1beta on long-term potentiation is coupled with increased activity of stress-activated protein kinases. J Neurosci 2000;20(18):6811–9.
26. Penninx BW, Geerlings SW, Deeg DJ, et al. Minor and major depression and the risk of death in older persons. Arch Gen Psychiatry 1999;56(10):889–95.
27. Mulsant BH, Ganguli M. Epidemiology and diagnosis of depression in late life. J Clin Psychiatry 1999;60(Suppl 20):9–15.
28. Jackson JC, Gordon SM, Hart RP, et al. The association between delirium and cognitive decline: a review of the empirical literature. Neuropsychol Rev 2004; 14(2):87–98.
29. Schneider EL. Demographics: aging in the third millennium. Science 1999; 283(5403):796–7.
30. Akira S, Takeda K. Toll-like receptor signalling. Nat Rev Immunol 2004;4(7): 499–511.
31. Konsman JP, Luheshi GN, Bluthe RM, et al. The vagus nerve mediates behavioural depression, but not fever, in response to peripheral immune signals; a functional anatomical analysis. Eur J Neurosci 2000;12(12):4434–46.
32. Goehler LE, Gaykema RP, Hammack SE, et al. Interleukin-1 induces c-Fos immunoreactivity in primary afferent neurons of the vagus nerve. Brain Res 1998;804(2):306–10.
33. Laflamme N, Lacroix S, Rivest S. An essential role of interleukin-1beta in mediating NF-kappaB activity and COX-2 transcription in cells of the blood-brain barrier in response to a systemic and localized inflammation but not during endotoxemia. J Neurosci 1999;19(24):10923–30.
34. Lacroix S, Feinstein D, Rivest S. The bacterial endotoxin lipopolysaccharide has the ability to target the brain in upregulating its membrane CD14 receptor within specific cellular populations. Brain Pathol 1998;8(4):625–40.
35. Banks WA. Physiology and pathology of the blood-brain barrier: implications for microbial pathogenesis, drug delivery and neurodegenerative disorders. J Neurovirol 1999;5(6):538–55.
36. Perry VH. The influence of systemic inflammation on inflammation in the brain: implications for chronic neurodegenerative disease. Brain Behav Immun 2004; 18(5):407–13.
37. Johnson RW. The concept of sickness behavior: a brief chronological account of four key discoveries. Vet Immunol Immunopathol 2002;87(3–4):443–50.
38. Gonzalez-Scarano F, Baltuch G. Microglia as mediators of inflammatory and degenerative diseases. Annu Rev Neurosci 1999;22:219–40.

39. Nicolle MM, Gonzalez J, Sugaya K, et al. Signatures of hippocampal oxidative stress in aged spatial learning- impaired rodents. Neuroscience 2001;107(3): 415–31.
40. Ogura K, Ogawa M, Yoshida M. Effects of ageing on microglia in the normal rat brain: immunohistochemical observations. Neuroreport 1994;5(10):1224–6.
41. Sheffield LG, Berman NE. Microglial expression of MHC class II increases in normal aging of nonhuman primates. Neurobiol Aging 1998;19(1):47–55.
42. Streit WJ, Sammons NW, Kuhns AJ, et al. Dystrophic microglia in the aging human brain. Glia 2004;45(2):208–12.
43. Streit WJ, Sparks DL. Activation of microglia in the brains of humans with heart disease and hypercholesterolemic rabbits. J Mol Med 1997;75(2):130–8.
44. Wong AM, Patel NV, Patel NK, et al. Macrosialin increases during normal brain aging are attenuated by caloric restriction. Neurosci Lett 2005;390(2):76–80.
45. Long JM, Kalehua AN, Muth NJ, et al. Stereological analysis of astrocyte and microglia in aging mouse hippocampus. Neurobiol Aging 1998;19(5):497–503.
46. Mouton PR, Long JM, Lei DL, et al. Age and gender effects on microglia and astrocyte numbers in brains of mice. Brain Res 2002;956(1):30–5.
47. Depino AM, Earl C, Kaczmarczyk E, et al. Microglial activation with atypical proinflammatory cytokine expression in a rat model of Parkinson's disease. Eur J Neurosci 2003;18(10):2731–42.
48. Perry VH, Cunningham C, Boche D. Atypical inflammation in the central nervous system in prion disease. Curr Opin Neurol 2002;15(3):349–54.
49. Mattiace LA, Davies P, Dickson DW. Detection of HLA-DR on microglia in the human brain is a function of both clinical and technical factors. Am J Pathol 1990;136(5):1101–14.
50. Sobel RA, Ames MB. Major histocompatibility complex molecule expression in the human central nervous system: immunohistochemical analysis of 40 patients. J Neuropathol Exp Neurol 1988;47(1):19–28.
51. Sheng JG, Mrak RE, Griffin WS. Enlarged and phagocytic, but not primed, interleukin-1 alpha-immunoreactive microglia increase with age in normal human brain. Acta Neuropathol (Berl) 1998;95(3):229–34.
52. Perry VH, Newman TA, Cunningham C. The impact of systemic infection on the progression of neurodegenerative disease. Nat Rev Neurosci 2003;4(2):103–12.
53. Cunningham C, Deacon R, Wells H, et al. Synaptic changes characterize early behavioural signs in the ME7 model of murine prion disease. Eur J Neurosci 2003;17(10):2147–55.
54. Nguyen MD, D'Aigle T, Gowing G, et al. Exacerbation of motor neuron disease by chronic stimulation of innate immunity in a mouse model of amyotrophic lateral sclerosis. J Neurosci 2004;24(6):1340–9.
55. Sibley WA, Bamford CR, Clark K. Clinical viral infections and multiple sclerosis. Lancet 1985;8441:1313–5.
56. Holmes C, El-Okl M, Williams AL, et al. Systemic infection, interleukin 1beta, and cognitive decline in Alzheimer's disease. J Neurol Neurosurg Psychiatry 2003; 74(6):788–9.
57. Brugg B, Dubreuil YL, Huber G, et al. Inflammatory processes induce beta-amyloid precursor protein changes in mouse brain. Proc Natl Acad Sci U S A 1995;92(7):3032–5.
58. Sly LM, Krzesicki RF, Brashler JR, et al. Endogenous brain cytokine mRNA and inflammatory responses to lipopolysaccharide are elevated in the Tg2576 transgenic mouse model of Alzheimer's disease. Brain Res Bull 2001;56(6):581–8.

59. Giulian D. Microglia and the immune pathology of Alzheimer disease. Am J Hum Genet 1999;65(1):13–8.

60. Xie Z, Morgan TE, Rozovsky I, et al. Aging and glial responses to lipopolysaccharide in vitro: greater induction of IL-1 and IL-6, but smaller induction of neurotoxicity. Exp Neurol 2003;182(1):135–41.

61. Ye SM, Johnson RW. An age-related decline in interleukin-10 may contribute to the increased expression of interleukin-6 in brain of aged mice. Neuroimmunomodulation 2001;9(4):183–92.

62. Kalehua AN, Taub DD, Baskar PV, et al. Aged mice exhibit greater mortality concomitant to increased brain and plasma TNF-alpha levels following intracerebroventricular injection of lipopolysaccharide. Gerontology 2000;46(3):115–28.

63. Terao A, Apte-Deshpande A, Dousman L, et al. Immune response gene expression increases in the aging murine hippocampus. J Neuroimmunol 2002;132(1-2):99–112.

64. Johnston M, Wakeling A, Graham N, et al. Cognitive impairment, emotional disorder and length of stay of elderly patients in a district general hospital. Br J Med Psychol 1987;60(Pt 2):133–9.

65. Wofford JL, Loehr LR, Schwartz E. Acute cognitive impairment in elderly ED patients: etiologies and outcomes. Am J Emerg Med 1996;14(7):649–53.

66. Janssens JP, Krause KH. Pneumonia in the very old. Lancet Infect Dis 2004;4(2):112–24.

67. George J, Bleasdale S, Singleton SJ. Causes and prognosis of delirium in elderly patients admitted to a district general hospital. Age Ageing 1997;26(6):423–7.

68. Rockwood K, Cosway S, Carver D, et al. The risk of dementia and death after delirium. Age Ageing 1999;28:551–6.

69. Dunn N, Mullee M, Perry VH, et al. Association between dementia and infectious disease: evidence from a case-control study. Alzheimer Dis Assoc Disord 2005;19(2):91–4.

70. Inouye SK, Rushing JT, Foreman MD, et al. Does delirium contribute to poor hospital outcomes? A three-site epidemiologic study. J Gen Intern Med 1998;13(4):234–42.

71. McCusker J, Cole M, Abrahamowicz M, et al. Delirium predicts 12-month mortality. Arch Intern Med 2002;162(4):457–63.

72. Kiecolt-Glaser JK, Preacher KJ, MacCallum RC, et al. Chronic stress and age-related increases in the proinflammatory cytokine IL-6. Proc Natl Acad Sci U S A 2003;100(15):9090–5.

73. Glaser R, Robles TF, Sheridan J, et al. Mild depressive symptoms are associated with amplified and prolonged inflammatory responses after influenza virus vaccination in older adults. Arch Gen Psychiatry 2003;60(10):1009–14.

74. Yirmiya R, Pollak Y, Morag M, et al. Illness, cytokines, and depression. Ann N Y Acad Sci 2000;917:478–87.

75. Kiecolt-Glaser JK, Glaser R. Depression and immune function: central pathways to morbidity and mortality. J Psychosom Res 2002;53(4):873–6.

76. Capuron L, Ravaud A, Miller AH, et al. Baseline mood and psychosocial characteristics of patients developing depressive symptoms during interleukin-2 and/or interferon-alpha cancer therapy. Brain Behav Immun 2004;18(3):205–13.

77. Levine J, Barak Y, Chengappa KN, et al. Cerebrospinal cytokine levels in patients with acute depression. Neuropsychobiology 1999;40(4):171–6.

78. Dentino AN, Pieper CF, Rao MK, et al. Association of interleukin-6 and other bio-logic variables with depression in older people living in the community. J Am Geriatr Soc 1999;47(1):6–11.

79. Penninx BW, Kritchevsky SB, Yaffe K, et al. Inflammatory markers and depressed mood in older persons: results from the Health, Aging and Body Composition study. Biol Psychiatry 2003;54(5):566–72.

80. Capuron L, Ravaud A, Gualde N, et al. Association between immune activation and early depressive symptoms in cancer patients treated with interleukin-2-based therapy. Psychoneuroendocrinology 2001;26(8):797–808.

81. Suarez EC, Lewis JG, Krishnan RR, et al. Enhanced expression of cytokines and chemokines by blood monocytes to in vitro lipopolysaccharide stimulation are associated with hostility and severity of depressive symptoms in healthy women. Psychoneuroendocrinology 2004;29(9):1119–28.

82. Lesch KP. Serotonergic gene expression and depression: implications for devel-oping novel antidepressants. J Affect Disord 2001;62(1–2):57–76.

83. Mattson MP, Maudsley S, Martin B. BDNF and 5-HT: a dynamic duo in age-related neuronal plasticity and neurodegenerative disorders. Trends Neurosci 2004;27(10):589–94.

84. Parnet P, Amindari S, Wu C, et al. Expression of type I and type II interleukin-1 receptors in mouse brain. Brain Res Mol Brain Res 1994;27(1):63–70.

85. Schobitz B, de Kloet ER, Sutanto W, et al. Cellular localization of interleukin 6 mRNA and interleukin 6 receptor mRNA in rat brain. Eur J Neurosci 1993; 5(11):1426–35.

86. Rothwell NJ. Annual review prize lecture. Cytokines—killers in the brain? J Phys-iol 1999;514(Pt 1):3–17.

87. Edoff K, Jerregard H. Effects of IL-1beta, IL-6 or LIF on rat sensory neurons co-cultured with fibroblast-like cells. J Neurosci Res 2002;67(2):255–63.

88. Li AJ, Katafuchi T, Oda S, et al. Interleukin-6 inhibits long-term potentiation in rat hippocampal slices. Brain Res 1997;748(1–2):30–8.

89. Vereker E, Campbell V, Roche E, et al. Lipopolysaccharide inhibits long term potentiation in the rat dentate gyrus by activating caspase-1. J Biol Chem 2000;275(34):26252–8.

90. Kelly A, Vereker E, Nolan Y, et al. Activation of p38 plays a pivotal role in the inhibitory effect of lipopolysaccharide and interleukin-1 beta on long term poten-tiation in rat dentate gyrus. J Biol Chem 2003;278(21):19453–62.

91. Lynch AM, Walsh C, Delaney A, et al. Lipopolysaccharide-induced increase in signalling in hippocampus is abrogated by IL-10–a role for IL-1 beta? J Neuro-chem 2004;88(3):635–46.

92. Neumann H, Schweigreiter R, Yamashita T, et al. Tumor necrosis factor inhibits neurite outgrowth and branching of hippocampal neurons by a rho-dependent mechanism. J Neurosci 2002;22(3):854–62.

93. Rozovsky I, Wei M, Morgan TE, et al. Reversible age impairments in neurite outgrowth by manipulations of astrocytic GFAP. Neurobiol Aging 2005;26(5): 705–15.

94. Gould E, Gross CG. Neurogenesis in adult mammals: some progress and prob-lems. J Neurosci 2002;22(3):619–23.

95. van Praag H, Schinder AF, Christie BR, et al. Functional neurogenesis in the adult hippocampus. Nature 2002;415(6875):1030–4.

96. Ekdahl CT, Claasen JH, Bonde S, et al. Inflammation is detrimental for neurogen-esis in adult brain. Proc Natl Acad Sci U S A 2003;100(23):13632–7.

97. Finch CE, Crimmins EM. Inflammatory exposure and historical changes in human life-spans. Science 2004;305(5691):1736–9.

98. Boisse L, Mouihate A, Ellis S, et al. Long-term alterations in neuroimmune responses after neonatal exposure to lipopolysaccharide. J Neurosci 2004; 24(21):4928–34.

99. Shanks N, Windle RJ, Perks PA, et al. Early-life exposure to endotoxin alters hypothalamic-pituitary-adrenal function and predisposition to inflammation. Proc Natl Acad Sci U S A 2000;97(10):5645–50.

100. Sternberg EM, Hill JM, Chrousos GP, et al. Inflammatory mediator-induced hypothalamic-pituitary-adrenal axis activation is defective in streptococcal cell wall arthritis-susceptible Lewis rats. Proc Natl Acad Sci U S A 1989;86(7): 2374–8.

101. Bilbo SD, Levkoff LH, Mahoney JH, et al. Neonatal infection induces memory impairments following an immune challenge in adulthood. Behav Neurosci 2005;119(1):293–301.

102. Murray CA, Clements MP, Lynch MA. Interleukin-1 induces lipid peroxidation and membrane changes in rat hippocampus: an age-related study. Gerontology 1999;45(3):136–42.

103. Ye S, Johnson RW. Regulation of interleukin-6 gene expression in brain of aged mice by nuclear factor kappaB. J Neuroimmunol 2001;117(1–2):87–96.

104. Ye SM, Johnson RW. Increased interleukin-6 expression by microglia from brain of aged mice. J Neuroimmunol 1999;93(1-2):139–48.

105. Fattori E, Lazzaro D, Musiani P, et al. IL-6 expression in neurons of transgenic mice causes reactive astrocytosis and increase in ramified microglial cells but no neuronal damage. Eur J Neurosci 1995;7(12):2441–9.

106. Bonni A, Sun Y, Nadal-Vicens M, et al. Regulation of gliogenesis in the central nervous system by the JAK-STAT signaling pathway. Science 1997;278(5337): 477–83.

107. Beckman KB, Ames BN. The free radical theory of aging matures. Physiol Rev 1998;78(2):547–81.

108. Mattson MP, Chan SL, Duan W. Modification of brain aging and neurodegenerative disorders by genes, diet, and behavior. Physiol Rev 2002;82(3):637–72.

109. Richwine AF, Godbout JP, Berg BM, et al. Improved psychomotor performance in aged mice fed diet high in antioxidants is associated with reduced ex vivo brain interleukin-6 production. Brain Behav Immun 2005;19(6):512–20.

110. Lee CK, Klopp RG, Weindruch R, et al. Gene expression profile of aging and its retardation by caloric restriction. Science 1999;285(5432):1390–3.

111. Blalock EM, Chen KC, Sharrow K, et al. Gene microarrays in hippocampal aging: statistical profiling identifies novel processes correlated with cognitive impairment. J Neurosci 2003;23(9):3807–19.

112. Lenczowski MJ, Bluthe RM, Roth J, et al. Central administration of rat IL-6 induces HPA activation and fever but not sickness behavior in rats. Am J Physiol 1999;276(3 Pt 2):R652–8.

113. Bluthe RM, Michaud B, Poli V, et al. Role of IL-6 in cytokine-induced sickness behavior: a study with IL-6 deficient mice. Physiol Behav 2000;70(3–4):367–73.

114. Godbout JP, Berg BM, Kelley KW, et al. Alpha-tocopherol reduces lipopolysaccharide-induced peroxide radical formation and interleukin-6 secretion in primary murine microglia and in brain. J Neuroimmunol 2004;149(1–2):101–9.

115. Berg BM, Godbout JP, Kelley KW, et al. Alpha-tocopherol attenuates lipopolysaccharide-induced sickness behavior in mice. Brain Behav Immun 2004; 18(2):149–57.

116. Berg BM, Godbout JP, Chen J, et al. (Alpha)-tocopherol and selenium facilitate recovery from lipopolysaccharide-induced sickness in aged mice. J Nutr 2005; 135(5):1157–63.

117. Godbout JP, Berg BM, Krzyszton C, et al. Alpha-tocopherol attenuates NFkappaB activation and pro-inflammatory cytokine production in brain and improves recovery from lipopolysaccharide-induced sickness behavior. J Neuroimmunol 2005;169:97–105.

118. Nadjar A, Bluthe RM, May MJ, et al. Inactivation of the cerebral NFkappaB pathway inhibits interleukin-1beta-induced sickness behavior and c-Fos expression in various brain nuclei. Neuropsychopharmacology 2005;30(8):1492–9.

119. Meydani SN, Leka LS, Fine BC, et al. Vitamin E and respiratory tract infections in elderly nursing home residents: a randomized controlled trial. JAMA 2004; 292(7):828–36.

Psychoneuroimmune Implications of Type 2 Diabetes: Redux

Jason C. O'Connor, PhD[a], Daniel R. Johnson, PhD[a],
Gregory G. Freund, MD[b],*

KEYWORDS

- Cytokine • Fever • Inflammation • Insulin resistance
- Macrophage • Mental health • Obesity • Sickness behavior

The pyschoneuroimmune (PNI) response can be broadly described as the "brain-based" component of innate immune activation. When the innate immune system is triggered, cytokines are elicited that orchestrate the physiologic, metabolic, behavioral, and psychological changes that occur in an individual as a result of infection. Then, like a counterweight, negative regulation of these pathways restores homeostatic balance. A sizable body of knowledge has arisen demonstrating that type 2 diabetes (T2D) is associated with alterations in the innate immune system. In addition, this proinflammatory-leaning imbalance is implicated in the development of secondary disease complications and comorbidities, such as delayed wound healing, accelerated progress of atherosclerosis, and retinopathy, in people who have T2D. The consequences of T2D-associated proinflammation on the PNI response has only of late become recognized. New experimental data and the results of recently published health-related quality-of-life surveys indicate that individuals who have T2D experience diminished feelings of happiness, well being, and satisfaction with life. These emotional and psychological consequences of T2D point to altered neuroimmunity as a previously unappreciated complication of T2D. This review article discusses recent data detailing the impact of T2D on a person's PNI response.

This article is a version of an article previously published in *Neurologic Clinics*: Roth J, Rummel C, Barth SW, Gerstberger R, Hubschle T. Molecular aspects of fever and hyperthermia. Neurol Clin 2006;24(3):421–39.

This research was supported by grants from the National Institutes of Health (DK64862 and NS58525, to G.G.F.) and University of Illinois Agricultural Experiment Station (to G.G.F.)

[a] Department of Animal Sciences, University of Illinois, 1201 West Gregory Drive, Urbana, IL 61801, USA

[b] Department of Pathology, 190 Medical Sciences Building, MC-714, 506 South Mathews Avenue, University of Illinois at Urbana-Champaign, Urbana, IL 61801, USA

* Corresponding author.

E-mail address: freun@illinois.edu (G.G. Freund).

TYPE 2 DIABETES

Diabetes is a widespread disease of impaired glucose metabolism that can be divided into two major categories. Type 1 diabetes (T1D) occurs when insulin, the primary hormone that increases tissue uptake of circulating blood glucose, is absent. Sometimes, T1D is referred to as insulin-dependent or juvenile-onset diabetes, and its cause is typically an autoimmune-based destruction of insulin-secreting pancreatic beta cells. T2D, also known as noninsulin dependent or adult-onset diabetes, is the more prevalent form of diabetes, affecting more than 23.6 million individuals in the United States.[1] T2D accounts for 85% to 90% of all cases of diabetes.[2] In fact, the prevalence of T2D is predicted to grow to affect upward of 300 million people globally during the next decade.[3] Typically, the onset of T2D occurs after age 30, and there is a significant genetic component. The concordance rate among identical twins is nearly 100%,[4] whereas first-degree relatives of people who have T2D have a 20% to 40% chance of developing T2D.[5]

T2D is a multifaceted disease that is associated with a number of maladies, and effective treatment of T2D and its associated complications is made difficult because of the complex and poorly understood disease progression. Data indicate that diabetes develops over the course of decades[2] and the elevated risk of complications begins many years before the clinical diagnosis of diabetes is made.[6] Overt T2D is preceded by a number of underlying conditions, such as insulin resistance, impaired glucose tolerance (IGT),[2,7] subclinical proinflammation,[8] and metabolic syndrome.[2] Developing diabetes, which is indicated by the presence of insulin resistance and IGT, often goes undetected because of the body's ability to compensate. Euglycemia is usually maintained for many years, even though a state of insulin resistance exists. When the ability of insulin-sensitive tissues to uptake glucose starts to decline, the pancreatic beta cells can increase their output of insulin to compensate for diminished tissue sensitivity and rising blood glucose. With increasing insulin resistance, beta cells are unable to compensate. Even at this extreme, normal fasting glucose levels are often maintained, but individuals begin to experience bouts of postprandial hyperglycemia, hence, IGT.[2]

T2D is strongly associated with a sedentary lifestyle and obesity.[9,10] In addition, a recent downward shift in onset age[2] and a rise in the incidence in Asian populations, which traditionally have lower rates of obesity,[2,11] suggest that other precipitating factors may be involved. Early detection of diabetes is paramount for reducing associated morbidity and mortality rates because progression of T2D often goes undetected as a result of a lack of routine screening during the "prediabetic" IGT period.

T2D is associated with a long list of complications, including increased risk of cerebrovascular and cardiovascular disease, impaired wound healing, increased susceptibility to infection, and increased incidence of Alzheimer disease.[1,12–19] The mechanism by which T2D accelerates and exacerbates the development of these conditions is not fully understood; however, the close relationship between these disease states and T2D suggests a shared common pathogenic precursor.[20] One likely suspect is chronic inflammation because many diabetic complications, including altered psychoneuroimmunity, have an inflammatory component to their pathology. Overall, T2D is now considered to be a proinflammatory disease involving chronic activation of the innate immune system,[3,21] likely impinging on quality of life. For people who have T2D, health-related quality-of-life assessments show lower satisfaction than for control subjects,[22] especially in regard to negative impact on the emotional attribute, which measures perceived happiness.[23] In sum, T2D not only debilitates physically but also depresses emotional health and well-being.

TYPE 2 DIABETES AS A PROINFLAMMATORY DISEASE

The relationship between T2D and the innate immune system is bidirectional. Dysregulated innate immunity characterized by persistent, subclinical, chronic inflammation is intimately associated with the insulin-resistant state, obesity, and T2D.[24–26] Most evidence indicates that chronic inflammation directly contributes to the pathogenesis of T2D.[8,24,26–32] Historically, the concept that inflammation is associated with insulin resistance has been explored for more than 20 years.[33,34] More recently, Pickup[21] and Crook[3] advanced the hypothesis that T2D is a disease of the innate immune system. This hypothesis was based on findings in a large number of individuals who had T2D and who showed subtle elevations in proinflammatory biomarkers and acute phase reactants, including interleukin-1β (IL-1β), tumor necrosis factor–α (TNFα), IL-6, sialic acid, serum amyloid, C-reactive protein, and cortisol.[3,21,29,35–37] In addition, prospective studies showed that alterations in C-reactive protein and IL-6 predict the development of T2D in human subjects,[37] as do elevations in the acute-phase reactants fibrinogen and plasminogen activator inhibitor (PAI)-1.[38]

Recent T2D work has solidified our understanding of the mechanism by which chronic inflammation can cause insulin resistance. Cai and colleagues[32] reported that NF-κB and inflammatory transcriptional targets are activated in the liver by both diet-induced obesity and genetic-onset obesity. Moreover, they were able to reproduce similar changes in the hepatic inflammatory profile by selectively expressing a constitutively active IKK-β in hepatocytes, which, in turn, caused mice to exhibit a T2D phenotype. The activation of the NF-κB pathway resulted in increased hepatic production of TNF-α, IL-1β, and IL-6. Also, Cai and colleagues[32] neutralized IL-6, systemically reversing the T2D phenotype. In support of Cai and colleagues, Arkan and colleagues[31] selectively knocked out IKK-β in either hepatocytes or myeloid cells. Hepatocyte-specific deletion of IKK-β preserved hepatic insulin sensitivity resulting from a high-fat diet, genetic obesity, or aging. However, deletion of IKK-β in myeloid cells resulted in global protection of insulin sensitivity resulting from a high-fat diet, genetic obesity, or aging.[31] These results underscore the potential importance of myeloid cells (monocytes and macrophages) to chronic inflammation-induced insulin resistance.

On the other hand, there is still some uncertainty as to whether chronic inflammation leads to insulin resistance or whether insulin insensitivity brings about a condition of chronic inflammation. Symptoms inherent to T2D, such as hyperglycemia, hyperinsulinemia, and insulin resistance, can independently induce proinflammation by way of dysregulation of macrophage activation. In diet-induced obesity, overnutrition and increased fat mass result in infiltration of macrophages into adipose tissue, where adipokines, low levels of oxygen, or adipocyte apoptosis may stimulate macrophages to secrete proinflammatory cytokines.[25,26,39] Proinflammatory cytokines such as TNF-α[36,40] and IL-6[41–44] induce insulin resistance in a number of tissues, and insulin resistance leads to IGT. In turn, hyperglycemia[45,46] and hyperinsulinemia[47] independently induce proinflammation, as measured by IL-6 secretion,[48] and heightened acute inflammatory responses to stimuli like lipopolysaccharide (LPS).[49] In healthy subjects, insulin inhibits acute-phase protein synthesis,[21] and, in animal models of T2D, the acute-phase response is increased by the relative insulin deficiency that results from insulin resistance.[21,50] Hyperglycemia has been postulated to play a role in the generation of acute-phase proteins and the inflammatory response[51,52] because treatments that both increase insulin sensitivity and lower blood glucose levels reduce the levels of serum acute-phase proteins.[52,53] Additionally, macrophage function, which plays a crucial role in the inflammatory response as an initiating event of the neuroimmune response, is altered by hyperinsulinemia and hyperglycemia.[49,54–59] Diabetes-associated alterations in the innate immune response have primarily been described within the context of the peripheral complications of T2D. Not only does the proinflammation observed with insulin resistance likely contribute to accelerated progression of T2D and its complications but it also likely exacerbates PNI-based sequelae, negatively impacting the emotional well-being and quality of life for patients who have diabetes.

THE PSYCHONEUROIMMUNE RESPONSE

The PNI response, or brain-based innate immune reaction, is initiated by infection with pathogenic microorganisms that trigger, in the host, a set of immunologic, physiologic, metabolic, and behavioral responses mediated by innate immune cells that recognize pathogen-associated molecular patterns by way of Toll-like receptors (TLRs). LPS is an archetypal, pathogen-associated molecular pattern and a component of gram-negative bacterial cell walls. LPS binds to TLR-4 and CD-14 on the surface membrane of monocytes and macrophages. The proinflammatory cytokines that are produced as a result of subsequent TLR-4–dependent NF-κB pathway activation are part of a cytokine network that includes both proinflammatory and anti-inflammatory cytokines. These anti-inflammatory cytokines can specifically inhibit a single proinflammatory cytokine. For instance, IL-1 receptor antagonist (IL-1ra) binds to the IL-1 receptor 1 to competitively block IL-1–mediated signaling, or these anti-inflammatory cytokines can nonspecifically down-regulate production or action of proinflammatory cytokines, for instance, IL-4 and IL-10, reduce the secretion of IL-1β, IL-6, and TNF-α by macrophages.[60] Importantly, dysregulated or excessive inflammation can exacerbate pre-existent disease states[61,62] and profoundly depress a person's mood and feeling of well-being,[63,64] The possible association between heightened peripheral inflammation and central inflammation has only recently been systematically tested in animal models of T2D, despite the obvious clinical implications.

FEVER

Fever is one of the host defense mechanisms against infection, injury, and inflammation. Fever is an adaptive homeostatic state that is characterized by an increased set point in body temperature.[65] Elevated body temperature stimulates the proliferation of immune cells and is unfavorable for the growth of many bacteria and viruses.[66] When exogenous pyrogens (experimentally represented by LPS) invade the organism, fever is caused through the activation of myeloid cells that subsequently release endogenous pyrogens, proinflammatory cytokines, prostaglandins, and free radicals. This is of clinical importance because cytokine immunotherapy, which can activate cytokine cascades, is also associated with fever.[67] Importantly, evidence indicates that both peripheral and brain-based IL-1β and TNF-α are involved directly in the pyrogenic response to inflammation.[68–70] In the periphery, IL-1β and TNF-α cause increased production of IL-6, the principal endogenous pyrogen.[69] The liver is the main clearance organ for circulating LPS.[71–73] Kupffer cells account for 80% to 90% of the total population of fixed tissue macrophages in the body[74,75] and are believed to be responsible for the liver's clearance of LPS. Additionally, Kupffer cells may be a principle producer of cytokines and, hence, the fever induced by LPS.[76] Therefore, altered peripheral macrophage function caused by T2D likely has a pronounced effect on the febrile response.

The effect of insulin resistance has been studied in the Zucker (fa/fa) rat model of obesity and T2D.[77] In this study, various cytokines were infused directly into the lateral ventricle of the brains by way of a surgically implanted cannula. The obese rats exhibited a differential febrile response to the pyrogenic cytokine IL-1. They reached a peak febrile temperature that was about 0.5°C higher than that of their lean counterparts, and interestingly, the febrile response of these obese rats persisted over a longer duration than did that of the control lean rats. A second independent study using both fa/fa rats and Otsuka Long-Evans Tokushima fatty rats (which are obese because of the absence of the cholecystokinin-A receptor) also demonstrated a febrile response to intravenous *Escherichia coli*–derived LPS, which trended higher in obese animals when compared with lean counterparts.[78] It is important to point out that some conflicting data have been reported regarding the effect of obesity and T2D on febrile responsiveness because changes in ambient temperature alter the fever response in fa/fa rats,[79] and IL-6 administered directly into the brain does not induce a higher fever in obese rats.[77] These findings underscore the importance of the experimental conditions, presence of specific exogenous pyrogen, and method of administration of the exogenous pyrogen in making an interpretation of data regarding an effect of T2D on febrile responsiveness.

In their laboratory, the authors used the *db/db* (C57BL/6 J-lepr^db/db^) mouse model of T2D. The *db/db* mouse displays characteristic hyperphagia, metabolic dysfunction, morbid obesity, and neuroendocrine abnormalities that parallel uncontrolled human T2D (**Table 1**). Using this model, the authors observed exacerbated febrile responsiveness to intraperitoneal LPS in diabetic mice compared with nondiabetic, heterozygote control (*db/+*) mice (**Fig 1**). When 8-week-old *db/db* mice and *db/+* mice were injected intraperitoneally with LPS, LPS-induced fever was significantly increased in *db/db* mice compared with *db/+* mice. The peak change in colonic temperature as measured using a rectally inserted thermocouple was 1.5°C for *db/db* mice but only 0.6°C for *db/+* mice. In addition, *db/db* mice had a marked extension in the duration of fever compared with *db/+* mice. Together, these results indicate that the febrile responsiveness, an important aspect of brain-based innate immunity is exacerbated in an experimental model of T2D.

SICKNESS BEHAVIOR

LPS is a potent activator of the neuroimmune system,[80] and LPS-induced sickness has been is a key tool in PNI research. Sickness behavior refers to a coordinated

Table 1
Comparisons of body weight, blood glucose levels, and serum insulin levels for db/+ mice and Db/db mice, with Db/db mice showing elevated body weight, blood glucose levels, and serum insulin levels

Characteristic (Measurement)	db/+ Mice	db/db Mice
Body weight (g)	27.6 ± 0.55	36.7 ± 0.57[a]
FBG (mg/dl)	115.2 ± 19.08	400.4 ± 15.35[a]
RBG (mg/dl)	169.8 ± 12.23	423.0 ± 17.84[a]
FSI (ng/ml)	1.3 ± 0.05	2.4 ± 0.05[a]
RSI (ng/ml)	2.2 ± 0.08	5.4 ± 0.09[a]

Results represent the average of n = 5 mice ± SEM.
Abbreviations: FBG, fasting blood glucose; FSI, fasting serum insulin; RBG, random blood glucose; RSI, random serum insulin.
[a] $P<.05$.
From O'Connor JC, Satpathy A, Hartman ME, et al. IL-1beta-mediated innate immunity is amplified in the db/db mouse model of type 2 diabetes. J Immunol 2005;174;4993; with permission. Copyright © 2005, The American Association of Immunologists, Inc.

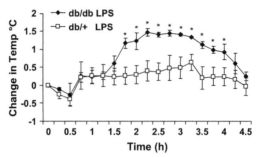

Fig. 1. Febrile response to lipopolysaccharide (LPS) in *db/db* mice. 8-week-old db/db and db/+ mice were injected intraperitoneally with LPS (100 μg/kg). Colonic temperature was measured at the times indicated. Data represent an average of five mice per group ± SEM. P<.05 *db/db* versus *db/+*.

set of nonspecific behavioral modifications that occur in individuals during an infection.[66,81–84] Sickness behavior is typically accompanied by fever and a variety of behavioral responses, including decreased appetite, fatigue, sleep disturbances, retardation of motor activity, reduced interest in the physical and social environment, loss of libido, impaired cognitive abilities, anhedonia, and depressed mood.[66,85,86] Although these behavioral changes are often interpreted to be an unavoidable consequence of a degraded state, increasing evidence suggests that these cytokine-mediated symptoms are part of an organized and evolutionarily conserved adaptive defense response to infection. Sickness behavior reflects motivational reorganization whereby the individual's priorities are restructured to maximize the immune system's efficiency in fighting infection. The main proinflammatory cytokines responsible for the initiation of the host's behavioral response to infection are IL-1β, IL-6, and TNF-α.[81,87] These cytokines are secreted by activated monocytes and macrophages. However, as in models of experimental stroke, brain IL-1β appears to be the predominant cytokine that mediates sickness behavior,[87,88] because intracerebroventricular administration of IL-1ra blocks some sickness behaviors caused by peripheral or central innate immune system activation.[89,90]

Of clinical importance, these behavioral responses have been observed during the course of infection and also during systemic or central administration of cytokines. Cancer therapies involving treatment using proinflammatory or antiviral cytokines (mainly IL-2, TNF-α, and IFN-α) have been associated with flu-like and depressive symptoms, and signs of cognitive impairment.[91] Administration of IFN-α, which has been used in the treatment of chronic hepatitis C, is associated with symptoms of cognitive impairment, behavioral despair, fatigue, and depressed mood.[91] The symptoms of sickness behavior almost immediately disappear after termination of cytokine administration, supporting a causal role for cytokines in the mediation of these behaviorally based sequelae. Therefore, patients who have T2D, or even some prediabetic risk factors, may not only experience more debilitating conditions during an illness or infection but also may not tolerate immunotherapy as well. The heightened PNI responses may also interfere with a patient's diabetes treatment regimen because depressed mood or loss of the feeling of well-being is also a strong predictor of patient noncompliance with a prescribed course of therapy.[92,93]

LPS-induced social withdrawal is a classic behavioral feature of the innate immune response that is routinely used as a quantitative measure in rodents because of a large and repeatable change in interaction patterns that is easy to measure.[66] When tested in the *db/db* mice, LPS-induced sickness behavior was significantly augmented compared with that of nondiabetic control mice. Consistent with the experimental results showing the impact of T2D on the febrile response, the *db/db* mice were more sensitive to the behavioral effects of intraperitoneal LPS. Using a weight-adjusted dose of LPS, both the magnitude and duration of sickness behavior were exacerbated in the *db/db* mice. However, although a dose of 100 µg/kg LPS is commonly used in the study of sickness in rodents, under these conditions the *db/db* mice would receive a significantly larger dose of LPS because of their obesity-associated increase in body weight.[49] Clearance of LPS from the peritoneal cavity occurs primarily by way of the peritoneal lymphatic system and hematogenously by way of the portal vein.[94] Because abdominally based inflammation uses the vagus nerve to communicate with the brain, locally elevated LPS levels in the peritoneum (resulting from a weight-based strategy of LPS administration) would likely artificially heighten sickness behavior in obese mice versus thin mice. Therefore, LPS-dependent behavioral changes using a fixed dose of LPS were examined. Interestingly, these data also showed an exacerbated sickness behavior response in the *db/db* mice in which recovery from sickness was significantly delayed.[49] The *db/db* mice, also, had a significant increase in peritoneal levels of IL-1β and diminished up-regulation of the important IL-1 negative regulatory molecules, IL-1ra and IL-1R2 (the IL-1 decoy receptor), in both the periphery and the brain.[49] The importance of these studies is that they were the first to show decreased ability to recover from brain-based innate immune activation in a mouse model of T2D.

Heightened brain-based immune responsiveness has been identified in the nonobese diabetic mouse (a model of T1D),[95] indicating that both T1D and T2D (ie, diabetes in general) are associated with dysregulated neuroimmunity. Hence, altered central innate immunity may be a common feature or possibly a complication of diabetes. The mechanism responsible for neuroimmune dysregulation in diabetes is likely hyperglycemia. The authors showed that in a mouse model of T1D, LPS-dependent social withdrawal was augmented and reliant on elevated blood glucose.[96] T1D was induced in mice using streptozotocin, a potent, pancreatic, beta-cell toxin that in 4 days causes blood glucose levels to exceed 400 mg/dL.[96] When T1D mice were challenged using LPS, LPS-induced social withdrawal was more than double that of nondiabetic mice. Examination of peritoneal proinflammatory cytokine levels 2 hours after LPS administration showed that diabetic mice had 4-, 2.5- and 3.6-fold greater concentrations of IL-1β, IL-6, and TNF-α, respectively, compared with nondiabetic mice. Control of blood glucose levels moderated the LPS-induced social withdrawal. Finally, administration of streptozotocin to hyperglycemic and hyperinsulinemic *db/db* mice did not alter the LPS-induced social withdrawal.[96] Together, these findings indicate that mice that have T1D have augmented sickness in response to innate immune challenge that is caused by hyperglycemia and not by hyperinsulinemia.

Overall, most conditions with an inflammatory component that is comorbid with diabetes are made more ominous by also having T2D. For example, delayed wound healing has long been recognized as a complication of T2D. In rodents, prolonged secretion of proinflammatory cytokines is identified at the wound site in T2D mice.[97] Likewise, in experimental animal models of cerebral ischemia, diabetic mice suffer more severe damage and have poorer outcomes compared with nondiabetic mice. The authors showed that acute hypoxia triggers neuroimmune system activation, causing loss of interest in the social environment, and that recovery from hypoxia-induced neuroimmune system activation was impaired in the *db/db* mouse model of T2D.[98] Importantly, recovery from the behavioral consequences of acute hypoxia was nearly ablated in mice that lack IL-1R1 signaling and in mice that were intracerebroventricularly administered a caspase-1 inhibitor that blocks conversion of pro-IL-1β to IL-1β. Diabetic mice had prolonged recovery from neuroimmune system activation caused by the loss of brain-based up-regulation of IL-1ra and IL-1R2, but the speed of behavioral recovery could be doubled by administration of subcutaneous IL-1ra to these mice.[98] Such results demonstrate that acute hypoxia activates the IL-1 arm of the neuroimmune system, which diabetes exacerbates because of brain-based loss of IL-1 counter-regulation, and that treatment with IL-1ra ameliorates that condition.

On the flip side, anti-inflammatory cytokines have effectively been used to attenuate the behavioral changes that occur during immune activation. Central administration of recombinant IL-1ra,[89] IL-10,[95] IL-4,[99] and insulin-like growth factor–1 (IGF-1)[100,101] dampens the sickness behavior response induced by activation of the innate immune system. Importantly, the authors found that IGF-1 attenuates sickness behavior in response to peripheral LPS challenge in db/+ mice.[101] Although db/db mouse perito-neal macrophages elaborate more proinflammatory cytokines, they also, as noted previously in this article, fail to up-regulate two key counter-regulators of IL-1 in response to LPS: IL-1ra and IL-1R2.[49] In addition, this failure to up-regulate IL-1ra and IL-1R2 occurs not only in microbial-based innate immune activation (ie, LPS) but also during nonmicrobial-based innate immune activation (ie, acute hypoxia).[98] Thus, an imbalance in IL-1–based proinflammation and anti-inflammation appears key to T2D-associated dysregulated neuroimmunity. However, the story is not quite so simple because of an important difference between T2D in humans and the db/db mouse model of T2D; the absence of functional leptin signaling in db/db mice. In a recent article, the authors reported that leptin is key to acute hypoxia recovery because it dramatically augments IL-1ra production in mice.[102] In fact, leptin appears to be a more potent inducer of IL-1ra than hypoxia. In leptin-receptor-defective (db/db) and leptin-deficient (ob/ob) mice, recovery from hypoxia was delayed, and in ob/ob mice, leptin administration completely reversed this delayed recovery. In addi-tion, leptin administration to normal mice cut recovery time from hypoxia by one third and, in turn, boosted levels of serum IL-1ra. Finally, administration of leptin failed to alter hypoxia recovery in IL-1ra knockout mice.[102] These results show that by enhancing IL-1ra production, administration of leptin promoted sickness recovery from hypoxia, but they also suggest that diabetes in humans may be different because it is often associated with up-regulation of IL-1ra.[103]

HUMORAL AND NEURAL ROUTES COMMUNICATE IMMUNE STATUS TO THE BRAIN

Activated macrophages are the primary cellular source of IL-1β, TNF-α, and IL-6, and these proinflammatory cytokines are key to the communication between the immune system and the brain.[104] There are a number of different routes by which the periph-erally-generated cytokines may communicate with the brain.[87] The first of these routes involves the circumventricular organs, those regions of the brain that lack a fully intact blood-brain barrier (BBB). In these organs, cytokines can freely diffuse from the blood into the brain parenchyma, where they then may interact with macrophages.[104] Another route by which cytokines communicate with the brain is across the intact BBB. Blood-borne cytokines may interact with endothelial cells, which, in turn, signal perivascular macrophages located on the brain side of the BBB. Cytokines can also be actively transported across the BBB by way of a saturable transporter mechanism.[105] Regardless of the signal, when activated, perivascular macrophages can communi-cate with microglia, which are the resident macrophages of the brain.

Another route facilitates communication between the periphery and brain. Locally, peripheral inflammation is initially communicated to the brain by way of afferent vagus nerve fibers, which results in up-regulation of glial cell–derived proinflammatory cytokines in the brain.[66] Sensory vagal afferent terminals express receptors for IL-1, and following peripheral activation of the innate immune system, increased expression of c-fos occurs in the brain in the projection areas of the vagus. Subdiaphragmatic vagotomy in rodents prevents both behavioral depression and activation of the limbic system following intraperitoneal administration of LPS or recombinant IL-1β.[106] Induction of central IL-1β expression by using peripheral LPS or IL-1β is blocked in vagotomized animals, but when IL-1β is injected centrally, vagotomy has no effect on the activation of the brain-based innate immune response.[106] Recently, the relative contribution of the humoral versus neural communication pathways in mediating PNI has been debated, because subdiaphagmatic vagotomy does not block all aspects of the PNI response.[107] Therefore, cytokines mediate immune-system-to-brain communication in a complex, and often redundant, network that involves both neural and humoral components.

The various cytokines affecting the brain have two possible origins. First, cytokines originating from the peripheral immune organs can cross the BBB. Stimulation of the peripheral immune system could signal the brain in both a local and a systemic manner. Cytokines can reach the central nervous system directly by crossing at accessible areas in the BBB through the circumventricular organs.[108] This was demonstrated by the appearance of significant quantities of human recombinant IL-1 in mouse cortex after its subcutaneous injection, without an elevation of mouse IL-1 levels.[109] In addition, there is convincing evidence for the active, saturable, and specific transport of certain cytokines across the BBB.[109,110] Second, cytokines can be produced by cells within the central nervous system. Most of the cytokines and their receptors have been identified in various cell types of the central nervous system in both healthy and diseased states. It is believed that cytokines produced by neurons and glial cells within the brain participate in the complex autonomic, neuroendocrine, metabolic, and behavioral responses to infection, inflammation, ischemia, and other brain injuries.[111–113]

TYPE 2 DIABETES AFFECTS THE BLOOD-BRAIN BARRIER

As one of the primary interfaces between cytokines and the brain, the BBB has also been shown, in a few reports, to be compromised in cases of T2D. Normally, the BBB refers to a specialized feature of the brain's capillary bed, in which capillaries are connected via tight junctions. Brain endothelial cells have a significantly lower rate of endocytosis and lack nearly all intracellular pores spanning the capillary walls. These features help prevent the uncontrolled entry of blood-borne molecules into the brain.[114] MRI has shown that patients who have T2D have increased BBB permeability compared with healthy controls subjects.[115] Experimentally, streptozotocin-induced diabetes in rats was recently shown to increase BBB permeability, and treatment of these diabetic rats using statins (a class of cholesterol-lowering pharmaceutics) reduced BBB permeability.[116] In animal models that had insulin deficiency and marked hyperglycemia, there was a regionally specific decrease in cerebral blood flow (CBF), which may be a compensatory or protective mechanism. Duckrow and colleagues[117] found that hindbrain blood flow was more reduced than forebrain blood flow. Moreover, decreased regional CBF was dependent acutely and chronically on the degree of hyperglycemia. In these studies, an osmotic effect as a possible cause was eliminated because control experiments using mannitol showed no CBF change.

The results of studies of CBF in people who had hyperglycemia and hypoglycemia are more inconsistent that those of animal studies, which may be the result of the extreme glucose ranges that are often seen in animal models. Although the impact of diabetes-associated BBB permeability, specifically on the PNI response, has not been systematically studied, it seems reasonable to hypothesize that compromised BBB integrity may be a pathologic contributor to exacerbated brain-based responses to peripheral immune challenge.

TYPE 2 DIABETES AFFECTS THE SOURCE OF PROINFLAMMATORY CYTOKINES

Macrophage activation, an initial step in cell-based innate immune activation, results in the elaboration of proinflammatory cytokines and has repeatedly been shown to be perturbed in both human and animal studies of T2D. Because cytokines secreted by activated macrophages help direct the brain-based response to infection, diabetes-associated alterations in cytokine secretion caused by macrophages would likely have significant impact on the concomitant metabolic and behavioral changes that ensue. However, in animal models of T2D, the specific model and the experimental conditions being used impacted macrophage bioaction. In human patients who had T2D, circulating monocytes were reported to have increased expression of CD14,[118] which is a coreceptor for LPS. The scavenger receptor, CD36, is also up-regulated in macrophages by T2D.[119] Moreover, data from the authors' laboratory indicate that resident peritoneal macrophages isolated from *db/db* mice elaborate more IL-1β in response to LPS than occurs in nondiabetic mice. The authors found that the peritoneal fluid of *db/db* mice, when exposed to a fixed dose of LPS, had a peak increase in IL-1β concentration more than double that of nondiabetic mice exposed to LPS, and that resident peritoneal macrophages isolated from *db/db* mice produced more IL-1β after LPS stimulation.[49] Naguib and colleagues[97] noted that the inflammatory response to bacteria is prolonged in *db/db* mice as the result of unresolved proinflammatory cytokine expression. Studies conducted using macrophage cell lines[59,120] and primary macrophages[121,122] indicate that the diabetic milieu heightens macrophage responsiveness to innate immune activators like LPS. Contrary reports also exist demonstrating that macrophage activity is diminished by T2D conditions. For example, Zykova and colleagues[123] showed that peritoneal macrophages elicited using thioglycollate from C57BL/KS-lepr-*db/db* mice had a diminished cytokine secretion response to LPS + IFNγ ex vivo.

Hyperglycemia appears to be the predominant factor in making macrophages more responsive to immune stimulation. Several studies involving streptozotocin-induced diabetes in laboratory rodents have found hyperglycemia to cause heightened macrophage activation in response to stimuli, such as LPS. However, in terms of PNI, proinflammatory cytokine expression in the brain is critical in making functional changes in the brain-based response. This has been demonstrated using cytokine receptor knockout mice. Specifically, IL-1 receptor knockout mice are resistant to the behavioral changes normally induced by direct central administration of IL-1 into the lateral ventricle. Studies have confirmed that the degree of hyperglycemia usually observed in cases of T2D does, in fact, augment microglia-mediated inflammatory responses. In the Ins2 (Akita) mouse model of diabetes, hyperglycemic conditions resulted in morphologic changes in retinal microglia consistent with an activated state,[124] and LPS in the presence of high-glucose conditions synergistically increased cytotoxicity in primary rat microglia as a result of increased free radical production.[122] In an experimental model of ischemic stroke, microglia of *db/db* mice exhibited delayed expression of bfl-1, which is an endogenous bcl-2–related inhibitor of apoptosis.[125]

The mechanism by which hyperglycemia enhances macrophage activation is likely the result of an increase in oxidative stress or advanced glycation end products. During states of hyperglycemia, proteins can become nonenzymatically glycosylated, and glycosylated proteins are known to activate macrophages and render cells more susceptible to subsequent cytotoxic events.[126] However, in some models of T2D, like the Ins2 (Akita) or *db/db* mouse, hyperglycemia is associated with an induction of insulin resistance characterized by diminished signal transduction by way of the insulin receptor and insulin receptor substrate (IRS) proteins.[124]

ANTI-INFLAMMATORY CYTOKINE RESISTANCE

As discussed previously in this article, experimental results from animal models of T2D suggest that negative regulation of inflammatory processes is impaired, and chronic inflammation appears to induce a state of insulin resistance, likely mediated through impaired IRS-mediated signaling and increased expression of inhibitory proteins called suppressors of cytokine signaling (SOCS). Normal counter-regulation of proinflammation involves anti-inflammatory cytokines, such as IGF-1, IL-4, IL-10, and IL-13. These cytokines reduce the secretion of proinflammatory cytokines by macrophages and stimulate the secretion of a number of anti-inflammatory molecules, such as IL-1ra, IL-1R2, and soluble TNF receptors. IGF-1, IL-4, IL-10, and IL-13 use IRS proteins as a component of their own tyrosine phosphorylation signaling pathways. Importantly, up-regulation of SOCS proteins would inhibit certain actions of these anti-inflammatory cytokines because SOCS proteins recognize and bind to tyrosine phosphorylated motifs on membrane receptors to inhibit downstream signal amplification. Therefore, it is likely that during insulin-resistant states, there also exists a degree of anti-inflammatory cytokine resistance, which compounds the inflammation inherent to diabetes-associated hyperglycemia.

In vivo data demonstrate the diminished ability of anti-inflammatory molecules to attenuate the PNI response.[101] The hypothesis of diabetes-induced resistance to anti-inflammatory cytokines was described by Hartman and colleagues.[54] In this study, T2D conditions resulted in impaired IRS-2–mediated signal transduction in both a macrophage cell line and primary macrophages. Interestingly, the anti-inflammatory molecules IL-4 and IGF-1 showed diminished ability to signal by way of this shared pathway. In turn, others researchers showed that IRS-2–deficient lymphocytes have a diminished capacity to secrete TH2 cytokines.[127] Although the specific impact of SOCS up-regulation on PNI is not clear, SOCS proteins likely play an important role in diabetes-associated resistance to the immunologic effects of IL-10, IL-4, and IGF-1. The ability of IGF-1 to attenuate LPS-induced sickness behavior is impaired in *db/db* mice,[101] and SOCS proteins are up-regulated in number of models of T2D.[128,129] In addition, the authors were the first to report the relevance of the IL-4/IRS-2/phosphatidylinositide (PI3 K) pathway in macrophages by showing that IL-4–dependent elaboration of IL-1ra requires IRS-2–mediated PI3 K activity in primary macrophages.[130] The authors also demonstrated that macrophages isolated from *db/db* mice have impaired IRS-2–mediated PI3 K activity and constitutively overexpress SOCS-3. Examination of IL-4 signaling in *db/db* macrophages revealed that IL-4–dependent IRS-2/PI3 K complex formation and IRS-2 tyrosine phosphorylation were reduced compared with that of *db/+* macrophages. SOCS-3/IL-4 receptor complexes, however, were increased in *db/db* mouse macrophages compared with those of *db/+* mouse macrophages, as was *db/db* mouse macrophage SOCS-3 expression. These results indicate that in the *db/db* mouse model of T2D, macrophage expression of SOCS-3 is increased, resulting in impaired IL-4–dependent IRS-2/PI3 K formation that induces a state of IL-4 resistance, disrupting IL-4–dependent production of IL-1ra. More studies, however, are needed to delineate the role of SOCS up-regulation in T2D-assocaited PNI because, as mentioned previously in this article, the *db/db* mouse model of T2D is significantly different than for people who have diabetes.

HYPOTHALAMIC–PITUITARY–ADRENAL AXIS

One of the methods of central nervous system regulation of innate immunity is by neuroendocrine control of immunocompetent cells by way of the hypothalamic–pituitary–adrenal (HPA) axis. In the HPA axis, the hypothalamus acts as a master gland, exhibiting control over the network. The bidirectional communication of the neuroendocrine and immune systems is achieved by the actions of proinflammatory cytokines such as IL-1β, TNF-α, and IL-6, which are potent triggers to the HPA axis. Receptors for IL-1 have been identified in the hypothalamus, and IL-1β has been shown to induce the release of adrenocorticotropic hormone (ACTH) indirectly via corticotropin releasing factor in a dose-dependent manner.[131] It has been suggested that a negative feedback loop on macrophage IL-1 secretion is mediated by the HPA axis and sympathetic nervous system by the actions of central IL-1β.[132] The primary route of HPA activation by the actions of peripheral IL-1β appears to be accomplished by the stimulation of vagal afferents.[133]

Glucocorticoids inhibit the production of IL-1β via a negative feedback loop.[134] In fact, glucocorticoids serve as critical negative regulators of all myeloid cells.[135] Glucocorticoids, which are often released in response to stress, have anti-inflammatory and immunosuppressive effects. They not only negatively regulate macrophages but also stimulate the secretion of IL-10.[136] Hypophysectomy, which is the surgical removal of the pituitary, has demonstrated the role of this gland in maintaining proper immune function. Hypophysectomy results in decreased numbers of lymphocytes, decreased antibody response, and reduced thymus and spleen weights.[137] Adrenalectomy results in elevated proinflammatory cytokine expression in both the spleen and the brain in response to LPS[138] and in increased mortality in response to LPS, IL-1β, TNF-α, and infection.[139,140]

A number of studies have identified impaired HPA responsiveness associated with T2D, as reviewed by Chan and colleagues[141] A recent study has shown that hyperinsulinemia, independent of glucose, increased the HPA response in rats and that diabetes significantly impaired the ability of the HPA response to appropriately match the potency of the stressor.[142] T2D is also associated with chronic activation of the HPA axis and hypersecretion of glucocorticoids.[143,144] Chronic elevation of glucocorticoids results in a state of resistance or glucocorticoid insensitivity, causing failure of glucocorticoid-dependent negative feedback.[143,144] Hyperinsulinemia and insulin resistance likely alter the same pathways in the brain that are impacted in peripheral macrophages and tissues.

SUMMARY

The idea that T2D is associated with augmented innate immune function characterized by increased circulating levels of acute phase reactants and altered macrophage biology is well established, even though the mechanisms involved in this complex interaction are still not entirely clear. Initially, the majority of studies investigating innate immune function in cases of T2D were limited to the context of wound healing, atherosclerosis, stroke, and other commonly identified comorbidities. Several important recurring themes, however, have come from these data. First, T2D is associated with a state of chronic, subclinical inflammation. Second, in macrophages, T2D conditions enhance proinflammatory reactions and impair anti-inflammatory responses. Third, recovery from innate immune activation and resolution of inflammation in T2D is impaired. In sum, the impact of diminished emotional well-being on the quality of life for people who have diabetes is significant, and given the importance of inflammation to T2D, PNI-based T2D sequelae should be considered a complication of diabetes that warrant serious clinical attention.

REFERENCES

1. Diabetes facts and figures. American Diabetes Association; 2008. Available at: http://www.diabetes.org/diabetes-statistics.jsp.
2. Zimmet P, Alberti KG, Shaw J. Global and societal implications of the diabetes epidemic. Nature 2001;414(6865):782–7.
3. Crook M. Type 2 diabetes mellitus: a disease of the innate immune system? An update. Diabet Med 2004;21(3):203–7.
4. Sherwin R. In: Bennet J, Plum F, editors. Cecil textbook of medicine. Philadelphia: WB Saunders Company; 1996. p. 1258–77.
5. Crawford JM, Cotran RS. In: Collins T, Kumar V, Cotran RS, editors. Robbins pathologic basis of disease. Philadelphia: W.B. Saunders Company; 1999. p. 913.
6. Zimmet PZ, Alberti KG. The changing face of macrovascular disease in non–insulin-dependent diabetes mellitus: an epidemic in progress. Lancet 1997; 350(Suppl 1):SI1–4.
7. Harris M, Zimmet P. In: Alberti K, Zimmet P, DeFronzo R, editors. International textbook of diabetes mellitus. Chichester: Wiley; 1999. p. 9–23.
8. Spranger J, Kroke A, Mohlig M, et al. Inflammatory cytokines and the risk to develop type 2 diabetes: results of the prospective population-based European Prospective Investigation into Cancer and Nutrition (EPIC)–Potsdam Study. Diabetes 2003;52(3):812–7.
9. Zimmet PZ. Diabetes epidemiology as a tool to trigger diabetes research and care. Diabetologia 1999;42(5):499–518.
10. Zimmet P. Globalization, coca-colonization and the chronic disease epidemic: can the Doomsday scenario be averted? J Intern Med 2000;247(3):301–10.
11. Kitagawa T, Owada M, Urakami T, et al. Increased incidence of non–insulin dependent diabetes mellitus among Japanese schoolchildren correlates with an increased intake of animal protein and fat. Clin Pediatr (Phila) 1998;37(2): 111–5.
12. Muller LM, Gorter KJ, Hak E, et al. Increased risk of common infections in patients with type 1 and type 2 diabetes mellitus. Clin Infect Dis 2005;41(3): 281–8.
13. Mastropaolo MD, Evans NP, Byrnes MK, et al. Synergy in polymicrobial infections in a mouse model of type 2 diabetes. Infect Immun 2005;73(9):6055–63.
14. Taylor SI. Deconstructing type 2 diabetes. Cell 1999;97(1):9–12.
15. Bertoni AG, Saydah S, Brancati FL. Diabetes and the risk of infection-related mortality in the U.S. Diabetes Care 2001;24(6):1044–9.
16. Shah BR, Hux JE. Quantifying the risk of infectious diseases for people with diabetes. Diabetes Care 2003;26(2):510–3.
17. Llorente L, De La Fuente H, Richaud-Patin Y, et al. Innate immune response mechanisms in non–insulin dependent diabetes mellitus patients assessed by flow cytoenzymology. Immunol Lett 2000;74(3):239–44.
18. Geerlings SE, Hoepelman AI. Immune dysfunction in patients with diabetes mellitus (DM). FEMS Immunol Med Microbiol 1999;26(3–4):259–65.

19. Taubes G. Neuroscience. Insulin insults may spur Alzheimer's disease. Science 2003;301(5629):40–1.
20. Kernan WN, Inzucchi SE, Viscoli CM, et al. Insulin resistance and risk for stroke. Neurology 2002;59(6):809–15.
21. Pickup JC. Inflammation and activated innate immunity in the pathogenesis of type 2 diabetes. Diabetes Care 2004;27(3):813–23.
22. Maddigan SL, Feeny DH, Johnson JA. Health-related quality of life deficits associated with diabetes and comorbidities in a Canadian National Population Health Survey. Qual Life Res 2005;14(5):1311–20.
23. Maddigan SL, Feeny DH, Johnson JA. A comparison of the health utilities indices Mark 2 and Mark 3 in type 2 diabetes. Med Decis Making 2003;23(6):489–501.
24. Weisberg SP, McCann D, Desai M, et al. Obesity is associated with macrophage accumulation in adipose tissue. J Clin Invest 2003;112(12):1796–808.
25. Wellen KE, Hotamisligil GS. Obesity-induced inflammatory changes in adipose tissue. J Clin Invest 2003;112(12):1785–8.
26. Xu H, Barnes GT, Yang Q, et al. Chronic inflammation in fat plays a crucial role in the development of obesity-related insulin resistance. J Clin Invest 2003; 112(12):1821–30.
27. Beckman JA, Creager MA, Libby P. Diabetes and atherosclerosis: epidemiology, pathophysiology, and management. JAMA 2002;287(19):2570–81.
28. Duncan BB, Schmidt MI, Pankow JS, et al. Low-grade systemic inflammation and the development of type 2 diabetes: the atherosclerosis risk in communities study. Diabetes 2003;52(7):1799–805.
29. Freeman DJ, Norrie J, Caslake MJ, et al. C-reactive protein is an independent predictor of risk for the development of diabetes in the West of Scotland Coronary Prevention Study. Diabetes 2002;51(5):1596–600.
30. Krein SL, Vijan S, Pogach LM, et al. Aspirin use and counseling about aspirin among patients with diabetes. Diabetes Care 2002;25(6):965–70.
31. Arkan MC, Hevener AL, Greten FR, et al. IKK-beta links inflammation to obesity-induced insulin resistance. Nat Med 2005;11(2):191–8.
32. Cai D, Yuan M, Frantz DF, et al. Local and systemic insulin resistance resulting from hepatic activation of IKK-beta and NF-kappaB. Nat Med 2005;11(2):183–90.
33. Baron SH. Salicylates as hypoglycemic agents. Diabetes Care 1982;5(1):64–71.
34. White MF. IRS proteins and the common path to diabetes. Am J Physiol Endocrinol Metab 2002;283(3):E413–22.
35. Hotamisligil GS, Peraldi P, Budavari A, et al. IRS-1–mediated inhibition of insulin receptor tyrosine kinase activity in TNF-alpha– and obesity-induced insulin resistance. Science 1996;271(5249):665–8.
36. Kanety H, Feinstein R, Papa MZ, et al. Tumor necrosis factor alpha–induced phosphorylation of insulin receptor substrate-1 (IRS-1). Possible mechanism for suppression of insulin-stimulated tyrosine phosphorylation of IRS-1. J Biol Chem 1995;270(40):23780–4.
37. Pradhan AD, Manson JE, Rifai N, et al. C-reactive protein, interleukin 6, and risk of developing type 2 diabetes mellitus. JAMA 2001;286(3):327–34.
38. Festa A, D'Agostino R Jr, Tracy RP, et al. Elevated levels of acute-phase proteins and plasminogen activator inhibitor-1 predict the development of type 2 diabetes: the insulin resistance atherosclerosis study. Diabetes 2002;51(4):1131–7.
39. Odegaard JI, Chawla A. Mechanisms of macrophage activation in obesity-induced insulin resistance. Nat Clin Pract Endocrinol Metab 2008;4(11): 619–26.

40. Peraldi P, Hotamisligil GS, Buurman WA, et al. Tumor necrosis factor (TNF)-alpha inhibits insulin signaling through stimulation of the p55 TNF receptor and activation of sphingomyelinase. J Biol Chem 1996;271(22):13018–22.

41. Klover PJ, Zimmers TA, Koniaris LG, et al. Chronic exposure to interleukin-6 causes hepatic insulin resistance in mice. Diabetes 2003;52(11):2784–9.

42. Mooney RA, Senn J, Cameron S, et al. Suppressors of cytokine signaling-1 and -6 associate with and inhibit the insulin receptor. A potential mechanism for cytokine-mediated insulin resistance. J Biol Chem 2001;276(28):25889–93.

43. Senn JJ, Klover PJ, Nowak IA, et al. Interleukin-6 induces cellular insulin resistance in hepatocytes. Diabetes 2002;51(12):3391–9.

44. Senn JJ, Klover PJ, Nowak IA, et al. Suppressor of cytokine signaling-3 (SOCS-3), a potential mediator of interleukin-6-dependent insulin resistance in hepatocytes. J Biol Chem 2003;278(16):13740–6.

45. Stratton IM, Adler AI, Neil HA, et al. Association of glycaemia with macrovascular and microvascular complications of type 2 diabetes (UKPDS 35): prospective observational study. BMJ 2000;321(7258):405–12.

46. Esposito K, Nappo F, Marfella R, et al. Inflammatory cytokine concentrations are acutely increased by hyperglycemia in humans: role of oxidative stress. Circulation 2002;106(16):2067–72.

47. Krogh-Madsen R, Plomgaard P, Keller P, et al. Insulin stimulates interleukin-6 and tumor necrosis factor–alpha gene expression in human subcutaneous adipose tissue. Am J Physiol Endocrinol Metab 2004;286(2):E234–8.

48. Bluher M, Fasshauer M, Tonjes A, et al. Association of interleukin-6, C-reactive protein, interleukin-10 and adiponectin plasma concentrations with measures of obesity, insulin sensitivity and glucose metabolism. Exp Clin Endocrinol Diabetes 2005;113(9):534–7.

49. O'Connor JC, Satpathy A, Hartman ME, et al. IL-1beta-mediated innate immunity is amplified in the db/db mouse model of type 2 diabetes. J Immunol 2005; 174(8):4991–7.

50. Pickup JC, Day C, Bailey CJ, et al. Plasma sialic acid in animal models of diabetes mellitus: evidence for modulation of sialic acid concentrations by insulin deficiency. Life Sci 1995;57(14):1383–91.

51. Lin Y, Rajala MW, Berger JP, et al. Hyperglycemia-induced production of acute phase reactants in adipose tissue. J Biol Chem 2001;276(45):42077–83.

52. Ebeling P, Teppo AM, Koistinen HA, et al. Troglitazone reduces hyperglycaemia and selectively acute-phase serum proteins in patients with Type II diabetes. Diabetologia 1999;42(12):1433–8.

53. Scott CL. Diagnosis, prevention, and intervention for the metabolic syndrome. Am J Cardiol 2003;92(1A):35i–42i.

54. Hartman ME, O'Connor JC, Godbout JP, et al. Insulin receptor substrate-2-dependent interleukin-4 signaling in macrophages is impaired in two models of type 2 diabetes mellitus. J Biol Chem 2004;279(27):28045–50.

55. Aronson D, Rayfield EJ. How hyperglycemia promotes atherosclerosis: molecular mechanisms. Cardiovasc Diabetol 2002;1(1):1.

56. Hill JR, Kwon G, Marshall CA, et al. Hyperglycemic levels of glucose inhibit interleukin 1 release from RAW 264.7 murine macrophages by activation of protein kinase C. J Biol Chem 1998;273(6):3308–13.

57. Iida KT, Suzuki H, Sone H, et al. Insulin inhibits apoptosis of macrophage cell line, THP-1 cells, via phosphatidylinositol-3-kinase-dependent pathway. Arterioscler Thromb Vasc Biol 2002;22(3):380–6.

58. Ceolotto G, Gallo A, Miola M, et al. Protein kinase C activity is acutely regulated by plasma glucose concentration in human monocytes in vivo. Diabetes 1999; 48(6):1316–22.

59. Iida KT, Shimano H, Kawakami Y, et al. Insulin up-regulates tumor necrosis factor-alpha production in macrophages through an extracellular-regulated kinase-dependent pathway. J Biol Chem 2001;276(35):32531–7.

60. Dantzer R. Cytokine-induced sickness behaviour: a neuroimmune response to activation of innate immunity. Eur J Pharmacol 2004;500(1–3):399–411.

61. Cesari M, Penninx BW, Newman AB, et al. Inflammatory markers and onset of cardiovascular events: results from the Health ABC study. Circulation 2003; 108(19):2317–22.

62. Yaffe K, Lindquist K, Penninx BW, et al. Inflammatory markers and cognition in well-functioning African-American and white elders. Neurology 2003;61(1):76–80.

63. Penninx BW, Kritchevsky SB, Yaffe K, et al. Inflammatory markers and depressed mood in older persons: results from the Health, Aging and Body Composition study. Biol Psychiatry 2003;54(5):566–72.

64. Sluzewska A, Rybakowski J, Bosmans E, et al. Indicators of immune activation in major depression. Psychiatry Res 1996;64(3):161–7.

65. Kluger M, Kozak W, Mayfield K. Fever and immunity. In: Ader R, Felton D, Cohen N, editors. Psychoneuroimmunology. San Diego (CA): Academic Press; 2001. p. 687–702.

66. Dantzer R. Cytokine-induced sickness behavior: where do we stand? Brain Behav Immun 2001;15(1):7–24.

67. Turrin NP, Plata-Salaman CR. Cytokine–cytokine interactions and the brain. Brain Res Bull 2000;51(1):3–9.

68. Cartmell T, Poole S, Turnbull AV, et al. Circulating interleukin-6 mediates the febrile response to localised inflammation in rats. J Physiol 2000;526(Pt 3):653–61.

69. Luheshi GN, Stefferl A, Turnbull AV, et al. Febrile response to tissue inflammation involves both peripheral and brain IL-1 and TNF-alpha in the rat. Am J Phys 1997;272(3 Pt 2):R862–8.

70. Nadeau S, Rivest S. Role of microglial-derived tumor necrosis factor in mediating CD14 transcription and nuclear factor kappa B activity in the brain during endotoxemia. J Neurosci 2000;20(9):3456–68.

71. Mathison JC, Ulevitch RJ, Fletcher JR, et al. The distribution of lipopolysaccharide in normocomplementemic and C3-depleted rabbits and rhesus monkeys. Am J Pathol 1980;101(2):245–63.

72. Fox ES, Broitman SA, Thomas P. Bacterial endotoxins and the liver. Lab Invest 1990;63(6):733–41.

73. Braude AI, Carey FJ, Zalesky M. Studies with radioactive endotoxin. II. Correlation of physiologic effects with distribution of radioactivity in rabbits injected with radioactive sodium chromate. J Clin Invest 1955;34(6):858–66.

74. Armbrust T, Ramadori G. Functional characterization of two different Kupffer cell populations of normal rat liver. J Hepatol 1996;25(4):518–28.

75. Bioulac-Sage P, Kuiper J, Van Berkel TJ, et al. Lymphocyte and macrophage populations in the liver. Hepatogastroenterology 1996;43(7):4–14.

76. Li Z, Blatteis CM. Fever onset is linked to the appearance of lipopolysaccharide in the liver. J Endotoxin Res 2004;10(1):39–53.

77. Plata-Salaman CR, Peloso E, Satinoff E. Cytokine-induced fever in obese (fa/fa) and lean (Fa/Fa) Zucker rats. Am J Phys 1998;275(4 Pt 2):R1353–7.

78. Ivanov AI, Kulchitsky VA, Romanovsky AA. Does obesity affect febrile responsiveness? Int J Obes Relat Metab Disord 2001;25(4):586–9.

79. Ivanov AI, Romanovsky AA. Fever responses of Zucker rats with and without fatty mutation of the leptin receptor. Am J Physiol Regul Integr Comp Physiol 2002;282(1):R311–6.

80. Dantzer R, Bluthe R, Castanon N, et al. Cytokine effects on behavior. In: Ader R, Felton D, Cohen N, editors. Psychoneuroimmunology. San Diego (CA): Academic Press; 2001. p. 703–27.

81. Dantzer R, Bluthe RM, Gheusi G, et al. Molecular basis of sickness behavior. Ann N Y Acad Sci 1998;856:132–8.

82. Dunn AJ, Swiergiel AH. The role of cytokines in infection-related behavior. Ann N Y Acad Sci 1998;840:577–85.

83. Aubert A. Sickness and behaviour in animals: a motivational perspective. Neurosci Biobehav Rev 1999;23(7):1029–36.

84. Hart BL. Biological basis of the behavior of sick animals. Neurosci Biobehav Rev 1988;12(2):123–37.

85. Yirmiya R, Pollak Y, Morag M, et al. Illness, cytokines, and depression. Ann N Y Acad Sci 2000;917:478–87.

86. Yirmiya R. Depression in medical illness: the role of the immune system. West J Med 2000;173(5):333–6.

87. Konsman JP, Parnet P, Dantzer R. Cytokine-induced sickness behaviour: mechanisms and implications. Trends Neurosci 2002;25(3):154–9.

88. Burgess W, Gheusi G, Yao J, et al. Interleukin-1beta–converting enzyme-deficient mice resist central but not systemic endotoxin-induced anorexia. Am J Phys 1998;274(6 Pt 2):R1829–33.

89. Bluthe RM, Dantzer R, Kelley KW. Central mediation of the effects of interleukin-1 on social exploration and body weight in mice. Psychoneuroendocrinology 1997;22(1):1–11.

90. Swiergiel AH, Dunn AJ. The roles of IL-1, IL-6, and TNFalpha in the feeding responses to endotoxin and influenza virus infection in mice. Brain Behav Immun 1999;13(3):252–65.

91. Schiepers OJ, Wichers MC, Maes M. Cytokines and major depression. Prog Neuropsychopharmacol Biol Psychiatry 2005;29(2):201–17.

92. Ciechanowski PS, Katon WJ, Russo JE, et al. The relationship of depressive symptoms to symptom reporting, self-care and glucose control in diabetes. Gen Hosp Psychiatry 2003;25(4):246–52.

93. McKellar JD, Humphreys K, Piette JD. Depression increases diabetes symptoms by complicating patients' self-care adherence. Diabetes Educ 2004; 30(3):485–92.

94. Romanovsky AA, Ivanov AI, Lenczowski MJ, et al. Lipopolysaccharide transport from the peritoneal cavity to the blood: is it controlled by the vagus nerve? Auton Neurosci 2000;85(1–3):133–40.

95. Bluthe RM, Castanon N, Pousset F, et al. Central injection of IL-10 antagonizes the behavioural effects of lipopolysaccharide in rats. Psychoneuroendocrinology 1999;24(3):301–11.

96. Lin K-I, Johnson DR, Freund GG. LPS-dependent suppression of social exploration is augmented in type 1 diabetic mice. Brain Behav Immun 2007;21(6):775–82.

97. Naguib G, Al-Mashat H, Desta T, et al. Diabetes prolongs the inflammatory response to a bacterial stimulus through cytokine dysregulation. J Invest Dermatol 2004;123(1):87–92.

98. Johnson DR, O'Connor JC, Hartman ME, et al. Acute hypoxia activates the neuroimmune system which diabetes exacerbates. J Neurosci 2007;27(5): 1161–6.

99. Bluthe RM, Lestage J, Rees G, et al. Dual effect of central injection of recombinant rat interleukin-4 on lipopolysaccharide-induced sickness behavior in rats. Neuropsychopharmacology 2002;26(1):86–93.

100. Bluthe R, Kelley K, Dantzer R. Effects of insulin-like growth factor-I on cytokine-induced sickness behavior in mice. Brain Behav Immun 2006;20(1):57–63.

101. Johnson DR, O'Connor JC, Dantzer R, et al. Inhibition of vagally mediated immune-to-brain signaling by vanadyl sulfate speeds recovery from sickness. Proc Natl Acad Sci U S A 2005;102(42):15184–9.

102. Sherry CL, Kramer JM, York JM, et al. Behavioral recovery from acute hypoxia is reliant on leptin. Brain Behav Immun 2008;23(2):169–75.

103. Meier CA, Bobbioni E, Gabay C, et al. IL-1 receptor antagonist serum levels are increased in human obesity: a possible link to the resistance to leptin? J Clin Endocrinol Metab 2002;87:1184–8.

104. Perry VH. The influence of systemic inflammation on inflammation in the brain: implications for chronic neurodegenerative disease. Brain Behav Immun 2004; 18(5):407–13.

105. Banks WA, Farr SA, Morley JE. Entry of blood-borne cytokines into the central nervous system: effects on cognitive processes. Neuroimmunomodulation 2002;10(6):319–27.

106. Bluthe RM, Michaud B, Kelley KW, et al. Vagotomy blocks behavioural effects of interleukin-1 injected via the intraperitoneal route but not via other systemic routes. Neuroreport 1996;7(15–17):2823–7.

107. Wieczorek M, Swiergiel AH, Pournajafi-Nazarloo H, et al. Physiological and behavioral responses to interleukin-1beta and LPS in vagotomized mice. Physiol Behav 2005;85(4):500–11.

108. Watkins LR, Maier SF, Goehler LE. Cytokine-to-brain communication: a review & analysis of alternative mechanisms. Life Sci 1995;57(11):1011–26.

109. Banks WA, Kastin AJ. Relative contributions of peripheral and central sources to levels of IL-1 alpha in the cerebral cortex of mice: assessment with species-specific enzyme immunoassays. J Neuroimmunol 1997;79(1):22–8.

110. Banks WA, Ortiz L, Plotkin SR, et al. Human interleukin (IL) 1 alpha, murine IL-1 alpha and murine IL-1 beta are transported from blood to brain in the mouse by a shared saturable mechanism. J Pharmacol Exp Ther 1991; 259(3):988–96.

111. Breder CD, Hazuka C, Ghayur T, et al. Regional induction of tumor necrosis factor alpha expression in the mouse brain after systemic lipopolysaccharide administration. Proc Natl Acad Sci U S A 1994;91(24):11393–7.

112. Sternberg EM. Neural–immune interactions in health and disease. J Clin Invest 1997;100(11):2641–7.

113. Woiciechowsky C, Asadullah K, Nestler D, et al. Sympathetic activation triggers systemic interleukin-10 release in immunodepression induced by brain injury. Nat Med 1998;4(7):808–13.

114. Banks WA. The source of cerebral insulin. Eur J Pharmacol 2004;490(1–3):5–12.

115. Starr JM, Wardlaw J, Ferguson K, et al. Increased blood-brain barrier permeability in type II diabetes demonstrated by gadolinium magnetic resonance imaging. J Neurol Neurosurg Psychiatr 2003;74(1):70–6.

116. Mooradian AD, Haas MJ, Batejko O, et al. Statins ameliorate endothelial barrier permeability changes in the cerebral tissue of streptozotocin-induced diabetic rats. Diabetes 2005;54(10):2977–82.

117. Duckrow RB, Beard DC, Brennan RW. Regional cerebral blood flow decreases during chronic and acute hyperglycemia. Stroke 1987;18(1):52–8.

118. Fogelstrand L, Hulthe J, Hulten LM, et al. Monocytic expression of CD14 and CD18, circulating adhesion molecules and inflammatory markers in women with diabetes mellitus and impaired glucose tolerance. Diabetologia 2004; 47(11):1948–52.

119. Cipolletta C, Ryan KE, Hanna EV, et al. Activation of peripheral blood CD14+ monocytes occurs in diabetes. Diabetes 2005;54(9):2779–86.

120. O'Rourke L, Gronning LM, Yeaman SJ, et al. Glucose-dependent regulation of cholesterol ester metabolism in macrophages by insulin and leptin. J Biol Chem 2002;277(45):42557–62.

121. Stoffels K, Overbergh L, Giulietti A, et al. NOD macrophages produce high levels of inflammatory cytokines upon encounter of apoptotic or necrotic cells. J Autoimmun 2004;23(1):9–15.

122. Wang JY, Yang JM, Tao PL, et al. Synergistic apoptosis induced by bacterial endotoxin lipopolysaccharide and high glucose in rat microglia. Neurosci Lett 2001;304(3):177–80.

123. Zykova SN, Jenssen TG, Berdal M, et al. Altered cytokine and nitric oxide secretion in vitro by macrophages from diabetic type II–like db/db mice. Diabetes 2000;49(9):1451–8.

124. Barber AJ, Antonetti DA, Kern TS, et al. The Ins2Akita mouse as a model of early retinal complications in diabetes. Invest Ophthalmol Vis Sci 2005;46(6):2210–8.

125. Zhang L, Nair A, Krady K, et al. Estrogen stimulates microglia and brain recovery from hypoxia-ischemia in normoglycemic but not diabetic female mice. J Clin Invest 2004;113(1):85–95.

126. Godbout JP, Pesavento J, Hartman ME, et al. Methylglyoxal enhances cisplatin-induced cytotoxicity by activating protein kinase Cdelta. J Biol Chem 2002; 277(4):2554–61.

127. Wurster AL, Withers DJ, Uchida T, et al. Stat6 and IRS-2 cooperate in interleukin 4 (IL-4)–induced proliferation and differentiation but are dispensable for IL-4-dependent rescue from apoptosis. Mol Cell Biol 2002;22(1):117–26.

128. Emanuelli B, Peraldi P, Filloux C, et al. SOCS-3 inhibits insulin signaling and is up-regulated in response to tumor necrosis factor–alpha in the adipose tissue of obese mice. J Biol Chem 2001;276(51):47944–9.

129. Ueki K, Kondo T, Kahn CR. Suppressor of cytokine signaling 1 (SOCS-1) and SOCS-3 cause insulin resistance through inhibition of tyrosine phosphorylation of insulin receptor substrate proteins by discrete mechanisms. Mol Cell Biol 2004;24(12):5434–46.

130. O'Connor JC, Sherry CL, Guest CB, et al. Type 2 diabetes impairs insulin receptor substrate-2–mediated phosphatidylinositol 3–kinase activity in primary macrophages to induce a state of cytokine resistance to IL-4 in association with overexpression of suppressor of cytokine signaling-3. J Immunol 2007;178(11): 6886–93.

131. Uehara A, Gottschall PE, Dahl RR, et al. Interleukin-1 stimulates ACTH release by an indirect action which requires endogenous corticotropin releasing factor. Endocrinology 1987;121(4):1580–2.

132. Brown R, Li Z, Vriend CY, et al. Suppression of splenic macrophage interleukin-1 secretion following intracerebroventricular injection of interleukin-1 beta: evidence for pituitary-adrenal and sympathetic control. Cell Immunol 1991; 132(1):84–93.

133. Gaykema RP, Dijkstra I, Tilders FJ. Subdiaphragmatic vagotomy suppresses endotoxin-induced activation of hypothalamic corticotropin-releasing hormone neurons and ACTH secretion. Endocrinology 1995;136(10):4717–20.

134. Pariante CM, Pearce BD, Pisell TL, et al. The proinflammatory cytokine, inter-leukin-1alpha, reduces glucocorticoid receptor translocation and function. Endocrinology 1999;140(9):4359–66.
135. Glezer I, Rivest S. Glucocorticoids: protectors of the brain during innate immune responses. Neuroscientist 2004;10(6):538–52.
136. Swain MG, Appleyard C, Wallace J, et al. Endogenous glucocorticoids released during acute toxic liver injury enhance hepatic IL-10 synthesis and release. Am J Phys 1999;276(1 Pt 1):G199–205.
137. Berczi I, Nagy E, de Toledo SM, et al. Pituitary hormones regulate c-myc and DNA synthesis in lymphoid tissue. J Immunol 1991;146(7):2201–6.
138. Goujon E, Parnet P, Laye S, et al. Adrenalectomy enhances pro-inflammatory cytokines gene expression, in the spleen, pituitary and brain of mice in response to lipopolysaccharide. Brain Res Mol Brain Res 1996;36(1):53–62.
139. Bertini R, Bianchi M, Ghezzi P. Adrenalectomy sensitizes mice to the lethal effects of interleukin 1 and tumor necrosis factor. J Exp Med 1988;167(5):1708–12.
140. Butler LD, Layman NK, Riedl PE, et al. Neuroendocrine regulation of in vivo cyto-kine production and effects: I. In vivo regulatory networks involving the neuroen-docrine system, interleukin-1 and tumor necrosis factor–alpha. J Neuroimmunol 1989;24(1–2):143–53.
141. Chan O, Inouye K, Riddell MC, et al. Diabetes and the hypothalamo-pituitary-adrenal (HPA) axis. Minerva Endocrinol 2003;28(2):87–102.
142. Chan O, Inouye K, Akirav E, et al. Insulin alone increases hypothalamo-pituitary-adrenal activity, and diabetes lowers peak stress responses. Endocrinology 2005;146(3):1382–90.
143. Inouye K, Chan O, Riddell MC, et al. Mechanisms of impaired hypothalamic-pitu-itary-adrenal (HPA) function in diabetes: reduced counterregulatory responsive-ness to hypoglycaemia. Diabetes Nutr Metab 2002;15(5):348–55 [discussion: 355–6, 362].
144. Chan O, Inouye K, Vranic M, et al. Hyperactivation of the hypothalamo-pituitary-adrenocortical axis in streptozotocin-diabetes is associated with reduced stress responsiveness and decreased pituitary and adrenal sensitivity. Endocrinology 2002;143(5):1761–8.

Psychoneuroimmunology of Stroke

Robert Skinner, BSc[a],*, Rachel Georgiou, MSc[b],
Peter Thornton, BSc[a], Nancy Rothwell, PhD[a]

KEYWORDS

• Stroke • Central nervous system • Immune mediators • CNS

Stroke is one of the most common causes of death and disability in the Western world, and the key underlying pathologic event, cerebral ischemia, contributes to many other neurologic and neurosurgical disorders including head injury, subarachnoid hemorrhage, birth asphyxia, and vascular dementia.

In spite of its frequency and severity, there are no widely effective treatments for stroke. Thrombolysis (using tissue plasminogen activator, tPA) is the only acute pharmacologic treatment; other approaches (eg, aspirin, statins, management of hypertension and diabetes, and lifestyle changes) focus attention on prevention. Several hundred compounds have been shown to limit experimental ischemic brain injury in rodents by neuroprotective mechanisms, but none has yet proven effective in humans, for reasons that have been discussed extensively.[1] Most of these putative therapies have attempted to protect neurons from delayed injury, for example by blocking excitoxicity or detrimental changes in intracellular ion concentrations.

The potential contribution of immune or inflammatory processes to ischemic brain damage has been realized gradually over the past 15 years. As with many other aspects of central nervous system (CNS) function or disease, the prevailing view of the brain as an immune-privileged organ somewhat hindered research into neuroimmune interactions and neuroinflammation, despite the widespread acceptance of the dependence of multiple sclerosis on such processes and the inflammatory component of many CNS infections.

The early focus of stroke research was on cardiovasculature and neuronal function and injury. In contrast, it now is recognized widely that glial cells play both beneficial and detrimental roles in ischemic brain damage and recovery. In addition the vascular endothelium, extracellular matrix, adherent or invading immune cells, and numerous physiologic, endocrine, and immune factors within and outside the CNS markedly

This issue is a repurpose of August 2006 issue of the Neurologic Clinics (NCL Volume 24, Issue 3).
[a] Faculty of Life Sciences, Michael Smith Building (C2210), University of Manchester, Acker Street, Manchester M13 9PT, UK
[b] Stroke Services, Clinical Sciences Building, Hope Hospital, Stott Lane Salford M6 8HD, UK
* Corresponding author.
E-mail address: r.a.skinner@postgrad.manchester.ac.uk (R. Skinner).

Immunol Allergy Clin N Am 29 (2009) 359–379
doi:10.1016/j.iac.2009.02.010
0889-8561/09/$ – see front matter © 2009 Elsevier Inc. All rights reserved.

influence the outcome after a cerebrovascular event. Elevated body temperature strongly correlates with worse damage, and fever, itself mediated by inflammatory molecules, is a key risk factor for poor outcome.[2] Even in the absence of an overt acute-phase response, peripheral systemic or local inflammation or infection is believed to be a causal factor in the development of stroke and adversely influences outcome, presumably by neural or humoral afferent signals. The precise mechanisms by which peripheral events influence ischemic brain damage are unknown but provide an interesting opportunity for therapeutic intervention.

Similarly endocrine status affects the incidence and impact of stroke and related conditions linked to cerebral ischemia. Many neuropeptides (eg, corticotrophin-releasing factor, corticotropin, thyrotropin-releasing hormone, orexin) have been implicated in the pathogenesis of stroke,[3–6] and the hypothalamic-pituitary-adrenal (HPA) axis[7] and gonadal steroids[8] also have been reported to influence stroke.

Although there is no reported evidence to suggest that psychologic state determines when a stroke occurs or the neurologic outcome in any individual patient, cerebral ischemia has a profound influence on behavior and mood, and depression and fatigue are common and debilitating conditions in patients who have suffered a stroke.

STROKE

Stroke occurs when there is a disruption of the blood supply to the brain either by occlusion (ischemic stroke) or rupture (hemorrhagic stroke) of a blood vessel. The majority of strokes are ischemic (80%); primary intracerebral hemorrhage (15%) and subarachnoid hemorrhage (5%) account for the other forms of the disorder.[9] It is a heterogeneous condition with a number of underlying causes.

Clinical Features

The clinical features of stroke vary according to the location and extent of resulting injury and may include disruption of consciousness, motor, cognitive, sensory function, or coordination. In clinical practice assessment of the presenting features of the stroke can be used to determine the vascular territory likely to be affected (Oxford Community Stroke Project Classification), and prognosis varies depending on classification of initial event. One-year mortality is 66% for total anterior circulation stroke, compared with 11% in patients after lacunar stroke.[10,11] Initial stroke severity,[12] age,[13] coexisting medical disorders,[14] and gender also influence outcome.[15]

Burden

Stroke is a major health problem. In the United Kingdom it is the most common cause of acquired disability in adults.[16] Worldwide it is predicted that mortality from stroke will almost double by 2020 because of an ageing population and smoking behavior.[17] Stroke affects between 174 and 216 people per 100,000 population in the United Kingdom.[18]

Only 25% of patients make a total recovery after stroke.[19,20] A third of sufferers die within 30 days of onset, and two thirds of survivors are left with residual effects. Of these, one third have severe disabilities and require daily assistance. After hospitalization most sufferers return home where they rely on informal caretakers (most often their spouses) for support;[20] four out of five families are affected by stroke.[21]

Pathology

Ninety-five percent of ischemic stroke events (transient ischemic attack and stroke) can be attributed to the consequences of atheroma (50% atherothromboembolism, 25% small vessel disease within the brain, 20% arising from emboli from the heart, 5% resulting from other causes).[9,13] Individuals who have this disease almost always have atheroma in other arteries. Many risk factors for the development of atheroma have been identified, and these risk factors apply to other disorders in which vascular occlusion occurs (eg, coronary heart disease, myocardial infarction, claudication) as well as to stroke.

Treatment

In recent years the treatment of patients after stroke has changed dramatically with the development of specialist stroke care, new treatments, and improved secondary prevention.[9] Recombinant tissue plasminogen activator (r-tPA) remains the only licensed treatment for acute ischemic stroke. r-tPA is given at approved centers within 3 hours of stroke onset once hemorrhage and other contraindications to treatment have been excluded. Further trials of r-tPA are in progress.[22]

A significant proportion of those who have a stroke will have a further vascular event (up to 12% risk of further stroke; 3% risk of myocardial infarction within a year). Secondary prevention is important. Aspirin, started soon after stroke prevents 9 deaths or further strokes per 1000 patients treated.[23] Both primary and secondary prevention strategies focus on the management of modifiable risk factors of stroke, which include lifestyle modification and drug therapies. Statins seem to have effects on reducing the risk of stroke independent of their actions on reducing cholesterol.[24] It is suggested that statins have neuroprotective properties that include amelioration of the cytokine response to cerebral ischemia.[25] A recent phase II trial found lower rates of delayed ischemic deficit in patients who had subarachnoid hemorrhage treated with pravastatin.[26] Angiotensin-converting enzyme inhibitors used in the management of hypertension also have anti-inflammatory actions including reduction in interleukin (IL)-6 levels.[27,28] Concomitant treatment with angiotensin-converting enzyme inhibitors at the time of stroke has been associated with lower levels of inflammatory response and improved outcome.[29]

CENTRAL NERVOUS SYSTEM IMMUNE/INFLAMMATORY RESPONSE TO INJURY
Unique Features of the Brain

Inflammation is an innate immune response involving complex cellular processes in response to injury or infection. The CNS traditionally has been considered an immune-privileged site, but although it is somewhat resistant to inflammation, it is by no means exempt. Studies in the mouse using *Bacillus Calmette Guerin* as an inflammatory challenge show a rapid and acute inflammatory response characterized by leukocyte infiltration in the periphery. The same challenge in the CNS induced a delayed response that was markedly curtailed.[30] These studies illustrate that (1) the CNS is maintained in an immunosuppressed state, blunting the response to inflammatory challenge, and (2) common molecular mechanisms exist in peripheral and central inflammation.

In addition to cellular and molecular mechanisms, several anatomic features of the CNS act to limit the scope of brain inflammation: The CNS is protected by the blood–brain barrier (BBB), which restricts the infiltration of leukocytes and macromolecules.[31] Edema in the brain is limited by the cranium, and there is no classic lymphatic drainage.[32] Akin to inflammation in peripheral tissues, however, immune/inflammatory processes in the CNS play an important role in maintaining tissue homeostasis. Uncontrolled or excessive inflammatory responses to injury or infection clearly are detrimental and can have particularly devastating results in the CNS where tissues lack the capacity to regenerate (**Fig. 1**).

Key Mediators of the Central Nervous System Inflammatory Response and Ischemic Brain Injury

Stroke is the consequence of a transient or permanent reduction in cerebral blood flow caused by an embolus, thrombosis, or hemorrhage resulting in energy depletion, loss of cellular membrane potentials, calcium overload, and brain infarction.[33] Endothelial and glial cells of the CNS respond rapidly (activation) to tissue injury by releasing inflammatory mediators (eg, cytokines, chemokines) that cause marked changes in BBB permeability.[34–36] Disruption of the BBB by this active process or mechanical means allows leukocytes to infiltrate the CNS. Once within the brain, leukocytes are triggered to release more proinflammatory cytokines, chemokines, elastases, free radicals, and matrix metalloproteinases (MMPs), which further exacerbate damage.[37]

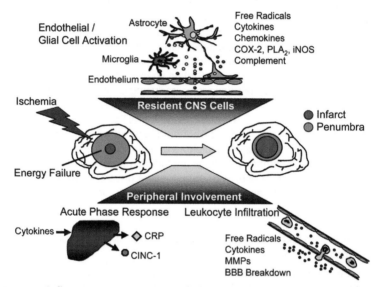

Fig. 1. Immune/inflammatory responses and their contribution to ischemic injury after stroke. Energy failure following a reduction in blood flow induces a region of cell death (*Infarct*) and a surrounding area of defective tissue (*Penumbra*). Over a course of days to weeks, inflammatory processes in resident and infiltrating cells in the penumbra exacerbate the infarct. Endothelial and glial cells become activated, release a plethora of mediators, including free radicals, cytokines, and chemokines, and increase the production of enzymes (eg, cyclooxygenase-2, phospholipase A$_2$, inducible nitric oxide synthetase). These enzymes can induce neuronal cell death and affect the blood–brain barrier, leading to leukocyte infiltration. Leukocytes cause further damage to the blood–brain barrier and parenchymal tissue through the production of free radicals and matrix metalloproteinases. Cytokines mediate the hepatic acute-phase response leading to the release of C-reactive protein and cytokine-induced neutrophil chemoattractant-1, which enhance the inflammatory process. BBB, blood–brain barrier; CINC-1, cytokine-induced neutrophil chemoattractant-1; COX-2, cyclooxygenase-2; CRP, C-reactive protein; iNOS, inducible nitric oxide synthetase; MMP, matrix metalloproteinase; PLA$_2$, phospholipase A$_2$.

Neutrophils are guided to the damaged CNS by chemokines (eg, cytokine-induced neutrophil chemoattractant, CINC-1)[38] and bind to adhesion molecules (eg, P-selectin, E-selectin, and intracellular adhesion molecule [ICAM]-1). The expression of these molecules is increased in brain endothelium following ischemia and in response to inflammatory mediators (eg, IL-1).[39-41] The expression of CD11a, a leukocyte glycoprotein that binds to adhesion molecules, aiding their infiltration across the intact BBB, also is increased in patients after stroke.[42] In addition to their contribution to parenchymal inflammation, neutrophils may exacerbate damage in other ways. (1) Endothelial attachment of these large cells can occlude vessels and further reduce blood flow and consequently hinder reperfusion.[43,44] (2) Binding of neutrophils can trigger an intracellular signaling cascade in endothelial cells that can increase BBB permeability,[45] enabling peripheral molecules to enter the injury site.

Free radicals such as nitric oxide and superoxide are produced locally in response to ischemia through diverse mechanisms, including mitochondrial dysfunction and neutrophil activation. They contribute significantly to ischemic inflammation by damaging cellular molecules[46] and the BBB[47] and by mediating edema.[48] Free radical production increases the expression of cytokines,[49] which in turn can induce free radical–producing enzymes, such as nitric oxide synthase.[50] The enzymatic activity of cyclooxygenase (COX) and phospholipase also induces free radical production.[51,52] Phospholipase A_2 activity yields arachidonic acid from membrane phospholipids, which can be metabolized by COX-1 and -2 to yield prostanoids. COX-1 is expressed constitutively and plays a role in the production of prostacyclin, a prostanoid with antiplatelet and vasodilatory actions. Mice lacking COX-1 have reduced cerebral blood flow in the penumbra following ischemia.[53] COX-2 is induced in neurons and glia by inflammatory stimuli and is thought to contribute to neurodegeneration through the production of prostaglandins.[54] Recent evidence indicates that prostaglandins have beneficial and detrimental effects depending on the receptor they activate. For example, prostaglandin E_2 enhances ischemic neurotoxicity through activation of the EP1 receptor[55] but can have protective effects through the EP2 receptor.[56]

Cytokines produced in the brain in response to ischemia include IL-1, IL-6, and tumor necrosis factor-α (TNF-α). These cytokines have pleiotropic effects that may be beneficial or harmful depending on the effector cell, the cytokine concentration, the extracellular composition, and the duration of action. Intracerebroventricular (ICV) administration of proinflammatory cytokines can induce neutrophil recruitment in naive rodents[57] and humans.[41] Besides their actions on the BBB, these cytokines can affect glial cell activation and neuronal cell viability directly.[58] IL-1 and IL-6 induce fever, which may exacerbate tissue injury.[36] IL-1 also has been implicated in the initiation of edema following hypoxic injury.[59] In addition, anti-inflammatory cytokines such as transforming growth factor-β (TGF-β) are expressed following stroke and may exert beneficial effects (eg, stimulating angiogenesis) during brain recovery.[60]

IL-1, IL-6, and TNF-α induce the release of hepatic acute phase proteins, such as C-reactive protein (CRP) and CINC-1.[61] Circulating CRP levels are elevated in patients after stroke,[62] and CRP can induce activation of the complement system.[63] The complement system is a cascade of proteins involved in the innate response to injury or infection that participates in phagocytosis, cytolysis, and immune reactions.[64] Complement production is increased by proinflammatory cytokines[35,66] and has been documented in patients after stroke.[67] Dysregulated activation of the complement system can lead to the production of a membrane attack complex (the terminal product of the cascade) that induces neuronal cell death.[68] Mice lacking an initiating component of the cascade have greatly reduced ischemic brain injury.[69] Recently it was shown that complement inhibition reduces the expression of proinflammatory cytokines and adhesion molecules in a murine model of ischemia-reperfusion injury.[70]

MMPs are a family of extracellular proteinases, and their role in cerebral ischemia, particularly in BBB breakdown, has attracted much attention in recent years.[71] Resident CNS cells and leukocytes are capable of producing MMP, and in a murine model of stroke leukocyte-derived MMP-9 contributes to BBB breakdown.[72] Furthermore, increased plasma MMP-9 levels correlate with hemorrhagic transformation in patients after stroke[73] and together with MMP-13 are indicative of infarct volume 24 hours after stroke.[74] MMP-9 is a key mediator of neuronal injury,[75] and its expression is induced by the proinflammatory cytokines IL-1 and TNF-α.[76,77]

EVIDENCE THAT IMMUNE MEDIATORS CONTRIBUTE TO STROKE

There is now substantial evidence that the expression of both proinflammatory (IL-1, IL-6, and TNF-α) and anti-inflammatory (IL-10 and TGF-β) cytokines is increased locally within the CNS in response to ischemia and contributes to subsequent injury. This section focuses on this evidence and the contribution of adhesion molecules as immune mediators whose expression is increased by cytokines.

Interleukin-1

IL-1 is an inflammatory cytokine with two well-characterized agonists, IL-1α and IL-1β, and a receptor antagonist (IL-1ra). In experimental rat model, cerebral ischemia IL-1β expression has been detected after only 30 minutes.[78] In this study, the cellular source was microglia and endothelial cells, but IL-1β also is expressed by invading macrophages and at a later time point by astrocytes.[79,80] IL-1 acts on astrocytes and endothelial cells that express IL-1 receptor type I, IL-1 receptor type II, and IL-1 receptor accessory protein; no data have demonstrated their expression on microglia.[81] Therefore endothelial cells and astrocytes are the likely targets of IL-1.

Several studies have revealed that ICV or systemic (**Fig. 2**) injection of IL-1β into rodents significantly exacerbates brain damage in animals exposed to cerebral ischemia.[82–84] In IL-1 knock-outs, infarct size is reduced 70% in the IL-1α/β knock-out compared with wild type, but no significant reduction is seen in the IL-1α or IL-1β single knock-outs,[85] suggesting a compensatory effect. IL-1β is secreted in

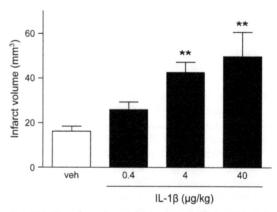

Fig. 2. Infarct sizes increase in a dose-dependant manner after systemic injection of IL-1β in mice with experimental cerebral ischemia (30-minute middle cerebral artery occlusion). (Courtesy of Barry McColl MD, Manchester, UK, with permission.)

an inactive proform; cleavage of this protein by caspase-1 releases the active form.[86] In caspase-1 knock-outs, ICAM-1 expression of the cerebral vasculature is greatly reduced,[87] and this reduction corresponds with reduction in injury.

IL-1 has a naturally occurring antagonist, IL-1ra, which binds the type I receptor but does not initiate signaling. When injected ICV, IL-1ra reduces infarct volume by as at least 50% in rodents exposed to cerebral ischemia.[82–84,88,89] IL-1ra injected systemically also reduces ischemic injury.[90–92] Antibodies raised against IL-1ra induce a significant increase in ischemic damage after cerebral ischemia, suggesting that endogenous IL-1ra is neuroprotective.[93]

The authors have completed a small randomized, placebo-controlled, double-blind phase II study.[94] Two hundred eighteen patients were screened, and 34 were accepted for the trial to receive either placebo or IL-1ra within 6 hours of onset of symptoms. IL-1ra was administered intravenously as a 100-mg loading dose over 60 seconds and 2 mg/kg/h administered over 72 hours. There were no serious adverse events associated with IL-1ra treatment. IL-1ra caused a significant reduction in circulating CRP (26%), IL-6 (23%), and white blood cell and leukocyte count (27%). These results show that IL-1ra has the potential to be a therapeutic drug for the treatment of stroke.

Tumor Necrosis Factor-α

In patients after acute cerebral stroke, the expression of proinflammatory cytokine TNF-α is increased in both the cerebrospinal fluid and serum.[95,96] TNF-α administered intracerebroventricularly exacerbates damage in a dose-dependent manner in cerebral ischemia in hypertensive rats.[97] Damage is reduced in animals injected with soluble TNF-α receptor or a monoclonal antibody raised against TNF-α,[97–99] suggesting TNF-α has a role similar to that of IL-1β. It has been observed, however, that mice deficient in TNF-α receptor have increased damage after ischemic brain injury,[100] suggesting that this cytokine also has neuroprotective properties. A further study found that TNF-α deficient mice have poorer chronic but improved acute outcome in cortical contusion injury,[101] suggesting its dual effects are time dependent.

Interleukin-6

IL-6 levels in the cerebrospinal fluid are significantly higher than serum levels in patients after stroke.[102] As with TNF-α, evidence supporting the role of IL-6 in stroke is conflicting. Administration of IL-6 is neuroprotective in rats exposed to experimental cerebral ischemia,[103] and this protection is thought to be mediated through the increased expression of IL-1ra and soluble TNF-α receptor.[104] Several studies, however, have indicated a detrimental role for IL-6 in other neurodegenerative diseases.[105] In contrast, injury induced by experimental cerebral ischemia in IL-6–deficient mice was the same as in the wild-type mice.[106]

Interleukin-10

Circulating leukocytes exhibit increased levels of IL-10 secretion in patients after ischemic or hemorrhagic stroke,[107] and clinical studies illustrate that low circulating levels of IL-10 correlate with worse outcome after stroke.[108] Administration of IL-10 reduces infarct volumes by 20% in rats after cerebral ischemia.[109]

Transforming Growth Factor-β

Clinical studies have shown that there is increased TGF-β mRNA and protein in the borders of the infarct in patients after stroke.[60] Several lines of evidence indicate that ICV administration of TGF-β attenuates damage induced by focal or global cerebral ischemia in rats.[110,111] Intracortical injection of soluble TGF-β receptor in rats increases neuronal death in cerebral ischemia.[112]

Thus studies of cytokines provide evidence that IL-1 is detrimental to outcome, and IL-10 and TGF-β are neuroprotective. Results for IL-6 and TNF-α are varied and suggest divergent responses to these mediators. These discrepancies could result from model variation and the associated differences in the spatial and temporal expression of cytokines after brain injury.

Adhesion Molecules

To investigate the contribution of leukocytes in experimental cerebral ischemia, studies targeting adhesion molecules have been performed in mice. Systemic administration of antibodies directed against adhesion molecules (CD11b/CD18) on neutrophils decreases infarct and the number of apoptotic cells in permanent cerebral ischemia.[113] Blocking leukocyte adhesion molecules, ICAM-1, on endothelial cells has a stronger effect, reducing infarct volume by 80%,[114] and mice in which ICAM-1 is deleted showed a fivefold decrease in ischemic injury.[115] Compared with the wild-type animals, P-selectin null mice have a significantly increased blood flow following reperfusion as well as a decrease in infarct size and infiltrating neutrophils.[116]

Enlimomab is a murine monoclonal antibody raised against ICAM-1 and has been observed to inhibit neutrophil adhesion to brain endothelium in vitro.[117] Administration of this antibody to rats and rabbits exposed to cerebral ischemia reduces infarct size and improves behavioral outcome.[118–120] After a successful safety study,[120] enlimbomab was used in a phase III clinical trial.[121] It was concluded that the use of mouse anti-ICAM-1 as a treatment for human stroke was not viable, because outcomes were significantly worse outcome than with placebo. A possible explanation for these results is that the murine antibody was recognized as a foreign antigen and caused an immune response. A major concern with anti-inflammatory therapy is the increased risk of peripheral infection, which is known to exacerbate brain damage.

COMMUNICATION BETWEEN THE BRAIN AND THE PERIPHERY

It is now evident that systemic inflammation is detrimental in the outcome and severity of stroke.[122,123] Increased peripheral markers of inflammation (neutrophil count, body temperature, and CRP levels) predict poor outcome after stroke.[95,124,125] The brain now is recognized as immunologically active and is in direct contact with the immune system; thus a systemic inflammatory response can influence brain function.

Cytokines play a local role at the point of infection in mediating immune defense in response to a pathogenic challenge, but they also signal the CNS, thereby initiating brain-mediated defenses such as fever.[126] Although it is clear that systemic cytokines such as IL-1 signal the brain, the exact mechanisms by which this signaling is accomplished remain unclear. Cytokines are not able to cross the BBB passively in significant quantities. There are four possible routes by which blood-borne cytokines, such as IL-1, can signal the brain: (1) by specific transporters;[127,128] (2) by binding to receptors on the cerebral vascular endothelium, which leads to the release of secondary messengers that can cross into the brain;[129] (3) by signaling at the regions of the brain where the BBB is weak or absent (circumventricular organs);[130] or (4) by a neural route.[131,132]

Risk factors for atherosclerosis, such as smoking, obesity, hypertension, and diabetes, do increase the risk of stroke and have been linked to inflammation. Circulating CRP and TNF-α levels increase with these risk factors,[133,134] and elevated levels of plasma IL-6, soluble ICAM-1, vascular adhesion cell molecule-1, and E-selectin have been correlated with increased blood pressure.[135,136] High levels of these inflammatory mediators increase the risk of stroke and enhance leukocyte attachment after cerebral ischemia.

Systemic administration of IL-1β increases cerebral infarct volumes in mice subjected to experimental cerebral ischemia (see **Fig. 2**), and this increased infarct volume is attenuated by administration of IL-1ra.[92] The exact mechanism by which these effects occur is largely unknown. Peripheral administration of IL-1 induces fever,[126] increases expression of adhesion molecules on brain endothelium,[137,138] and triggers release of BBB-permeable mediators such as nitric oxide,[139] all of which worsen ischemic brain injury. In patients after stroke, plasma levels of IL-6 are increased[62] and are associated with poor outcome, and the production of cytokines in circulating mononuclear cells has been documented.[140]

IL-1, IL-6, and TNF-α can each activate the HPA axis, a homeostatic stress response (for review see[141]), and subsequent release of cortisol inhibits the innate inflammatory response and further HPA activation.[142] Glucocorticoids can reduce ischemic injury in rats,[143] but there is also evidence that endogenous glucocorticoid production exacerbates ischemic brain damage.[144,145] Activation of the HPA axis can play a major role in CNS injury–induced immunodepression, shutting down the systemic immune response and leaving the patient prone to infection.[146]

After experimental stroke in mice, activated spleen cells secrete significantly enhanced levels of TNF-α, IL-6, interferon-γ, IL-2, and chemokines such as macrophage inflammatory protein-2.[147] Severe head injury induces chemokine release in the brain from astrocytes and microglia, but the levels seem insufficient to mobilize peripheral leukocyte populations.[148] In fact, leukocyte mobilization and infiltration in response to brain injury depend on the hepatic release of the chemokine CINC-1.[61] IL-1β injected into the brain causes increased expression of CINC-1 from the liver and controls the subsequent mobilization, attachment, and infiltration of neutrophils to the brain.[61] The mechanism by which expression of CINC-1 is increased in the liver after brain injury is still unclear.

PSYCHOLOGIC RESPONSE

Psychologic factors may influence the onset of stroke and initiation of disease processes associated with the risk of stroke. This section focuses on the psychologic responses that result from stroke in humans. The psychologic response to stroke is complex and includes changes in cognition, affective state, and behavior.[149] Symptoms such as fatigue, depression, sleep disturbance, loss of appetite, emotional changes, and cognitive disturbances are common after stroke and in other neurologic disorders.[150–152] The great variation in response to stroke among individual patients does not seem to depend on the characteristics of the ischemic insult. Psychosocial factors, including previous mood state and social support, are known to be important in determining the consequences of stroke to the individual and the quality of survival.[153] Psychologic responses to stroke are likely to be mediated by multiple mechanisms including immune function. As outlined earlier, there is bidirectional communication between the immune system and the brain. Behavioral, affective, and cognitive functions may be driven by the immune response.[154,155]

Stroke, as does any other form of acute injury or infection, initiates a constellation of physiologic, behavioral, and psychologic changes that have been characterized as the acute-phase response[156] or sickness behavior.[157,158] In noncompromised individuals, such behavioral change may be adaptive, serving to limit energy expenditure and promote recovery. Sickness behavior has been characterized as malaise, reduced appetite, weakness, fatigue, sleep disturbance, disinterest for usual activities and social interactions, and changes in pain perception.[157] Exogenous proinflammatory cytokines or endotoxin challenge that induces cytokine production causes sickness behavior in both humans (**Table 1**) and experimental animals.[159,160]

Psychologic responses to stroke are reported well beyond the acute phase of injury and may persist for months or years after the initial event.[171] For many patients such responses are perceived as problematic, being pathologic rather than adaptive. They are important consequences of stroke that represent a huge burden on patients, and some are associated with poorer recovery and increased mortality.

Poststroke Fatigue

Poststroke fatigue differs from normal fatigue (general tiredness caused by exertion that resolves with rest) in that it is not associated with exertion and is characterized as pervasive, abnormal, persistent, and excessive weariness.[172] Approximately half of all survivors experience some degree of fatigue following stroke,[173] and stroke is

Table 1		
Evidence for the role of cytokines in psychologic responses in humans		
Cytokine	**Evidence for Role in Psychologic Response**	**Reference**
TNF-α	Increased levels in response to endotoxin challenge in healthy volunteers with verbal and nonverbal memory function, depressed mood (also IL-6, IL-1ra)	161
	Increased levels in response to endotoxin challenge in healthy male volunteers associated with changes in sleep (decreased non—rapid eye movement sleep) and increased sleepiness (also IL-6, IL-1ra)	162
	Direct relationship of production and cognitive deterioration in AIDS patients	163
IL-1	Increased levels in patients with major depression given endotoxin challenge and associated suppression of rapid eye movement sleep and improved mood (transient < 24 hours) (also IL-6 and TNF)	164
	Increased levels of IL-1 have been associated with disruption of cognitive function (attentional and mnemonic deficits) in volunteers independent of the effects of fever	157
IL-2	Depressive symptoms, impairments of memory attention and executive functions in patients	165
	Fatigue, depression, cognitive disturbances reported by treated cancer patients	161
IL-6	Negative association between circulating levels and cognitive function in volunteers receiving a low dose of endotoxin	166
INF-α	Healthy volunteers show decreased reasoning speed, cancer and Hepatitis C patients report fatigue, sleepiness, anorexia, difficultly in concentration	167
	Difficulty in concentration leading to poor performance in psychometric testing	168
	Mood disturbances in treated patients coinciding with cytokine treatment that increase with dose and duration and disappear within 2 weeks of end of treatment	169
	80% of patients who had cancer and were treated with cytokines reported moderate to severe fatigue	170
	Fatigue, depression, cognitive disturbances are commonly reported	

associated with increased physical and mental "fatigability," leading to poor concentration, memory difficulties, irritability, and emotional lability and adversely affecting daily functioning. In a study of younger patients poststroke fatigue was described as overwhelming and uncontrollable.[174] It currently is poorly understood and is a neglected area of stroke care,[175] possibly because of its hidden nature which sufferer's themselves find difficult to describe.[176] In a long-term follow-up study, poststroke fatigue independently predicted decreased functional independence, institutionalization, and mortality even after adjustment for age.[177]

Poststroke fatigue is associated with sleep disturbance and depression, but although these problems often occur concurrently, it is clear that for many stroke patients fatigue is a separate problem.[178,179] The severity and duration of poststroke fatigue has not been associated with stroke-related variables such as lesion location.[180] Fatigue has been reported as an independent risk factor for first-ever stroke.[181] Physical activity has been linked with the IL-6 system, and through this system regular activity influences mood, performance, and cognitive function.[182]

Depression After Stroke

Physical and cognitive symptoms of depression and other psychologic consequences of stroke overlap with the physical effects of stroke, making diagnosis, measurement, and estimate of incidence difficult to establish.[183] The consequences of brain injury may be indistinguishable for psychologic and physical consequences of stroke. Depression is estimated to occur in 19% to 40% of patients after stroke.[184] The presence of depression 1 month after stroke is associated with higher rates of mortality at 12 and 24 months independent of initial stroke severity.[185] Although a relationship between site of injury within the brain and depression has been demonstrated,[186] the relationship does not explain most depressive symptoms.

Sleep Disturbances

Sleep-wake disorders are common after stroke (20%–40% of patients) and include insomnia, increased sleep needs (hypersomnia), and excessive daytime sleeping.[187] These effects may be caused by the area of the brain affected by the stroke (eg, thalamic or brainstem involvement) or result from multiple factors.

Other Psychologic Responses

In addition to the responses already outlined, patients experience many other problems after stroke that are analogous to components of sickness behavior.

Emotional lability, irritability, changes in cognitive function including memory difficulties, change in appetite, decrease in social activities and contacts, and altered pain sensation are common.[171]

Possible Mechanisms of Psychologic Responses to Stroke

It has been suggested that psychologic effects associated with both acute and chronic neurologic disorders share at least some underlying immunologic mechanisms.[172] How inflammation and immune response to injury such as stroke might influence longer-term psychologic responses to stroke has not been fully elucidated. In cancer, excessive activation of the central cytokine systems is thought to be responsible for the persistent symptoms associated with the disease.[188] Stroke is associated with inflammation, and IL-1 clearly is implicated in the pathogenesis of damage following ischemia.[189,190] Inflammatory markers including IL-6 (measured as a surrogate for IL-1, which is rarely detected in peripheral circulation) are elevated in plasma for many months after stroke and correlate with stroke severity.[65] Such cytokine activation may be responsible for or contribute to longer-term psychologic responses following stroke.

SUMMARY

There is now considerable evidence from both experimental and clinical studies that immune and inflammatory processes can contribute to the onset of stroke and the neurologic and psychologic outcomes. Several specific therapeutic targets have been identified that may significantly improve the devastating impact of stroke.

REFERENCES

1. Cheng YD, Al-Khoury L, Zivin JA. Neuroprotection for ischemic stroke: two decades of success and failure. NeuroRx 2004;1:36–45.
2. Reith J, Jorgensen HS, Pedersen PM, et al. Body temperature in acute stroke: relation to stroke severity, infarct size, mortality, and outcome. Lancet 1996; 347:422–5.
3. De Michele M, Touzani O, Foster AC, et al. Corticotropin-releasing factor: effect on cerebral blood flow in physiologic and ischaemic conditions. Exp Brain Res 2005;165:375–82.
4. Katsumata T, Katayama Y, Yonemori H, et al. Delayed administration of JTP-2942, a novel thyrotropin-releasing hormone analogue, improves cerebral blood flow and metabolism in rat postischaemic brain. Clin Exp Pharmacol Physiol 2001;28:48–54.
5. Nakamachi T, Endo S, Ohtaki H, et al. Orexin-1 receptor expression after global ischemia in mice. Regul Pept 2005;126:49–54.
6. Schwarz S, Schwab S, Klinga K, et al. Neuroendocrine changes in patients with acute space occupying ischaemic stroke. J Neurol Neurosurg Psychiatry 2003; 74:725–7.
7. Fassbender K, Schmidt R, Mossner R, et al. Pattern of activation of the hypothalamic-pituitary-adrenal axis in acute stroke. Relation to acute confusional state, extent of brain damage, and clinical outcome. Stroke 1994;25:1105–8.
8. Zeitoun K, Carr BR. Is there an increased risk of stroke associated with oral contraceptives? Drug Saf 1999;20:467–73.
9. Warlow C, Sudlow C, Dennis M, et al. Stroke. Lancet 2003;362:1211–24.
10. Bamford J, Sandercock P, Dennis M, et al. A prospective study of acute cerebrovascular disease in the community: the Oxfordshire Community Stroke Project 1981–86. 1. Methodology, demography and incident cases of first-ever stroke. J Neurol Neurosurg Psychiatry 1988;51:1373–80.
11. Bamford J, Sandercock P, Dennis M, et al. Classification and natural history of clinically identifiable subtypes of cerebral infarction. Lancet 1991;337:1521–6.
12. Lyden P, Lu M, Jackson C, et al. Underlying structure of the National Institutes of Health Stroke Scale: results of a factor analysis. NINDS tPA Stroke Trial Investigators. Stroke 1999;30:2347–54.
13. Warlow C, Dennis M, Van Gijn J, et al. Stroke: a practical guide to management. Oxford (UK): Blackwell Science; 2001.
14. Ostir GV, Goodwin JS, Markides KS, et al. Differential effects of premorbid physical and emotional health on recovery from acute events. J Am Geriatr Soc 2002; 50:713–8.
15. Wyller TB, Sodring KM, Sveen U, et al. Are there gender differences in functional outcome after stroke? Clin Rehabil 1997;11:171–9.
16. Wolfe CD. The impact of stroke. Br Med Bull 2000;56:275–86.

17. Murray CJL, Lopez AD. The global burden of disease: a comprehensive assessment of mortality and disability from diseases, injuries and risk factors in 1990 and projected to 2020. Boston: Harvard University Press; 2005.
18. Mant J, Wade D, Winner S. Health care needs assessment: stroke. In: Health care needs assessment: the epidemiologically based needs assessment reviews. Oxford (UK): Radcliffe Medical Press; 2004.
19. Anderson CS, Linto J, Stewart-Wynne EG. A population-based assessment of the impact and burden of caregiving for long-term stroke survivors. Stroke 1995;26:843–9.
20. Smout S, Koudstaal PJ, Ribbers GM, et al. Struck by stroke: a pilot study exploring quality of life and coping patterns in younger patients and spouses. Int J Rehabil Res 2001;24:261–8.
21. Burman ME. Family caregiver expectations and management of the stroke trajectory. Rehabil Nurs 2001;26:94–9.
22. Frey JL. Recombinant tissue plasminogen activator (rtPA) for stroke. The perspective at 8 years. Neurologist 2005;11:123–33.
23. Chen ZM, Sandercock P, Pan HC, et al. Indications for early aspirin use in acute ischemic stroke: a combined analysis of 40 000 randomized patients from the Chinese Acute Stroke Trial and the International Stroke Trial. On behalf of the CAST and IST collaborative groups. Stroke 2000;31: 1240–9.
24. Ruland SD. Lifestyle modification, antihypertensives, and cholesterol-lowering medication for primary and secondary stroke prevention. Continuum 2005;19: 47–60.
25. Sterzer P, Meintzschel F, Rosler A, et al. Pravastatin improves cerebral vasomotor reactivity in patients with subcortical small-vessel disease. Stroke 2001; 32:2817–20.
26. Tseng MY, Czosnyka M, Richards H, et al. Effects of acute treatment with pravastatin on cerebral vasospasm, autoregulation, and delayed ischemic deficits after aneurysmal subarachnoid hemorrhage: a phase II randomized placebo-controlled trial. Stroke 2005;36:1627–32.
27. Berg AH, Scherer PE. Adipose tissue, inflammation, and cardiovascular disease. Circ Res 2005;96:939–49.
28. Schieffer B, Bunte C, Witte J, et al. Comparative effects of AT1-antagonism and angiotensin-converting enzyme inhibition on markers of inflammation and platelet aggregation in patients with coronary artery disease. J Am Coll Cardiol 2004;44:362–8.
29. Di NM, Papa F. Angiotensin-converting enzyme inhibitor use is associated with reduced plasma concentration of C-reactive protein in patients with first-ever ischemic stroke. Stroke 2003;34:2922–9.
30. Matyszak MK. Inflammation in the CNS: balance between immunological privilege and immune responses. Prog Neurobiol 1998;56:19–35.
31. Deli MA, Abraham CS, Kataoka Y, et al. Permeability studies on in vitro blood-brain barrier models: physiology, pathology, and pharmacology. Cell Mol Neurobiol 2005;25:59–127.
32. Hickey WF. Basic principles of immunological surveillance of the normal central nervous system. Glia 2001;36:118–24.
33. Dirnagl U, Iadecola C, Moskowitz MA. Pathobiology of ischaemic stroke: an integrated view. Trends Neurosci 1999;22:391–7.
34. del Zoppo GJ, Mabuchi T. Cerebral microvessel responses to focal ischemia. J Cereb Blood Flow Metab 2003;23:879–94.

35. Lynch NJ, Willis CL, Nolan CC, et al. Microglial activation and increased synthesis of complement component C1q precedes blood-brain barrier dysfunction in rats. Mol Immunol 2004;40:709–16.

36. Rothwell NJ, Hopkins SJ. Cytokines and the nervous system II: actions and mechanisms of action. Trends Neurosci 1995;18:130–6.

37. Kochanek PM, Hallenbeck JM. Polymorphonuclear leukocytes and monocytes/macrophages in the pathogenesis of cerebral ischemia and stroke. Stroke 1992; 23:1367–79.

38. Yamasaki Y, Matsuo Y, Matsuura N, et al. Transient increase of cytokine-induced neutrophil chemoattractant, a member of the interleukin-8 family, in ischemic brain areas after focal ischemia in rats. Stroke 1995;26:318–22.

39. Haring HP, Berg EL, Tsurushita N, et al. E-selectin appears in nonischemic tissue during experimental focal cerebral ischemia. Stroke 1996;27:1386–91.

40. Love S, Barber R. Expression of P-selectin and intercellular adhesion molecule-1 in human brain after focal infarction or cardiac arrest. Neuropathol Appl Neurobiol 2001;27:465–73.

41. Schoning B, Elepfandt P, Daberkow N, et al. Differences in immune cell invasion into the cerebrospinal fluid and brain parenchyma during cerebral infusion of interleukin-1beta. Neurol Sci 2002;23:211–8.

42. Kim JS, Chopp M, Chen H, et al. Adhesive glycoproteins CD11a and CD18 are upregulated in the leukocytes from patients with ischemic stroke and transient ischemic attacks. J Neurol Sci 1995;128:45–50.

43. del Zoppo GJ, Schmid-Schonbein GW, Mori E, et al. Polymorphonuclear leukocytes occlude capillaries following middle cerebral artery occlusion and reperfusion in baboons. Stroke 1991;22:1276–83.

44. Schmid-Schonbein GW. Capillary plugging by granulocytes and the no-reflow phenomenon in the microcirculation. Fed Proc 1987;46:2397–401.

45. Maier CM, Hsieh L, Yu F, et al. Matrix metalloproteinase-9 and myeloperoxidase expression: quantitative analysis by antigen immunohistochemistry in a model of transient focal cerebral ischemia. Stroke 2004;35:1169–74.

46. Lipton P. Ischemic cell death in brain neurons. Physiol Rev 1999;79:1431–568.

47. Inglis VI, Jones MP, Tse AD, et al. Neutrophils both reduce and increase permeability in a cell culture model of the blood-brain barrier. Brain Res 2004;998: 218–29.

48. Heo JH, Han SW, Lee SK. Free radicals as triggers of brain edema formation after stroke. Free Radic Biol Med 2005;39:51–70.

49. Crack PJ, Taylor JM. Reactive oxygen species and the modulation of stroke. Free Radic Biol Med 2005;38:1433–44.

50. Taylor BS, de Vera ME, Ganster RW, et al. Multiple NF-kappaB enhancer elements regulate cytokine induction of the human inducible nitric oxide synthase gene. J Biol Chem 1998;273:15148–56.

51. Bonventre JV. Roles of phospholipase A2 in brain cell and tissue injury associated with ischemia and excitotoxicity. J Lipid Mediat Cell Signal 1997;16: 199–208.

52. Pepicelli O, Fedele E, Bonanno G, et al. In vivo activation of N-methyl-D-aspartate receptors in the rat hippocampus increases prostaglandin E(2) extracellular levels and triggers lipid peroxidation through cyclooxygenase-mediated mechanisms. J Neurochem 2002;81:1028–34.

53. Iadecola C, Sugimoto K, Niwa K, et al. Increased susceptibility to ischemic brain injury in cyclooxygenase-1-deficient mice. J Cereb Blood Flow Metab 2001;21: 1436–41.

54. Manabe Y, Anrather J, Kawano T, et al. Prostanoids, not reactive oxygen species, mediate COX-2-dependent neurotoxicity. Ann Neurol 2004;55: 668–75.
55. Ahmad A, Saleem S, Ahmad M, et al. Prostaglandin EP1 receptor contributes to excitotoxicity and focal ischemic brain damage. Toxicol Sci 2006;89(1):265–70.
56. McCullough L, Wu L, Haughey N, et al. Neuroprotective function of the PGE2 EP2 receptor in cerebral ischemia. J Neurosci 2004;24:257–68.
57. Anthony DC, Bolton SJ, Fearn S, et al. Age-related effects of interleukin-1 beta on polymorphonuclear neutrophil-dependent increases in blood-brain barrier permeability in rats. Brain 1997;120(Pt 3):435–44.
58. Allan SM, Rothwell NJ. Inflammation in central nervous system injury. Philos Trans R Soc Lond B Biol Sci 2003;358:1669–77.
59. Lazovic J, Basu A, Lin HW, et al. Neuroinflammation and both cytotoxic and vasogenic edema are reduced in interleukin-1 type 1 receptor-deficient mice conferring neuroprotection. Stroke 2005;36:2226–31.
60. Krupinski J, Kumar P, Kumar S, et al. Increased expression of TGF-beta 1 in brain tissue after ischemic stroke in humans. Stroke 1996;27:852–7.
61. Campbell SJ, Hughes PM, Iredale JP, et al. CINC-1 is an acute-phase protein induced by focal brain injury causing leukocyte mobilization and liver injury. FASEB J 2003;17:1168–70.
62. Smith CJ, Emsley HC, Gavin CM, et al. Peak plasma interleukin-6 and other peripheral markers of inflammation in the first week of ischaemic stroke correlate with brain infarct volume, stroke severity and long-term outcome. BMC Neurol 2004;4:2.
63. Pedersen ED, Waje-Andreassen U, Vedeler CA, et al. Systemic complement activation following human acute ischaemic stroke. Clin Exp Immunol 2004; 137:117–22.
64. Van Beek J. Complement activation: beneficial and detrimental effects in the CNS. Ernst Schering Res Found Workshop 2004;47:67–85.
65. Emsley HC, Smith CJ, Gavin CM, et al. An early and sustained peripheral inflammatory response in acute ischaemic stroke: relationships with infection and atherosclerosis. J Neuroimmunol 2003;139:93–101.
66. Veerhuis R, Janssen I, De Groot CJ, et al. Cytokines associated with amyloid plaques in Alzheimer's disease brain stimulate human glial and neuronal cell cultures to secrete early complement proteins, but not C1-inhibitor. Exp Neurol 1999;160:289–99.
67. Lindsberg PJ, Ohman J, Lehto T, et al. Complement activation in the central nervous system following blood-brain barrier damage in man. Ann Neurol 1996;40:587–96.
68. Singhrao SK, Neal JW, Rushmere NK, et al. Spontaneous classical pathway activation and deficiency of membrane regulators render human neurons susceptible to complement lysis. Am J Pathol 2000;157:905–18.
69. Ten VS, Sosunov SA, Mazer SP, et al. C1q-deficiency is neuroprotective against hypoxic-ischemic brain injury in neonatal mice. Stroke 2005;36:2244–50.
70. Storini C, Rossi E, Marrella V, et al. C1-inhibitor protects against brain ischemia-reperfusion injury via inhibition of cell recruitment and inflammation. Neurobiol Dis 2005;19:10–7.
71. Cunningham LA, Wetzel M, Rosenberg GA. Multiple roles for MMPs and TIMPs in cerebral ischemia. Glia 2005;50:329–39.
72. Gidday JM, Gasche YG, Copin JC, et al. Leukocyte-derived matrix metalloproteinase-9 mediates blood-brain barrier breakdown and is proinflammatory after

transient focal cerebral ischemia. Am J Physiol Heart Circ Physiol 2005;289: H558–68.

73. Castellanos M, Leira R, Serena J, et al. Plasma metalloproteinase-9 concentration predicts hemorrhagic transformation in acute ischemic stroke. Stroke 2003; 34:40–6.

74. Rosell A, varez-Sabin J, Arenillas JF, et al. A matrix metalloproteinase protein array reveals a strong relation between MMP-9 and MMP-13 with diffusion-weighted image lesion increase in human stroke. Stroke 2005;36:1415–20.

75. Gu Z, Kaul M, Yan B, et al. S-nitrosylation of matrix metalloproteinases: signaling pathway to neuronal cell death. Science 2002;297:1186–90.

76. Kauppinen TM, Swanson RA. Poly(ADP-ribose) polymerase-1 promotes microglial activation, proliferation, and matrix metalloproteinase-9-mediated neuron death. J Immunol 2005;174:2288–96.

77. Vecil GG, Larsen PH, Corley SM, et al. Interleukin-1 is a key regulator of matrix metalloproteinase-9 expression in human neurons in culture and following mouse brain trauma in vivo. J Neurosci Res 2000;61:212–24.

78. Hillhouse EW, Kida S, Iannotti F. Middle cerebral artery occlusion in the rat causes a biphasic production of immunoreactive interleukin-1beta in the cerebral cortex. Neurosci Lett 1998;249:177–9.

79. Buttini M, Sauter A, Boddeke HW. Induction of interleukin-1 beta mRNA after focal cerebral ischaemia in the rat. Brain Res Mol Brain Res 1994;23:126–34.

80. Sairanen TR, Lindsberg PJ, Brenner M, et al. Global forebrain ischemia results in differential cellular expression of interleukin-1beta (IL-1beta) and its receptor at mRNA and protein level. J Cereb Blood Flow Metab 1997;17:1107–20.

81. Pinteaux E, Parker LC, Rothwell NJ, et al. Expression of interleukin-1 receptors and their role in interleukin-1 actions in murine microglial cells. J Neurochem 2002;83:754–63.

82. Yamasaki Y, Matsuura N, Shozuhara H, et al. Interleukin-1 as a pathogenetic mediator of ischemic brain damage in rats. Stroke 1995;26:676–80.

83. Loddick SA, Rothwell NJ. Neuroprotective effects of human recombinant interleukin-1 receptor antagonist in focal cerebral ischaemia in the rat. J Cereb Blood Flow Metab 1996;16:932–40.

84. Stroemer RP, Rothwell NJ. Exacerbation of ischemic brain damage by localized striatal injection of interleukin-1beta in the rat. J Cereb Blood Flow Metab 1998; 18:833–9.

85. Boutin H, LeFeuvre RA, Horai R, et al. Role of IL-1alpha and IL-1beta in ischemic brain damage. J Neurosci 2001;21:5528–34.

86. Thornberry NA, Bull HG, Calaycay JR, et al. A novel heterodimeric cysteine protease is required for interleukin-1 beta processing in monocytes. Nature 1992;356:768–74.

87. Huang FP, Wang ZQ, Wu DC, et al. Early NFkappaB activation is inhibited during focal cerebral ischemia in interleukin-1beta-converting enzyme deficient mice. J Neurosci Res 2003;73:698–707.

88. Relton JK, Rothwell NJ. Interleukin-1 receptor antagonist inhibits ischaemic and excitotoxic neuronal damage in the rat. Brain Res Bull 1992;29:243–6.

89. Stroemer RP, Rothwell NJ. Cortical protection by localized striatal injection of IL-1ra following cerebral ischemia in the rat. J Cereb Blood Flow Metab 1997; 17:597–604.

90. Garcia JH, Liu KF, Relton JK. Interleukin-1 receptor antagonist decreases the number of necrotic neurons in rats with middle cerebral artery occlusion. Am J Pathol 1995;147:1477–86.

91. Lin MT, Kao TY, Jin YT, et al. Interleukin-1 receptor antagonist attenuates the heat stroke-induced neuronal damage by reducing the cerebral ischemia in rats. Brain Res Bull 1995;37:595–8.
92. Relton JK, Martin D, Thompson RC, et al. Peripheral administration of interleukin-1 receptor antagonist inhibits brain damage after focal cerebral ischemia in the rat. Exp Neurol 1996;138:206–13.
93. Loddick SA, Wong ML, Bongiorno PB, et al. Endogenous interleukin-1 receptor antagonist is neuroprotective. Biochem Biophys Res Commun 1997;234:211–5.
94. Emsley HC, Smith CJ, Georgiou RF, et al. A randomised phase II study of interleukin-1 receptor antagonist in acute stroke patients. J Neurol Neurosurg Psychiatry 2005;76:1366–72.
95. Vila N, Filella X, Deulofeu R, et al. Cytokine-induced inflammation and long-term stroke functional outcome. J Neurol Sci 1999;162:185–8.
96. Zaremba J, Skrobanski P, Losy J. Tumour necrosis factor-alpha is increased in the cerebrospinal fluid and serum of ischaemic stroke patients and correlates with the volume of evolving brain infarct. Biomed Pharmacother 2001;55:258–63.
97. Barone FC, Arvin B, White RF, et al. Tumor necrosis factor-alpha. A mediator of focal ischemic brain injury. Stroke 1997;28:1233–44.
98. Dawson DA, Martin D, Hallenbeck JM. Inhibition of tumor necrosis factor-alpha reduces focal cerebral ischemic injury in the spontaneously hypertensive rat. Neurosci Lett 1996;218:41–4.
99. Hosomi N, Ban CR, Naya T, et al. Tumor necrosis factor-alpha neutralization reduced cerebral edema through inhibition of matrix metalloproteinase production after transient focal cerebral ischemia. J Cereb Blood Flow Metab 2005;25:959–67.
100. Bruce AJ, Boling W, Kindy MS, et al. Altered neuronal and microglial responses to excitotoxic and ischemic brain injury in mice lacking TNF receptors. Nat Med 1996;2:788–94.
101. Scherbel U, Raghupathi R, Nakamura M, et al. Differential acute and chronic responses of tumor necrosis factor-deficient mice to experimental brain injury. Proc Natl Acad Sci U S A 1999;96:8721–6.
102. Tarkowski E, Rosengren L, Blomstrand C, et al. Early intrathecal production of interleukin-6 predicts the size of brain lesion in stroke. Stroke 1995;26:1393–8.
103. Loddick SA, Turnbull AV, Rothwell NJ. Cerebral interleukin-6 is neuroprotective during permanent focal cerebral ischemia in the rat. J Cereb Blood Flow Metab 1998;18:176–9.
104. Tilg H, Trehu E, Atkins MB, et al. Interleukin-6 (IL-6) as an anti-inflammatory cytokine: induction of circulating IL-1 receptor antagonist and soluble tumor necrosis factor receptor p55. Blood 1994;83:113–8.
105. Campbell IL, Abraham CR, Masliah E, et al. Neurologic disease induced in transgenic mice by cerebral overexpression of interleukin 6. Proc Natl Acad Sci U S A 1993;90:10061–5.
106. Clark WM, Rinker LG, Lessov NS, et al. Lack of interleukin-6 expression is not protective against focal central nervous system ischemia. Stroke 2000;31:1715–20.
107. Pelidou SH, Kostulas N, Matusevicius D, et al. High levels of IL-10 secreting cells are present in blood in cerebrovascular diseases. Eur J Neurol 1999;6:437–42.
108. Van Exel E, Gussekloo J, de Craen AJ, et al. Inflammation and stroke: the Leiden 85-Plus Study. Stroke 2002;33:1135–8.

109. Spera PA, Ellison JA, Feuerstein GZ, et al. IL-10 reduces rat brain injury following focal stroke. Neurosci Lett 1998;251:189–92.

110. Henrich-Noack P, Prehn JH, Krieglstein J. TGF-beta 1 protects hippocampal neurons against degeneration caused by transient global ischemia. Dose-response relationship and potential neuroprotective mechanisms. Stroke 1996;27:1609–14.

111. Prehn JH, Backhauss C, Krieglstein J. Transforming growth factor-beta 1 prevents glutamate neurotoxicity in rat neocortical cultures and protects mouse neocortex from ischemic injury in vivo. J Cereb Blood Flow Metab 1993;13: 521–5.

112. Ruocco A, Nicole O, Docagne F, et al. A transforming growth factor-beta antagonist unmasks the neuroprotective role of this endogenous cytokine in excitotoxic and ischemic brain injury. J Cereb Blood Flow Metab 1999;19:1345–53.

113. Chopp M, Li Y, Jiang N, et al. Antibodies against adhesion molecules reduce apoptosis after transient middle cerebral artery occlusion in rat brain. J Cereb Blood Flow Metab 1996;16:578–84.

114. Jiang N, Moyle M, Soule HR, et al. Neutrophil inhibitory factor is neuroprotective after focal ischemia in rats. Ann Neurol 1995;38:935–42.

115. Soriano SG, Lipton SA, Wang YF, et al. Intercellular adhesion molecule-1-deficient mice are less susceptible to cerebral ischemia-reperfusion injury. Ann Neurol 1996;39:618–24.

116. Connolly ES Jr, Winfree CJ, Prestigiacomo CJ, et al. Exacerbation of cerebral injury in mice that express the P-selectin gene: identification of P-selectin blockade as a new target for the treatment of stroke. Circ Res 1997;81:304–10.

117. Smith CW, Rothlein R, Hughes BJ, et al. Recognition of an endothelial determinant for CD 18-dependent human neutrophil adherence and transendothelial migration. J Clin Invest 1988;82:1746–56.

118. Clark WM, Madden KP, Rothlein R, et al. Reduction of central nervous system ischemic injury by monoclonal antibody to intercellular adhesion molecule. J Neurosurg 1991;75:623–7.

119. Bowes MP, Rothlein R, Fagan SC, et al. Monoclonal antibodies preventing leukocyte activation reduce experimental neurologic injury and enhance efficacy of thrombolytic therapy. Neurology 1995;45:815–9.

120. Schneider D, Berrouschot J, Brandt T, et al. Safety, pharmacokinetics and biological activity of enlimomab (anti-ICAM-1 antibody): an open-label, dose escalation study in patients hospitalized for acute stroke. Eur Neurol 1998;40:78–83.

121. Enlimomab Acute Stroke Trial Investigators. Use of anti-ICAM-1 therapy in ischemic stroke: results of the Enlimomab Acute Stroke Trial. Neurology 2001; 57:1428–34.

122. Rost NS, Wolf PA, Kase CS, et al. Plasma concentration of C-reactive protein and risk of ischemic stroke and transient ischemic attack: the Framingham study. Stroke 2001;32:2575–9.

123. Ridker PM, Cushman M, Stampfer MJ, et al. Inflammation, aspirin, and the risk of cardiovascular disease in apparently healthy men. N Engl J Med 1997;336: 973–9.

124. Muir KW, Weir CJ, Alwan W, et al. C-reactive protein and outcome after ischemic stroke. Stroke 1999;30:981–5.

125. Azzimondi G, Bassein L, Nonino F, et al. Fever in acute stroke worsens prognosis. A prospective study. Stroke 1995;26:2040–3.

126. Hashimoto M, Ishikawa Y, Yokota S, et al. Action site of circulating interleukin-1 on the rabbit brain. Brain Res 1991;540:217–23.

127. Banks WA, Ortiz L, Plotkin SR, et al. Human interleukin (IL) 1 alpha, murine IL-1 alpha and murine IL-1 beta are transported from blood to brain in the mouse by a shared saturable mechanism. J Pharmacol Exp Ther 1991;259:988–96.
128. Banks WA, Kastin AJ. Blood to brain transport of interleukin links the immune and central nervous systems. Life Sci 1991;48:L117–21.
129. Van Dam AM, de Vries HE, Kuiper J, et al. Interleukin-1 receptors on rat brain endothelial cells: a role in neuroimmune interaction? FASEB J 1996;10:351–6.
130. Blatteis CM. Role of the OVLT in the febrile response to circulating pyrogens. Prog Brain Res 1992;91:409–12.
131. Goehler LE, Relton JK, Dripps D, et al. Vagal paraganglia bind biotinylated inter-leukin-1 receptor antagonist: a possible mechanism for immune-to-brain communication. Brain Res Bull 1997;43:357–64.
132. Goehler LE, Gaykema RP, Hammack SE, et al. Interleukin-1 induces c-Fos immunoreactivity in primary afferent neurons of the vagus nerve. Brain Res 1998;804:306–10.
133. Bruunsgaard H, Skinhoj P, Pedersen AN, et al. Ageing, tumour necrosis factor-alpha (TNF-alpha) and atherosclerosis. Clin Exp Immunol 2000;121:255–60.
134. Mendall MA, Patel P, Ballam L, et al. C reactive protein and its relation to cardio-vascular risk factors: a population based cross sectional study. BMJ 1996;312:1061–5.
135. Blann AD, Tse W, Maxwell SJ, et al. Increased levels of the soluble adhesion molecule E-selectin in essential hypertension. J Hypertens 1994;12:925–8.
136. DeSouza CA, Dengel DR, Macko RF, et al. Elevated levels of circulating cell adhesion molecules in uncomplicated essential hypertension. Am J Hypertens 1997;10:1335–41.
137. Osborn L. Leukocyte adhesion to endothelium in inflammation. Cell 1990;62:3–6.
138. Springer TA. Adhesion receptors of the immune system. Nature 1990;346:425–34.
139. Morin AM, Stanboli A. Nitric oxide synthase localization in cultured cerebrovas-cular endothelium during mitosis. Exp Cell Res 1994;211:183–8.
140. Kostulas N, Pelidou SH, Kivisakk P, et al. Increased IL-1beta, IL-8, and IL-17 mRNA expression in blood mononuclear cells observed in a prospective ischemic stroke study. Stroke 1999;30:2174–9.
141. Chrousos GP. The hypothalamic-pituitary-adrenal axis and immune-mediated inflammation. N Engl J Med 1995;332:1351–62.
142. Glezer I, Rivest S. Glucocorticoids: protectors of the brain during innate immune responses. Neuroscientist 2004;10:538–52.
143. Felszeghy K, Banisadr G, Rostene W, et al. Dexamethasone downregulates che-mokine receptor CXCR4 and exerts neuroprotection against hypoxia/ischemia-induced brain injury in neonatal rats. Neuroimmunomodulation 2004;11:404–13.
144. Sugo N, Hurn PD, Morahan MB, et al. Social stress exacerbates focal cerebral ischemia in mice. Stroke 2002;33:1660–4.
145. Smith-Swintosky VL, Pettigrew LC, Sapolsky RM, et al. Metyrapone, an inhibitor of glucocorticoid production, reduces brain injury induced by focal and global ischemia and seizures. J Cereb Blood Flow Metab 1996;16:585–98.
146. Meisel C, Schwab JM, Prass K, et al. Central nervous system injury induced immune deficiency syndrome. Nat Rev Neurosci 2005;6(10):775–86.
147. Offner H, Subramanian S, Parker SM, et al. Experimental stroke induces massive, rapid activation of the peripheral immune system. J Cereb Blood Flow Metab 2005;8.

148. Ott L, McClain CJ, Gillespie M, et al. Cytokines and metabolic dysfunction after severe head injury. J Neurotrauma 1994;11:447–72.

149. Bogousslavsky J. William Feinberg lecture 2002: emotions, mood, and behavior after stroke. Stroke 2003;34:1046–50.

150. Chaudhuri A, Behan PO. Fatigue in neurological disorders. Lancet 2004;363: 978–88.

151. Eskesen V, Sorensen EB, Rosenorn J, et al. The prognosis in subarachnoid hemorrhage of unknown etiology. J Neurosurg 1984;61:1029–31.

152. Powell J, Kitchen N, Heslin J, et al. Psychosocial outcomes at 18 months after good neurological recovery from aneurysmal subarachnoid haemorrhage. J Neurol Neurosurg Psychiatry 2004;75:1119–24.

153. Clark MS, Smith DS. Psychological correlates of outcome following rehabilitation from stroke. Clin Rehabil 1999;13:129–40.

154. Maier SF, Watkins LR. Cytokines for psychologists: implications of bidirectional immune-to-brain communication for understanding behavior, mood, and cognition. Psychol Rev 1998;105:83–107.

155. Maier SF. Bi-directional immune-brain communication: implications for understanding stress, pain, and cognition. Brain Behav Immun 2003;17:69–85.

156. Baumann H, Gauldie J. The acute phase response. Immunol Today 1994;15: 74–80.

157. Dantzer R. Cytokine-induced sickness behavior: mechanisms and implications. Ann N Y Acad Sci 2001;933:222–34.

158. Kent S, Bluthe RM, Kelley KW, et al. Sickness behavior as a new target for drug development. Trends Pharmacol Sci 1992;13:24–8.

159. Capuron L, Dantzer R. Cytokines and depression: the need for a new paradigm. Brain Behav Immun 2003;17(Suppl 1):S119–24.

160. Larson SJ, Dunn AJ. Behavioral effects of cytokines. Brain Behav Immun 2001; 15:371–87.

161. Reichenberg A, Yirmiya R, Schuld A, et al. Cytokine-associated emotional and cognitive disturbances in humans. Arch Gen Psychiatry 2001;58:445–52.

162. Hermann DM, Mullington J, Hinze-Selch D, et al. Endotoxin-induced changes in sleep and sleepiness during the day. Psychoneuroendocrinology 1998;23: 427–37.

163. Seilhean D, Kobayashi K, He Y, et al. Tumor necrosis factor-alpha, microglia and astrocytes in AIDS dementia complex. Acta Neuropathol (Berl) 1997;93: 508–17.

164. Bauer J, Hohagen F, Gimmel E, et al. Induction of cytokine synthesis and fever suppresses REM sleep and improves mood in patients with major depression. Biol Psychiatry 1995;38:611–21.

165. Capuron L, Ravaud A, Miller AH, et al. Baseline mood and psychosocial characteristics of patients developing depressive symptoms during interleukin-2 and/ or interferon-alpha cancer therapy. Brain Behav Immun 2004;18:205–13.

166. Krabbe KS, Reichenberg A, Yirmiya R, et al. Low-dose endotoxemia and human neuropsychological functions. Brain Behav Immun 2005;19:453–60.

167. Neurological effects of recombinant human interferon. Br Med J (Clin Res Ed) 1983;286:1054–5.

168. Pavol MA, Meyers CA, Rexer JL, et al. Pattern of neurobehavioral deficits associated with interferon alfa therapy for leukemia. Neurology 1995;45:947–50.

169. Adams F, Quesada JR, Gutterman JU. Neuropsychiatric manifestations of human leukocyte interferon therapy in patients with cancer. JAMA 1984;252:938–41.

170. Wichers M, Maes M. The psychoneuroimmuno-pathophysiology of cytokine-induced depression in humans. Int J Neuropsychopharmacol 2002;5:375–88.
171. Anderson R. The aftermath of stroke: the experience of patients and their families. 1992.
172. De Groot MH, Phillips SJ, Eskes GA. Fatigue associated with stroke and other neurologic conditions: implications for stroke rehabilitation. Arch Phys Med Rehabil 2003;84:1714–20.
173. Carlsson GE, Moller A, Blomstrand C. Consequences of mild stroke in persons < 75 years—a 1-year follow-up. Cerebrovasc Dis 2003;16:383–8.
174. Roding J, Lindstrom B, Malm J, et al. Frustrated and invisible—younger stroke patients' experiences of the rehabilitation process. Disabil Rehabil 2003;25:867–74.
175. Morley W, Jackson K, Mead GE. Post-stroke fatigue: an important yet neglected symptom. Age Ageing 2005;34:313.
176. Carlsson GE, Moller A, Blomstrand C. A qualitative study of the consequences of hidden dysfunctions' one year after a mild stroke in persons < 75 years. Disabil Rehabil 2004;26:1373–80.
177. Glader EL, Stegmayr B, Asplund K. Poststroke fatigue: a 2-year follow-up study of stroke patients in Sweden. Stroke 2002;33:1327–33.
178. Staub F, Bogousslavsky J. Fatigue after stroke: a major but neglected issue. Cerebrovasc Dis 2001;12:75–81.
179. Choi-Kwon S, Kim HS, Kwon SU, et al. Factors affecting the burden on caregivers of stroke survivors in South Korea. Arch Phys Med Rehabil 2005;86:1043–8.
180. Ingles JL, Eskes GA, Phillips SJ. Fatigue after stroke. Arch Phys Med Rehabil 1999;80:173–8.
181. Schuitemaker GE, Dinant GJ, Van Der Pol GA, et al. Vital exhaustion as a risk indicator for first stroke. Psychosomatics 2004;45:114–8.
182. Pedersen BK, Febbraio M. Muscle-derived interleukin-6—a possible link between skeletal muscle, adipose tissue, liver, and brain. Brain Behav Immun 2005;19:371–6.
183. De Coster L, Leentjens AF, Lodder J, et al. The sensitivity of somatic symptoms in post-stroke depression: a discriminant analytic approach. Int J Geriatr Psychiatry 2005;20:358–62.
184. Turner-Stokes L, Hassan N. Depression after stroke: a review of the evidence base to inform the development of an integrated care pathway. Part 2: treatment alternatives. Clin Rehabil 2002;16:248–60.
185. House A, Knapp P, Bamford J, et al. Mortality at 12 and 24 months after stroke may be associated with depressive symptoms at 1 month. Stroke 2001;32:696–701.
186. Robinson RG. Poststroke depression: prevalence, diagnosis, treatment, and disease progression. Biol Psychiatry 2003;54:376–87.
187. Bassetti CL. Sleep and stroke. Semin Neurol 2005;25:19–32.
188. Cleeland CS, Bennett GJ, Dantzer R, et al. Are the symptoms of cancer and cancer treatment due to a shared biologic mechanism? A cytokine-immunologic model of cancer symptoms. Cancer 2003;97:2919–25.
189. Arvin B, Neville LF, Barone FC, et al. The role of inflammation and cytokines in brain injury. Neurosci Biobehav Rev 1996;20:445–52.
190. Emsley HC, Tyrrell PJ. Inflammation and infection in clinical stroke. J Cereb Blood Flow Metab 2002;22:1399–419.

Exercise, Inflammation, and Innate Immunity

Jeffrey A. Woods, PhD[a,b,c,]*, Victoria J. Vieira, MS[a,c], K. Todd Keylock, MS[a]

KEYWORDS

• Innate immunity • Exercise • Macrophages

It is well known that physically fit individuals are at a lower risk of developing age-related diseases and are likely to experience greater longevity.[1] Epidemiologic studies have shown that physical exercise is an effective means of preventing several chronic diseases, such as heart disease and type 2 diabetes.[2,3] Some studies also have shown that physically active individuals are less susceptible than sedentary individuals to viral and bacterial infections, suggesting that exercise improves overall immune function.[4,5] Physical exercise also has been shown to protect against cognitive impairment and depression.[6] Unfortunately, the mechanisms behind these favorable effects of exercise are not understood fully.

Determining the exact mechanism by which exercise exerts its range of health benefits has proven to be a challenge, especially in human studies, because of individual variability, the heterogeneous nature of exercise, and the numerous systems that exercise affects. Several factors need to be taken into account, including human genetic variability, the subjective nature of defining differing levels of exercise intensity, differences in training duration, and the relationship between exercise and other lifestyle factors. There is evidence to support a variety of mechanisms, including a decrease in age-associated immunosenescence,[7] an increase in innate immune function,[5] a decrease in chronic inflammation,[8] an increase in stress resistance,[9] a decrease in adiposity,[10] and more global physiologic changes such as lower blood pressure, an improved lipid profile, and decreased insulin resistance.[3,11–13] This article focuses on how exercise may affect the innate immune system, highlighting its role in regulating the inflammatory process, which recently has been found to be an underlying contributor to many chronic diseases.[14–16] It also discusses potential mechanisms whereby exercise may affect the innate immune system.

This issue is a repurpose of August 2006 issue of the Neurologic Clinics (NCL Volume 24, Issue 3).
[a] Department of Kinesiology and Community Health, University of Illinois at Urbana-Champaign, 906 South Goodwin Avenue, Urbana, IL 6180, USA
[b] Department of Pathology, University of Illinois at Urbana-Champaign, 506 South Mathews Avenue, Urbana, IL 6180, USA
[c] Division of Nutritional Science, University of Illinois at Urbana-Champaign, 905 South Goodwin Avenue, Urbana, IL 6180, USA
* Corresponding author. Department of Kinesiology and Community Health, University of Illinois at Urbana-Champaign, 906 South Goodwin Avenue, Urbana, IL 6180, USA.
E-mail address: woods1@uiuc.edu (J.A. Woods).

Immunol Allergy Clin N Am 29 (2009) 381–393
doi:10.1016/j.iac.2009.02.011
0889-8561/09/$ – see front matter

THE EMERGING IMPORTANCE OF INNATE IMMUNITY IN DISEASE

The initial phases of an organism's response to infection depend on the innate immune response.[17] This response encompasses a variety of mechanisms that recognize and respond to pathogens. The innate immune system may be activated by several different mechanisms including exposure to microorganisms, food ingestion, or any other situation in which human beings are exposed to their external environment.[18] Moreover, tissue necrosis and extracellular release of cellular contents including heat shock proteins (HSP) also can activate innate immunity.[9] Normal aging is associated with reductions in T-lymphocyte function[5] and changes in innate immunity,[19] making older individuals more susceptible to infection. The dysregulation in immune function termed "immunosenescence" is thought to contribute to many age-related diseases.

Inflammation

The term "inflammation" is used to describe the environment produced by activated macrophages, including a milieu of chemokines, cytokines, and other proteins that are a central aspect of the innate immune response. The inflammatory response may be acute, as in a transitory physical injury or infection, or it may be low grade and chronic, as in long-term infections and autoimmune diseases.[20] Chronic, low-level inflammation is defined as two- to fourfold elevation in circulating levels of proinflammatory and anti-inflammatory cytokines and acute-phase proteins such as C-reactive protein (CRP), as well as minor increases in counts of neutrophils and natural killer cells.[8]

Recently, it has been appreciated that low-level inflammatory mechanisms are involved in the pathogenesis of several chronic diseases, including ischemic cardiovascular disease, colorectal cancer, stroke, type 2 diabetes, chronic obstructive pulmonary disease, and Alzheimer's disease.[8] A low-grade inflammatory profile also has been associated recently with ageing and obesity and is predictive of the development of several chronic diseases.

Macrophages

Macrophages, acting as central mediators of the innate immune response, provide a first line of defense against many common microorganisms. Tissue-resident macrophages are activated during an inflammatory response or are recruited to the host tissue from the blood by chemokines. Although they traditionally are considered cells that secrete inflammatory proteins and phagocytose pathogens, it is now understood that macrophages are quite a bit more complex. For example, they act differently depending on their activation status, which is influenced largely by the microenvironment in which they reside. That is, a macrophage may be classically activated for bacterial killing if it is exposed to the cytokine interferon-gamma (IFN-γ) as well as an immune activator, such as lipopolysaccharide (LPS). These cells are proinflammatory in that they produce interleukin (IL)-1, TNF-α, IL-6, and IL-12.[21] Macrophages also may be alternatively activated when they are exposed to cytokines such as IL-4, IL-13, or transforming growth factor-beta.[22] When macrophages are alternatively activated, they secrete the anti-inflammatory cytokines IL-10 and IL-1 receptor antagonist (ra) and produce other factors such as transforming growth factor-beta and vascular endothelial growth factor that promote healing and repair. These alternatively activated macrophages have anti-inflammatory effects and may have roles in tissue healing and repair by promoting angiogenesis or stabilizing atherosclerotic plaques.[23] They also have been implicated in accelerating tumor growth by secretion of growth factors and inhibition of anti-tumor T1 helper cells.[22]

Many studies from the author's laboratory and others have demonstrated dysregulation in macrophage function as a consequence of aging and disease. Moreover, it has been suggested that dysregulated macrophage function may contribute to the increased susceptibility to infection[24] and reductions in wound healing[25] seen in aged and diseased people. The author and others have demonstrated that aging results in a decrease in the ability of macrophages to become acutely classically activated when presented with agents such as IFN-γ or LPS.[26–29] This effect may be mediated by reduced IFN-γ signaling through stat-1 protein.[26] These findings suggest that, with aging, the ability of macrophages to kill microbes becomes impaired. Unfortunately, little is known about the effects of aging or chronic disease on alternative macrophage activation.

Cytokines

The innate inflammatory response is orchestrated predominantly by cytokines. Cytokines have many important functions in regard to immunity. Cytokine production, like many aspects of immune function, is dysregulated in aged individuals.[30] Thus, age-associated shifts in cytokine profiles affect the immune response and pathogen resistance. In general, aging is associated with an increase in proinflammatory cytokines, such as TNF-α and IL-6, and a decrease in anti-inflammatory cytokines.[30]

Several chronic conditions are orchestrated by inflammatory cytokines. For example, TNF-α is increased in many chronic conditions such as obesity, atherosclerosis, and type 2 diabetes.[15,31,32] TNF-α has been shown to cause insulin resistance and has been suggested as a mechanistic link between obesity and inflammatory diseases such as heart disease and type 2 diabetes.[16,33] Additionally, proinflammatory cytokines such as TNF-α produce a dyslipidemic state[34] and activate endothelial cells, resulting in vasoconstriction and hemostasis.[35]

EXERCISE, MACROPHAGES, AND INFLAMMATION

Both epidemiologic and longitudinal data suggest that increasing physical activity is an effective means of reducing systemic low-level inflammation in conditions such as obesity, metabolic syndrome, and diabetes, as well as in healthy aged individuals. Moreover, there is evidence indicating that exercise can also reduce acute inflammation.

Exercise Reduces Acute Inflammation

In both human and animal models, acute inflammation can be reduced with exhaustive or even moderate exercise. Using a mouse model, the authors' laboratory showed that daily strenuous exercise had an anti-inflammatory effect on allogeneic tumor growth by decreasing the number of infiltrating macrophages and neutrophils.[36] The exercise did not have an effect on maximal tumor size but did delay tumor growth and lead to a more rapid regression of the tumor. The stress of the exhaustive exercise may have had an anti-inflammatory effect through activation of the hypothalamic-pituitary-adrenal (HPA) axis resulting in glucocorticoid suppression of immune response. It also has been shown that moderate-intensity exercise can decrease inflammatory responses, including leukocyte infiltration and activation of nuclear factor κB, in a mouse model of ovalbumin-sensitized pulmonary inflammation.[37] This anti-inflammatory effect was brought about by exercise-released glucocorticoids and could be blocked by the glucocorticoid antagonist RU486.

An organism usually responds to infection and the presence of LPS with inflammation, such as TNF-α production. Exercise may modulate this response. Bagby and colleagues[38] reported that exhaustively exercised rats had markedly decreased TNF production in response to LPS administration for up to 6 hours. The authors suggest that increased corticosterone in response to exercise suppressed macrophage function, thereby leading to the blunted inflammatory response. In a human study using exhaustive exercise, Starkie and colleagues[39] administered an LPS challenge to young males who rested, exercised exhaustively, or were administered IL-6. After the LPS challenge, both the exercise and IL-6 groups had significantly decreased plasma TNF-α compared with the rest group. This study suggested that exercise-induced production of IL-6 acted as an anti-inflammatory cytokine, blocking TNF-α production. These studies indicate that factors released by exercise, such as glucocorticoids or other stress hormones (eg, epinephrine, IL-6), lead to an acute decrease of inflammation in response to specific inflammatory challenges.

Exercise Reduces Chronic Inflammation: Cross-Sectional Data

At least 17 cross-sectional studies have evaluated the effects of various forms of exercise or physical activity on serum CRP, a marker of inflammation produced by the liver as part of the acute phase response.[40] In all these studies, the average CRP in the highest category of physical activity was significantly lower than in the lowest level of physical activity.[40] Three recent cross-sectional studies demonstrated that physical fitness, assessed either indirectly by self rating[41,42] or directly by maximum oxygen uptake (VO_{2max}),[43] was inversely associated with CRP in middle-aged healthy adults, even after adjusting for potential confounds including age, body composition, diabetes, and pharmacologic interventions.[41-43] Jankord and Jemiolo[44] studied 12 extremely healthy older men who were either very active or less active and found that the most active participants had significantly lower levels of the inflammatory cytokine IL-6 and higher levels of the anti-inflammatory cytokine IL-10. This finding suggests an anti-inflammatory effect of exercise and the possibility of a dose response, such that greater levels of fitness are more associated with an anti-inflammatory profile than are lower degrees of physical fitness.[44] The findings of this study illustrate that this relationship is true for extremely healthy older adults and suggest that exercise may be an effective way to decrease the inflammatory profile that accompanies normal aging.

Another cross-sectional study conducted by Pischon and colleagues[45] noted that the inverse relationship between physical activity and inflammatory markers was virtually abolished when the authors adjusted for the effect of body mass index (BMI), suggesting that the anti-inflammatory effect of exercise may be mediated by a reduction in adiposity. A significant negative relationship remained between leptin and physical activity, however. Leptin has been shown to have several important immunologic roles and to be associated with inflammation. Thus, an independent exercise-associated reduction in circulating leptin levels may help explain the mechanism behind exercise's anti-inflammatory role.

Although the cross-sectional nature of these studies prevents the determination of a cause–effect relationship, the large sample sizes and care taken to adjust for several lifestyle factors clearly indicate that exercise has an independent anti-inflammatory effect. The effect seems to be active in individuals who have metabolic syndrome, heart disease, and insulin resistance as well as in healthy individuals.

Exercise Reduces Chronic Inflammation: Longitudinal Data

Given the abundance of cross-sectional evidence suggesting a link between exercise and inflammation, some investigators have conducted longitudinal studies to test whether exercise training is associated with a reduction in inflammation in subgroups of the population. Adamopoulos and colleagues[46] conduced a 12-week training study with a randomized crossover design and found that moderate exercise training reduced peripheral markers of inflammation (granulocyte macrophage colony-stimulating factor, monocyte chemoattractant protein [MCP-1], soluble intracellular adhesion molecule-1, and soluble vascular adhesion molecule-1) in 12 patients who had stable chronic heart failure.[46] Another group conducted a randomized 2 × 2 factorial trial of 12 weeks of exercise training using a group of sedentary adult men who had metabolic syndrome and found that individuals who exercised and took the 3-hydroxy-3-methylglutaryl coenzyme A reductase inhibitor, pravastatin, had significant reductions in the inflammatory markers MCP-1 and IL-8 compared with individuals who took the drug without exercising.[47] In terms of the lowering of the inflammatory marker MCP-1, there was no statistical difference between the individuals who took the drug and exercised and those who exercised and took a placebo. This finding suggests that the anti-inflammatory effect of exercise was stronger than that of this particular statin drug in terms of lowering MCP-1 levels. Similarly, Goldhammer and colleagues[48] studied 28 patients who had coronary heart disease and who underwent a 12-week intense aerobic training program; they found that many proinflammatory mediators (eg, CRP, IL-1, IL-6, and IFN-γ) were reduced after the training program. They also showed that levels of the anti-inflammatory cytokine IL-10 increased, suggesting that the mechanism of exercise's anti-inflammatory effect may involve increased expression of anti-inflammatory proteins. These authors reported that levels of inflammatory cytokines decreased after exercise, even in the absence of significant weight reductions.

Anti-inflammatory effects of exercise have been observed in children and adolescents as well as in healthy adults. Balogopal and colleagues[49] investigated the impact of a diet and exercise intervention on inflammatory markers in 21 obese, insulin-resistant adolescents. The intervention was associated with reductions in body fat, insulin resistance, and levels of the inflammatory markers CRP, fibrinogen, and IL-6. Kelly and colleagues[50] also studied an overweight adolescent population to determine the effects of an 8-week exercise-training regimen on indices of subclinical inflammation, endothelial function, and insulin sensitivity. In that study, aerobic exercise improved fitness and endothelial function but was not associated with a reduction in CRP. Possibly, the 8-week training protocol was too short to determine effects attributable to exercise training.

Okita and colleagues[51] tested whether 2 months of exercise training was associated with reductions in weight and serum CRP levels in 199 healthy adult women. The subjects lost an average of 3 kg ($P < .01$), and CRP levels decreased by an average of 0.22 mg/L ($P < .01$). Interestingly, the largest weight-reduction quartile did not show significant decreases in CRP levels, whereas the moderate weight-reduction quartile showed remarkable CRP decreases. The authors suggest that the strenuous exercise routine used may have had a negative effect in the quartile of the greatest weight reduction. That is, this particular group may have experienced overtraining, which has been shown to lead to muscle damage and increased inflammation. This particular quartile did experience the greatest increase in serum levels of uric acid, an indicator of vigorous exercise training.[51] These findings suggest an anti-inflammatory effect of exercise independent of weight loss. In the 16-week longitudinal trial conducted by Marcell and colleagues,[52] exercise training was not associated with improved levels of CRP or adiponectin in a population of middle-aged overweight adults. These researchers studied the effects of either moderate or intense exercise on plasma levels of CRP and adiponectin and found that, although fitness improved in both groups compared with the control group, no major differences in inflammatory markers were found after the exercise-training period. At baseline, however, fitness (assessed by a VO_{2max} test) was correlated with lower CRP levels (r = -0.38; P = .006).[52]

With few exceptions, longitudinal studies have indicated that exercise training has an anti-inflammatory effect for individuals who have chronic diseases such as heart disease and metabolic syndrome and for overweight but otherwise healthy children and adults. The studies conducted have varied in the duration of the training protocols, but most have been between 8 and 12 weeks long. The duration of the training protocol seems to affect whether differences in inflammatory markers are observed. The shorter studies, such as the 8-week study conducted by Balogpal,[49] tend not to show significant reductions in inflammatory markers. A possible explanation is that the anti-inflammatory effect of exercise requires a longer duration of training. The strength of the reciprocal relationship between fitness and inflammation observed in cross-sectional studies would support this possibility. Although virtually all the 12-week training studies reported decreases in inflammatory markers, the 16-week study conducted by Marcell and colleagues[52] did not result in improvements in the inflammatory protein CRP. In that study, however, the sample size was rather small, with only 17 individuals in each group (low-intensity training, high-intensity training, or no training). Further long-term studies using larger samples are needed before any conclusions can be made regarding the long-term effects of exercise training on markers of inflammation.

POTENTIAL MECHANISMS RESPONSIBLE FOR THE ANTI-INFLAMMATORY EFFECT OF EXERCISE
Exercise Reduces Adiposity

Adipose tissue now is classified as an endocrine organ, because it secretes a wide variety of hormones and inflammatory mediators.[53] Accordingly, it has been hypothesized that the negative relationship between exercise training and systemic inflammation might result from the weight loss (eg, fat loss) effect of exercise. In fact, BMI[54,55] and, more specifically, percentage fat mass[56–58] have been associated positively with several of the inflammatory markers (ie, TNF-α, IL-6, CRP) that also have been shown to be reciprocally related to physical activity.[2,48,54,59] Some studies, however, report that the relationships between inflammatory markers and physical activity are independent of differential levels of obesity,[10,41,60] suggesting that exercise has an independent anti-inflammatory effect. One drawback of these previous studies is that only a few have assessed adiposity directly by measuring percentage body fat.[52,60] Most have used BMI to assess body fatness indirectly, which may have prevented the proper statistical adjustment for total adiposity in population studies.[61] For example, Nicklas and colleagues[62] conducted a large clinical trial including sedentary older individuals who were randomly assigned to one of four treatments: control, diet-induced weight loss, exercise, or diet plus exercise, for 18 months. They found that the diet-induced weight loss resulted in significant reductions in inflammatory markers compared with the groups that had no weight loss, but the effect of exercise was no stronger than the effect of diet alone. They concluded that the exercise effect resulted from weight loss. These authors did not assess body fat directly; thus, it is possible that the exercise group lost a greater percentage fat mass then did the diet-only group, although the total weight reductions were similar. On the other hand, You and colleagues[60] found that exercise plus diet, but not diet alone (which produced a similar fat reduction), was associated with a significant reduction in all the inflammatory markers measured, including IL-6, TNF-α, and

CRP, in that population of obese postmenopausal women. These authors did measure the percentage of body fat directly. Additional large-scale studies using a direct assessment of total body adiposity are needed before the mechanistic effect of exercise on inflammation can be evaluated properly.

Exercise Reduces Macrophage Accumulation

Recent studies have shown that macrophages accumulate in white adipose tissue of obese humans[63] and rodents.[64] It has been shown that a large portion of the inflammatory response associated with obesity is derived from macrophages residing in the stromovascular portion of fat tissue.[64] That is, although adipocytes produce inflammatory cytokines such as TNF-α and IL-6 and hormones such as leptin, most of the inflammatory cells in the adipose tissue are produced by macrophages that were drawn to the adipose tissue.[65] Moreover, the number of macrophages present in adipose tissue is directly correlated with both adiposity and adipocyte size.[53] This macrophage population is classically activated[63] and contributes significantly to the inflammatory state associated with obesity and its comorbidities.[65] What is not known is how or why macrophages are attracted to adipose tissue in obesity. A recent study by Cinti and colleagues[66] suggested that obesity-associated adipocyte necrosis is mechanistically responsible for the macrophage accumulation and ensuing inflammatory response. Adipose tissue has been shown to secrete MCP-1,[67] a chemokine that attracts macrophages. Exercise has been shown to decrease the expression of MCP-1 in individuals who have metabolic syndrome.[47] Thus, by limiting the growth and subsequent necrosis of adipocytes, exercise may serve to decrease macrophage accumulation in fat tissue and thus decrease inflammation. This suggestion has not yet been tested.

The Interleukin-6 Paradox

Like adipose tissue, skeletal muscle acts as an endocrine organ, secreting mediators that have the ability to reduce or enhance systemic low-level inflammation. Through the production of myokines, skeletal muscle links physical activity to several physiologic processes, including metabolism, endocrine control, and immune function.[8] This activity is exemplified best by the findings that skeletal muscle is a major source of the cytokine IL-6 during exercise. Both mRNA and circulating levels of IL-6 increase with exercise and correlate with the increase in IL-6 gene expression in skeletal muscle cells after exercise.[8] Moreover, IL-6 increases in proportion to exercise duration, intensity, number of muscle fibers recruited, and individual fitness level.[68]

Although traditionally considered a proinflammatory cytokine, IL-6 recently has been suggested to have anti-inflammatory properties.[69] Thus, the mechanism behind the anti-inflammatory effect of exercise may in fact be an increase in the level of IL-6. Mechanistically, IL-6 may work to antagonize the proinflammatory effects of TNF-α.[70] Starkie and colleagues[39] tested this hypothesis by conducting three experiments using human volunteers who rested, rode a bicycle for 3 hours, or were infused with IL-6 for 3 hours while they rested. After 2.5 hours, all participants received an immune-system stimulus (LPS) to induce low-grade inflammation. In the control group, LPS-stimulated TNF-α production increased in the control group but was prevented completely in the exercise group (which resulted in elevations in circulating IL-6) and in the nonexercised IL-6-infusion group. These data provide circumstantial evidence that exercise-induced increases in IL-6 may prevent inflammation-induced elevations in TNF-α. Definitive evidence to support this hypothesis is needed, however.

The Cholinergic Anti-Inflammatory Pathway

Recently, Pavlov and Tracey[71] described what they refer to as "the cholinergic anti-inflammatory pathway." They suggest that stimulation of the parasympathetic nervous system, by way of the efferent vagus nerve, inhibits proinflammatory cytokine release and protects against systemic inflammation. What they describe is a central homeostatic mechanism by which the sympathetic division of the autonomic nervous system stimulates the inflammatory response through the release of epinephrine and norepinephrine, while the parasympathetic nervous system works reciprocally to suppress this release of proinflammatory cytokine. The authors note, "[T]he bi-directional brain-periphery communication, which occurs through reciprocal autonomic nervous system mechanisms, hormones and humoral factors, is vital for regulating visceral functions and maintaining homeostasis." One of the major functions of the efferent vagus nerve is to control heart rate. One of the long-term responses to exercise training is a decrease in heart rate variability[72] so the parasympathetic nervous system becomes more efficient in stimulating the reciprocating sympathetic nervous system. Thus, exercise training may increase efferent vagus nerve activity, and this increased activity may contribute to the anti-inflammatory effect of exercise. To the author's knowledge, this hypothesis has not yet been investigated.

Exercise: A Unique Stressor

Although chronic exercise is associated with a decrease in systemic inflammation, acute exercise results in varying degrees of microtrauma to the muscle, connective tissue, or bones and joints, especially in unaccustomed subjects. These microtraumas lead to a mild inflammatory response to repair the damaged tissue. This inflammatory response is a normal phenomenon that occurs with exercise training and, over time, leads to adaptation and improved fitness. Without adequate rest, the damaged tissue does not have time to repair, and a chronic inflammatory condition, overtraining syndrome, may develop.[73] Systemic inflammation is proposed as the central feature of over-training syndrome, for which symptoms include generalized fatigue, depression, muscle and joint pain, or loss of appetite.

Stress may be defined as a stimulus that activates the HPA axis or the sympathetic nervous system to help an organism adapt physiologically to deal with a threat.[74] Although paradoxical, it is likely that the acute stress associated with exercise eventually leads to a decrease in chronic inflammation. Certain stressors, such as exercise, might enhance some aspects of immune function by enhancing the organism's ability to adapt. It has been shown that increased aerobic fitness is associated with a lower HPA axis response to psychologic stress in humans.[75] A cross-sectional study was recently conducted using older and young unfit women (based on a VO_{2max} test $\leq$ the average for the respective age group) compared with older fit women (who had a $VO_{2max} >$ than the average of their age group). All participants underwent a stress test battery that combined mental and physical challenges as well as a psychosocial stressor. The older unfit women had greater cortisol responses to the challenge than both the young-unfit and the older-fit women. Thus, these findings suggest that higher aerobic fitness among older women is associated with a reduction in age-related changes in the response to stress and may be an effective means of modifying age-related neuroendocrine changes.[75] Animal studies also have shown that trained rats exhibit stress resistance. For example, Greenwood and colleagues[76] found that 4 to 6 weeks of voluntary wheel running prevented stress-induced norepinephrine depletion in certain body tissues. They suggest that the mechanism may have to do with adaptations in peripheral sympathetic nerve synthesis/release rates and central sympathetic circuit activation.[76]

Another mechanism by which exercise increases stress resistance may be through increases in endogenous antioxidant defenses and increased expression of HSP. One study conducted in diabetic rats showed that endurance exercise increased tissue HSP expression, suggesting that exercise training may be protective against oxidative stress.[77] Campisi and colleagues[78] also conducted a study to determine whether prior voluntary wheel running increased the stress-induced induction in HSP72 in the brain as well as in peripheral and immune tissues. These investigators conducted experiments using Fischer 344 rats, which were housed with an active running wheel or an immobilized running wheel for 8 weeks before tail-shock stress exposure. Although both groups of rats underwent a normal stress response (an increase in serum corticosterone), the active rats responded to this stress with a greater and faster HSP72 response, supporting the hypothesis that exercise training is associated with increased stress resistance.

De la Fuente and colleagues[79] suggest that the favorable effects of exercise on disease prevention probably involve increased expression of intracellular antioxidants. Although heavy exercise is associated with an increase in the inflammatory response and in the production of reactive oxygen species, it has been suggested that adaptation to regular exercise training is modulated by free radicals produced during exercise. That is, regular exercise training leads to an adaptation of antioxidative mechanisms.[80] If oxidative stress is related causally to chronic low-level inflammation, it stands to reason that regular exercise might reduce such inflammation by increasing endogenous antioxidant defenses.

SUMMARY

Regular exercise is protective against several chronic diseases ranging from physiologic diseases such as cardiovascular disease to neurologic diseases such as dementia and depression. Exciting recent research points to chronic inflammation as an underlying contributor to many age-related chronic diseases. Cross-sectional and longitudinal studies in animals and humans have shown both an acute and a chronic anti-inflammatory effect. Because innate immunity is a key regulator of inflammatory processes, and chronic inflammation contributes to many illnesses, the effect of regular exercise on innate immunity, most importantly macrophages, holds much promise in terms of defining these mechanisms. Unfortunately, the mechanisms responsible for the observed anti-inflammatory effect of regular exercise have not been elucidated. This article presents several compelling potential mechanisms for the anti-inflammatory effect of exercise, including loss of body fat, reductions in macrophage accumulation in adipose tissue, altered macrophage phenotype in adipose tissue, exercise-induced muscle production of IL-6, or alterations in the balance between the sympathetic and parasympathetic nervous systems. Further investigation to confirm or reject these testable hypotheses will allow better application of exercise therapy to treat and prevent illnesses associated with chronic inflammation.

REFERENCES

1. Blair SN, Cheng Y, Holder JS. Is physical activity or physical fitness more important in defining health benefits? Med Sci Sports Exerc 2001;33(6 Suppl):S379–99 [discussion: S419–20].

2. Colbert LH, Visser M, Simonsick EM, et al. Physical activity, exercise, and inflammatory markers in older adults: findings from the Health, Aging and Body Composition Study. J Am Geriatr Soc 2004;52(7):1098–104.

3. Stewart KJ. Role of exercise training on cardiovascular disease in persons who have type 2 diabetes and hypertension. Cardiol Clin 2004;22(4):569–86.

4. DiPenta JM, Johnson JG, Murphy RJ. Natural killer cells and exercise training in the elderly: a review. Can J Appl Physiol 2004;29(4):419–43.

5. Kohut ML, Senchina DS. Reversing age-associated immunosenescence via exercise. Exerc Immunol Rev 2004;10:6–41.

6. Resnick B. Research review: exercise interventions for treatment of depression. Geriatr Nurs 2005;26(3):196.

7. Woods JA, Lowder TW, Keylock KT. Can exercise training improve immune function in the aged? Ann N Y Acad Sci 2002;959:117–27.

8. Bruunsgaard H. Physical activity and modulation of systemic low-level inflammation. J Leukoc Biol 2005;(Jul):20.

9. Fleshner M. Physical activity and stress resistance: sympathetic nervous system adaptations prevent stress-induced immunosuppression. Exerc Sport Sci Rev 2005;33(3):120–6.

10. Nicklas BJ, You T, Pahor M. Behavioural treatments for chronic systemic inflammation: effects of dietary weight loss and exercise training. CMAJ 2005;172(9):1199–209.

11. Tamura Y, Tanaka Y, Sato F, et al. Effects of diet and exercise on muscle and liver intracellular lipid contents and insulin sensitivity in type 2 diabetic patients. J Clin Endocrinol Metab 2005;90(6):3191–6.

12. Yokoyama H, Emoto M, Fujiwara S, et al. Short-term aerobic exercise improves arterial stiffness in type 2 diabetes. Diabetes Res Clin Pract 2004;65(2):85–93.

13. Nishida Y, Tokuyama K, Nagasaka S, et al. Effect of moderate exercise training on peripheral glucose effectiveness, insulin sensitivity, and endogenous glucose production in healthy humans estimated by a two-compartment-labeled minimal model. Diabetes 2004;53(2):315–20.

14. Wellen KE, Hotamisligil GS. Inflammation, stress, and diabetes. J Clin Invest 2005;115(5):1111–9.

15. Spranger J, Kroke A, Mohlig M, et al. Inflammatory cytokines and the risk to develop type 2 diabetes: results of the prospective population-based European Prospective Investigation into Cancer and Nutrition (EPIC)-Potsdam Study. Diabetes 2003;52(3):812–7.

16. Schmidt MI, Duncan BB. Diabesity: an inflammatory metabolic condition. Clin Chem Lab Med 2003;41(9):1120–30.

17. Frantz S, Bauersachs J, Kelly RA. Innate immunity and the heart. Curr Pharm Des 2005;11(10):1279–90.

18. Duncan BB, Schmidt MI. Chronic activation of the innate immune system may underlie the metabolic syndrome. Sao Paulo Med J 2001;119(3):122–7.

19. Hasler P, Zouali M. Immune receptor signaling, aging, and autoimmunity. Cell Immunol 2005;233(2):102–8.

20. Janeway C, Travers P, Walport M, et al. Immunobiology. New York: Garland Publishing; 2001.

21. Mosser DM. The many faces of macrophage activation. J Leukoc Biol 2003;73(2):209–12.

22. Goerdt S, Politz O, Schledzewski K, et al. Alternative versus classical activation of macrophages. Pathobiology 1999;67(5–6):222–6.

23. Gordon S. Alternative activation of macrophages. Nat Rev Immunol 2003;3(1):23–35.

24. Chelvarajan RL, Collins SM, Doubinskaia IE, et al. Defective macrophage function in neonates and its impact on unresponsiveness of neonates to polysaccharide antigens. J Leukoc Biol 2004;75(6):982–94.

25. Martin P, D'Souza D, Martin J, et al. Wound healing in the PU.1 null mouse–tissue repair is not dependent on inflammatory cells. Curr Biol 2003;13(13):1122–8.

26. Yoon P, Keylock KT, Hartman ME, et al. Macrophage hypo-responsiveness to interferon-gamma in aged mice is associated with impaired signaling through Jak-STAT. Mech Ageing Dev 2004;125(2):137–43.

27. Lu Q, Ceddia MA, Price EA, et al. Chronic exercise increases macrophage-mediated tumor cytolysis in young and old mice. Am J Physiol 1999;276(2 Pt 2):R482–9.

28. Ding A, Hwang S, Schwab R. Effect of aging on murine macrophages. Diminished response to IFN-gamma for enhanced oxidative metabolism. J Immunol 1994;153(5):2146–52.

29. Boehmer ED, Meehan MJ, Cutro BT, et al. Aging negatively skews macrophage TLR2- and TLR4-mediated pro-inflammatory responses without affecting the IL-2-stimulated pathway. Mech Ageing Dev 2005;(Sep):7.

30. Han SN, Meydani SN. Antioxidants, cytokines, and influenza infection in aged mice and elderly humans. J Infect Dis 2000;182(Suppl 1):S74–80.

31. Hotamisligil GS, Spiegelman BM. Tumor necrosis factor alpha: a key component of the obesity-diabetes link. Diabetes 1994;43(11):1271–8.

32. Hotamisligil GS, Arner P, Caro JF, et al. Increased adipose tissue expression of tumor necrosis factor-alpha in human obesity and insulin resistance. J Clin Invest 1995;95(5):2409–15.

33. Hotamisligil GS. Inflammatory pathways and insulin action. Int J Obes Relat Metab Disord 2003;27(Suppl 3):S53–5.

34. Chu NF, Spiegelman D, Hotamisligil GS, et al. Plasma insulin, leptin, and soluble TNF receptors levels in relation to obesity-related atherogenic and thrombogenic cardiovascular disease risk factors among men. Atherosclerosis 2001;157(2):495–503.

35. Scalera F. Intracellular glutathione and lipid peroxide availability and the secretion of vasoactive substances by human umbilical vein endothelial cells after incubation with TNF-alpha. Eur J Clin Invest 2003;33(2):176–82.

36. Zielinski MR, Muenchow M, Wallig MA, et al. Exercise delays allogeneic tumor growth and reduces intratumoral inflammation and vascularization. J Appl Physiol 2004;96(6):2249–56.

37. Pastva A, Estell K, Schoeb TR, et al. RU486 blocks the anti-inflammatory effects of exercise in a murine model of allergen-induced pulmonary inflammation. Brain Behav Immun 2005;19(5):413–22.

38. Bagby GJ, Sawaya DE, Crouch LD, et al. Prior exercise suppresses the plasma tumor necrosis factor response to bacterial lipopolysaccharide. J Appl Physiol 1994;77(3):1542–7.

39. Starkie R, Ostrowski SR, Jauffred S, et al. Exercise and IL-6 infusion inhibit endotoxin-induced TNF-alpha production in humans. FASEB J 2003;17(8):884–6.

40. Kasapis C, Thompson PD. The effects of physical activity on serum C-reactive protein and inflammatory markers: a systematic review. J Am Coll Cardiol 2005; 45(10):1563–9.

41. Katja B, Tiina L, Veikko S, et al. Associations of leisure time physical activity, self-rated physical fitness, and estimated aerobic fitness with serum C-reactive protein among 3803 adults. Atherosclerosis 2005;(Jul):23.

42. Pitsavos C, Panagiotakos DB, Chrysohoou C, et al. The associations between physical activity, inflammation, and coagulation markers, in people with metabolic syndrome: the ATTICA study. Eur J Cardiovasc Prev Rehabil 2005;12(2):151–8.

43. Kondo N, Nomura M, Nakaya Y, et al. Association of inflammatory marker and highly sensitive C-reactive protein with aerobic exercise capacity, maximum oxygen uptake and insulin resistance in healthy middle-aged volunteers. Circ J 2005;69(4):452–7.
44. Jankord R, Jemiolo B. Influence of physical activity on serum IL-6 and IL-10 levels in healthy older men. Med Sci Sports Exerc 2004;36(6):960–4.
45. Pischon T, Hankinson SE, Hotamisligil GS, et al. Leisure-time physical activity and reduced plasma levels of obesity-related inflammatory markers. Obesity Research 2003;11(9):1055–64.
46. Adamopoulos S, Parissis J, Kroupis C, et al. Physical training reduces peripheral markers of inflammation in patients with chronic heart failure. Eur Heart J 2001;22(9):791–7.
47. Troseid M, Lappegard KT, Claudi T, et al. Exercise reduces plasma levels of the chemokines MCP-1 and IL-8 in subjects with the metabolic syndrome. Eur Heart J 2004;25(4):349–55.
48. Goldhammer E, Tanchilevitch A, Maor I, et al. Exercise training modulates cytokines activity in coronary heart disease patients. Int J Cardiol 2005;100(1):93–9.
49. Balagopal P, George D, Patton N, et al. Lifestyle-only intervention attenuates the inflammatory state associated with obesity: a randomized controlled study in adolescents. J Pediatr 2005;146(3):342–8.
50. Kelly AS, Wetzsteon RJ, Kaiser DR, et al. Inflammation, insulin, and endothelial function in overweight children and adolescents: the role of exercise. J Pediatr 2004;145(6):731–6.
51. Okita K, Nishijima H, Murakami T, et al. Can exercise training with weight loss lower serum C-reactive protein levels? Arterioscler Thromb Vasc Biol 2004; 24(10):1868–73.
52. Marcell TJ, McAuley KA, Traustadottir T, et al. Exercise training is not associated with improved levels of C-reactive protein or adiponectin. Metabolism 2005;54(4):533–41.
53. Fantuzzi G. Adipose tissue, adipokines, and inflammation. J Allergy Clin Immunol 2005;115(5):911–9 [quiz: 920].
54. Esposito K, Pontillo A, Di Palo C, et al. Effect of weight loss and lifestyle changes on vascular inflammatory markers in obese women: a randomized trial. JAMA 2003;289(14):1799–804.
55. Ziccardi P, Nappo F, Giugliano G, et al. Reduction of inflammatory cytokine concentrations and improvement of endothelial functions in obese women after weight loss over one year. Circulation 2002;105(7):804–9.
56. Ryan AS, Nicklas BJ. Reductions in plasma cytokine levels with weight loss improve insulin sensitivity in overweight and obese postmenopausal women. Diabetes Care 2004;27(7):1699–705.
57. Vozarova B, Weyer C, Hanson K, et al. Circulating interleukin-6 in relation to adiposity, insulin action, and insulin secretion. Obes Res 2001;9(7):414–7.
58. Laimer M, Ebenbichler CF, Kaser S, et al. Markers of chronic inflammation and obesity: a prospective study on the reversibility of this association in middle-aged women undergoing weight loss by surgical intervention. Int J Obes 2002; 26:659–62.
59. Mattusch F, Dufaux B, Heine O, et al. Reduction of the plasma concentration of C-reactive protein following nine months of endurance training. Int J Sports Med 2000;21(1):21–4.
60. You T, Berman DM, Ryan AS, et al. Effects of hypocaloric diet and exercise training on inflammation and adipocyte lipolysis in obese postmenopausal women. J Clin Endocrinol Metab 2004;89(4):1739–46.

61. Movsesyan L, Tanko LB, Larsen PJ, et al. Variations in percentage of body fat within different BMI groups in young, middle-aged and old women. Clin Physiol Funct Imaging 2003;23(3):130–3.
62. Nicklas BJ, Ambrosius W, Messier SP, et al. Diet-induced weight loss, exercise, and chronic inflammation in older, obese adults: a randomized controlled clinical trial. Am J Clin Nutr 2004;79(4):544–51.
63. Weisberg SP, McCann D, Desai M, et al. Obesity is associated with macrophage accumulation in adipose tissue. J Clin Invest 2003;112(12):1796–808.
64. Xu H, Barnes GT, Yang Q, et al. Chronic inflammation in fat plays a crucial role in the development of obesity-related insulin resistance. J Clin Invest 2003;112(12):1821–30.
65. Bouloumie A, Curat CA, Sengenes C, et al. Role of macrophage tissue infiltration in metabolic diseases. Curr Opin Clin Nutr Metab Care 2005;8(4):347–54.
66. Cinti S, Mitchell G, Barbatelli G, et al. Adipocyte death defines macrophage localization and function in adipose tissue of obese mice and humans. J Lipid Res 2005;46(11):2347–55.
67. Christiansen T, Richelsen B, Bruun JM. Monocyte chemoattractant protein-1 is produced in isolated adipocytes, associated with adiposity and reduced after weight loss in morbid obese subjects. Int J Obes (Lond) 2005;29(1):146–50.
68. Pedersen BK, Febbraio M. Muscle-derived interleukin-6—a possible link between skeletal muscle, adipose tissue, liver, and brain. Brain Behav Immun 2005;19(5):371–6.
69. Keller P, Keller C, Carey AL, et al. Interleukin-6 production by contracting human skeletal muscle: autocrine regulation by IL-6. Biochem Biophys Res Commun 2003;310(2):550–4.
70. Pedersen BK, Steensberg A, Keller P, et al. Muscle-derived interleukin-6: lipolytic, anti-inflammatory and immune regulatory effects. Pflugers Arch 2003;446(1):9–16.
71. Pavlov VA, Tracey KJ. The cholinergic anti-inflammatory pathway. Brain Behav Immun 2005;19:413–22.
72. Rosenwinkel ET, Bloomfield DM, Arwady MA, et al. Exercise and autonomic function in health and cardiovascular disease. Cardiol Clin 2001;19(3):369–87.
73. Smith LL. Cytokine hypothesis of overtraining: a physiological adaptation to excessive stress? Med Sci Sports Exerc 2000;32(2):317–31.
74. Glaser R, Kiecolt-Glaser JK. Stress-induced immune dysfunction: implications for health. Nat Rev Immunol 2005;5(3):243–51.
75. Traustadottir T, Bosch PR, Matt KS. The HPA axis response to stress in women: effects of aging and fitness. Psychoneuroendocrinology 2005;30(4):392–402.
76. Greenwood BN, Kennedy S, Smith TP, et al. Voluntary freewheel running selectively modulates catecholamine content in peripheral tissue and c-Fos expression in the central sympathetic circuit following exposure to uncontrollable stress in rats. Neuroscience 2003;120(1):269–81.
77. Atalay M, Oksala NK, Laaksonen DE, et al. Exercise training modulates heat shock protein response in diabetic rats. J Appl Physiol 2004;97(2):605–11.
78. Campisi J, Leem TH, Greenwood BN, et al. Habitual physical activity facilitates stress-induced HSP72 induction in brain, peripheral, and immune tissues. Am J Physiol Regul Integr Comp Physiol 2003;284(2):R520–30.
79. De la Fuente M, Hernanz A, Vallejo MC. The immune system in the oxidative stress conditions of aging and hypertension: favorable effects of antioxidants and physical exercise. Antioxid Redox Signal 2005;7(9–10):1356–66.
80. Niess AM, Dickhuth HH, Northoff H, et al. Free radicals and oxidative stress in exercise–immunological aspects. Exerc Immunol Rev 1999;5:22–56.

Index

Note: Page numbers of article titles are in **boldface** type.

Immunol Allergy Clin N Am 29 (2009) 395–404
doi:10.1016/S0889-8561(09)00022-8
0889-8561/09/$ – see front matter © 2009 Elsevier Inc. All rights reserved.

immunology.theclinics.com

Moving?

Make sure your subscription moves with you!

To notify us of your new address, find your **Clinics Account Number** (located on your mailing label above your name), and contact customer service at:

E-mail: elspcs@elsevier.com

800-654-2452 (subscribers in the U.S. & Canada)
314-453-7041 (subscribers outside of the U.S. & Canada)

Fax number: 314-523-5170

Elsevier Periodicals Customer Service
11830 Westline Industrial Drive
St. Louis, MO 63146

*To ensure uninterrupted delivery of your subscription, please notify us at least 4 weeks in advance of move.

Printed and bound by CPI Group (UK) Ltd, Croydon, CR0 4YY

03/10/2024

01040450-0020